The
Natural
Year

Also by Jane Alexander

SUPERTHERAPIES
THE DETOX PLAN

The
Natural
Year

A SEASONAL GUIDE

TO ALTERNATIVE

HEALTH & BEAUTY

Jane Alexander

AVON BOOKS ◆ NEW YORK

NOTE TO READER: The author of this book is not a physician, and the ideas, procedures, and suggestions in the book are intended to supplement, not replace, the medical and legal advice of trained professionals. All matters regarding your health require medical supervision. Consult your medical practitioner before adopting the suggestions in this book, as well as about any condition that may require diagnosis or medical attention.

AVON BOOKS, INC.
1350 Avenue of the Americas
New York, New York 10019

Copyright © 1997 by Jane Alexander
Cover illustration by Faranak
Interior design by Kellan Peck
Published by arrangement with Bantam Books
Visit our website at **http://www.AvonBooks.com**
Library of Congress Catalog Card Number: 98-94789
ISBN: 0-380-73143-6

First Avon Books Trade Paperback Printing: February 1999

AVON TRADEMARK REG. U.S. PAT. OFF. AND IN OTHER COUNTRIES, MARCA REGISTRADA, HECHO EN U.S.A.

Printed in the U.S.A.

OPM   10   9   8   7   6   5   4   3   2   1

For Adrian—my seasonal soul

ACKNOWLEDGMENTS

My debts of gratitude, given in full, would run longer than this book itself. As always, deep thanks and love to all my family and friends who share the joys of the seasons with me and support me in all my endeavors. Special thanks in particular to Jane Rayson for introducing me to Monty (the bouncing boxer) without whom I would not have come to enjoy (and endure) the countryside in all its seasonal phases—from blazing sun to sleeting rain. The seasonal observations that run through *The Natural Year* have all come from first-hand experience of tramping the fields and lanes of Somerset each and every day.

My sincere and grateful thanks too to all the therapists and experts who have given so freely of their time, knowledge and healing throughout the genesis of this book. If I started listing names we'd be here forever, but every time I mention you within the pages of this book rest assured my thoughts and thanks have gone out to you.

My continuing thanks and admiration to my exceedingly wonderful agent Judith Chilcote who turned me from a jobbing journalist into an author. And gratitude to all the team at Bantam who transform reams of unruly paper into a solid book and then scatter it far and wide into bookshops across the land. In particular, my heartfelt thanks go to Francesca Liversidge—I'm very lucky to have her as my editor.

CONTENTS

April
76
Boosting your health with tonics • The big stretch: gaining flexibility in your body • The ultimate stretch • Celebrating Easter

May
96
Beltane: the wild and wonderful festival of May • A time for cleansing • Detoxing • Looking after your lymph • The mystery of the Moor • Manual lymph drainage • Living with the dance

SUMMER: The Season of the Emotions
123
The season of fire and the evil heat • Exercise revisited • Watch the sun • Shifting your diet into summer • Tibetan medicine: a brief introduction • Losing weight and the Mind Diet • The "eat masses and still lose weight" healthy eating plan

June
149
Looking at your emotions • The most effective bodywork systems for freeing emotions

July
167
Boosting self-esteem • Sing yourself happy • The power of play • Holidays, health, and happiness

August
189
The joy of juice • Living your life with passion • Biodynamic therapy and watsu: two unusual ways of touching your emotions

Contents xi

AUTUMN: The Season of the Mind
205
Indian summer: the harbinger of autumn • The season of metal, air and the dry evil • The autumn diet • Exercise for autumn • Looking at your life path

September
228
Feng shui: esoteric interior design • From managing space to managing time • NLP: the master communicator

October
251
The mid-autumn cleanse: strengthening your body for winter • Halloween: pulling back the veil between the worlds • Divination: how the future can help you with the present

November
274
Stress: the penalty for being superpeople • Quindo: banishing stress and boosting assertiveness • Art therapy: unleashing the inner artist • The mystery of the night: working with your dreams

WINTER: The Season of the Soul
295
The season of water and the evil cold • The winter diet: fortifying and strengthening • Winter tonics • Sweet and spicy scents for winter • Exercise and winter • A dose of light: keeping spirits bright • The quietness of winter: a time for reflection and growth • Mindfulness

December
318
Coping with Christmas • Handling hangovers • The natural first-aid kit for Christmas • Life after Christmas • Using affirmations

The
Natural
Year

Introduction

Starting to Live Your Life with the Seasons

Do you sometimes feel as if life is racing past you? As if you are running up a down escalator that is picking up speed by the second? Is life an uphill struggle where everything seems an incredible effort? Perhaps you have trouble losing weight; or maybe your energy levels seem to flag lower and lower? Do you ever despair of getting your life on track? And do you beat up on yourself because sometimes all you want to do is hide away and tell the world to carry on without you?

If you've answered yes to all or any of these questions it's no great surprise. Most people feel nowadays as if they have to live life on an endless treadmill, permanently racing to go nowhere fast. Society expects so much of us. We are supposed to be cheery, bright, successful superpeople—all the time. And if we get ill or feel depressed, we are branded failures.

It simply isn't fair and it certainly isn't realistic. It comes about because we are almost all living very unnatural lives—pitting ourselves against the natural rhythms of the year. What we have lost in recent years is this concept of natural cycles in life. That there are times to be bright and cheerful but, equally, times when

1

it is fine to be withdrawn and inward-looking. As human beings we may be intellectually and technologically advanced but we are still governed by the natural world. And the natural world is a seasonal world, a never-ending succession of highs and lows, ups and downs. It is ruled by a perpetual sequence of birth, growth, maturation, decay, death and rebirth. All around us, nature follows its regular rhythm: it has a time for energy, growth and vitality; a time for relaxation and plenty; a time of storing and harvesting and a time of withdrawal and solitude.

So why is it that we humans manage to completely ignore the natural cycle of life? If we, too, were to regulate our lives by our natural clock we would find life a much easier ride. Our bodies would be healthier, our emotions more balanced, and our hopes and aspirations might stand a better chance of becoming reality. Living by the seasons, learning through the seasons, we could get back into balance with the natural scheme of life.

Losing weight can become easy if we pick the right time to do it, with the right preparation. Relationships become less fraught when we understand that our emotions have cycles, too, that there are times to be close and loving but equally times to get away from each other and venture into the wider world. Choose the right time to change your job, and your whole career path could transform overnight. And your soul will rejoice if you give it back its rightful sojourn of solitude and contemplation. This book aims to return you gently to the natural wheel of life, living in tune and in balance with the seasons, with the ever-shifting cycle of life.

In the past there would have been no need for a book such as this. Nobody would need lessons in how to live in tune with nature—our ancestors knew its cycles and patterns like the backs of their own hands. They lived close to the land and, if they dared ignore the seasonal progress of the year, it was at their peril. Yet in our modern world we have moved ourselves out of sync with nature and its cycles. We no longer need to watch the earth, the skies, the rivers and sea to pick the best times for sowing and reaping, the time to bring our herds and flocks back from the high pastures into the home fold because so few of us earn our living by the land. We have spent the last century desperately running away from the domination of nature. We have sought to control the natural world, to bend it to our will, to allow ourselves to live free of its implacable dictates. And we have succeeded to a large degree.

We can sit warm and snug in our centrally heated homes while the rain and hail storm outside. We can work in a cool breeze in our offices while the summer sun beats down on the parched earth. We can eat strawberries at Christmas and, if we choose, winter stews and casseroles at the height of summer. We have comfort and we have choice—and isn't it wonderful!

Not for one moment am I suggesting we throw it all in and head back to the fields to become born-again peasants. I've lived without central heating in winter and I have absolutely no desire to do it again. I've spent nights tossing and turning, unable to sleep through muggy heatwaves and positively yearned for an air conditioner. Let's be under no illusions—life before technology could be tough and unpleasant. When we think fondly of "the good old days" we conveniently blank out nasties like frozen taps, chilblains and frostbite; hunger when a harvest failed; misery when the rain fell too much or too little. No one in their right mind wants to turn the clock right back.

However, we are in danger of moving too far in the opposite direction. In our quest for comfort and ease we are losing many of our natural allies; we are forgetting many deep truths about life and living. We push our bodies to extraordinary lengths and expect them to perform like robots, permanently fit and full of energy. We feel under pressure to spend our lives perpetually happy and full of joy. And so, when we feel tired and in need of rest; when we feel down or depressed, we blame ourselves. In our fast-moving consumer society we are expected always to be in top form, to be constantly bright and breezy, happy and contented. And if we aren't we beat ourselves up over it.

Living with the seasons *isn't* about a permanent feel-good factor—that would be as artificial as a stick of candy floss. It isn't about having nonstop, super-powered energy all the time. Living with the seasons is about balance. It's about recognizing the right time to be bright and bouncy, the right time to storm out into the world, to take it by the horns and shake it. But equally, it is about accepting that there are times when you will gain nothing by charging the hill except exhaustion and disappointment. It's about remembering that there are times to retreat and focus inward rather than outward.

In winter it's perfectly natural to feel more quiet and contemplative; it's even normal to feel slightly sad and depressed. It's our "soul time," a time to escape and muse, to ponder and retreat. It's the natural time of the year for soul-searching, for devoting time to our inner lives, our deepest needs and desires. Yet nowadays we are told all too often to "snap out of it"; we're taught techniques to banish the big bad blues, to deny the dark side of our souls. This book, on the other hand, will show you how to work with your down periods, to welcome the opportunity to give your inner life its time. Everything has its place, and even the seemingly nasty side of life can help you change and grow.

I pondered long and hard over which season I should start this book and after much thought. I decided upon spring. The "new year" that we celebrate on January 1 is a new year on calendar only. As far as the seasons go it is the heart of winter, a mid-season celebration. It's the time when we should be looking within rather than without. No wonder so many of us have such problems with New Year resolutions. I've lost count of the number of diets I've started on January 1 which have fallen by the wayside by January 3; how many times I've promised myself I'll go to the gym four times a week and then not been able to tear myself away from the fire and a good book. It's hardly surprising: midwinter is exactly the wrong time to be launching yourself into wildly energetic new pursuits; precisely the wrong time to be restricting or depriving yourself.

The old Celtic calendar, on the other hand, claims the end of autumn as the new year—and with good reason. This is the point at which everything has grown, come to fruit, been harvested and gathered in. The old year is dead and the new one can now begin. However, this is a period of initial quiet, a time of slumber. Although there is life, softly germinating under ground, it is still a quiet time.

For our purposes, the best point to jump into the natural year is with the upsurge of spirits that the first sunny days of spring bring. Spring starts with the bursting of new life, the optimism that comes with lengthening days and increased sunlight. We awake from the mystical soul-time of winter into a season which is unashamedly about the physical. It's a good time to start out on a new life-plan because your mood should be lifting, your energy levels rising, and you should be feeling responsive to change. Sticking to resolutions should be much easier in spring than in the depths of winter. However, if you buy this book in summer, autumn or winter you certainly shouldn't feel you have to wait until next spring to start. The year is a cycle and it really doesn't matter when you leap in. The important point is to move yourself back into working *with* the seasons rather than against them. Another important point is that you don't have to do it all—or certainly not all at once. Just do what feels comfortable to you. Experiment, try things out, see what suits you and what doesn't. You might wait until next year before trying some things.

Above all, remember that we are all individuals, with our own, vastly differing cycles and rhythms. This book is a general guide only—don't take it as gospel. If it makes sense and feels good, try it. But if the book is telling you to withdraw and contemplate when you are wild with energy, then follow your body. As you become more attuned to the way the external world affects your inner self you will begin to just "feel" what is right and what is wrong for you at any given time. The main purpose of this book is to guide you back into an understanding of what your body needs and what your mind and emotions crave.

At the beginning of each seasonal section I give the basic information for that period: how to adapt your diet, your exercise program and the kinds of issues you might address in your personal or professional life. To my mind, the seasons each have a different focus, a different series of tasks. So spring, to me at least, is the Season of the Body, a time when we need to look at our relationship with the physical, with our health, with how we see our bodies. It's an energetic time, a time to start new projects.

In summer the emphasis shifts to the emotional. It's a time to look at our relationship with our feelings and also to consider how we relate to other people. This doesn't mean that we shouldn't work with our bodies in the summer. Most certainly we should. One point I will continue to make throughout this book is that everything is connected. Our bodies affect our minds, but equally our minds affect our bodies. Both affect our psyches and our souls. And our external environment and the people around us will affect us too, in body, mind and spirit. So really the four seasons are just different ways of looking at the whole. It's as if the year offered us a selection of ways to grow

and change. You might start with the body and find your career
or relationships shift. Likewise, making changes in your psyche
could quite literally alter your body.

Autumn is the time I call the Season of the Mind. It's also a
time to view our relationship with the environment around us
and our path, our purpose in life. Autumn is a dynamic season
which has a powerful effect on almost everyone, and represents
another big shift in the year. For children, the year begins in
September with the return to school after the long summer break.
Colleges and universities follow the pattern. It makes good seasonal sense as autumn ushers in fresh thoughts, a new impetus
for learning, for using the mind.

Winter sees a deep plunge into the Season of the Soul. It mirrors
our relationship with spirit, with the divine, with something larger
and greater than ourselves. This is a section which might cause
some people problems. When it comes to spirits and souls, many
of us rush into denial. Why? Maybe we have been put off spiritual
matters by early religious experiences. Maybe we feel we simply
don't have the time, the luxury, the indulgence, to become "spiritual." Or maybe we are frightened of what would happen if we
delved deep enough into our truer essence. Whatever the reason,
rest assured that the winter section isn't all about spirituality and
it most certainly isn't about religion, so just try it and see. If
anything feels uncomfortable or ridiculous, just read it through
and let it go.

The individual chapters on each month of the year develop
the themes of the season and provide a loose framework for
action. This isn't a precise guidebook, more of a seasonal "pick
and mix" bag which outlines the kinds of activities, treatments,
and therapies that are particularly attuned to that time of year.
Please don't feel constrained by their order in the book. If you
feel like launching into Rolfing in January, that's fine. You don't
have to wait until the "right" month. See what appeals and give
it a go. Even making the tiniest change, taking on board just one
small point, instigating one new ritual or routine in your life will
make a difference and you'll notice a change. It's like throwing
a tiny pebble into a pool—the ripples spread out and touch every
part of the water. Even the smallest change in your actions or
even your thoughts can have much larger consequences.

The whole idea of seasonal health is to make change gently,

naturally; to work with the ebb and flow of the year. Working with this program means looking to long-term change—and constant change. Nothing stays the same in nature and so we can hardly expect ourselves to stay the same month after month, year after year. We mature, we grow, we learn new skills and seek different goals. You can't stop the clock and you shouldn't want to. When energy stays still, it easily turns stagnant; when it flows freely but in a controlled manner, it stays healthy, vibrant, alive.

Hopefully, this book will help you get back in touch with your natural self, to find yourself moving with the flow of life. And once you manage that, suddenly you *will* find that your life changes. The world will become, quite literally, a different place.

The Long-Lost Wisdom of the Seasons

Much of the information in this book is not new. It dates back decades, centuries, even millennia. Seasonal living is not some fresh fad dreamt up by marketing people or put under the microscope by scientists—it is living wisdom that has been used for thousands of years. Most of the advice in this book has been tried and tested by literally millions of people and it has been handed down from generation to generation for one simple reason: it works. The ancient Indians, Tibetans and Chinese were highly advanced in science, technology and medicine. Their ultimate quest was for immortality and, if they didn't quite achieve that, at the very least they succeeded in living very long lives, in exceptionally good health.

Throughout this book I have drawn on a very wide variety of disciplines and therapies but the mainstays are the great ancient healing systems of traditional Chinese medicine (TCM) and Ayurveda from India, backed up by the Western system of naturopathy. I also pay a lot of attention to the old festivals of the Celtic year which have been passed down and form the basis of modern paganism. Seasonal rituals are just as important as what you eat or how you exercise.

If you are serious about your health and well-being, I would truly recommend you put yourself in the care of a good natural health-care practitioner. Throughout the book I will be talking about hoards of different natural therapies, but at this stage you really need to find someone who will act as your complementary GP. Not someone to take the place of a medical practitioner but who can look at all aspects of your life and put you in the peak of health. I have described all the major therapies in my first book, *Supertherapies,* and which you choose is totally up to you. But I would suggest you might look to a practitioner of either naturopathy, Ayurveda or TCM. All these disciplines are used to working with the seasons and will help you adapt yourself to the shifts and changes of the year. Their practitioners will be able to advise you on adjusting your diet, your exercise and your mindset—to fine-tune the information in this book especially for you. I have outlined these three disciplines below and suggest you pick whichever seems most appealing. However, throughout the book, I shall be using information from them all.

The Five Energies: The Chinese Approach to the Seasons

The Chinese have followed the wisdom of the seasons for millennia. While more primitive cultures merely watched the passing year and adapted their lives to fit in with the rigors of each season, the Chinese evaluated and experimented, gradually building up a vast storehouse of knowledge. They made a precise study of the nature of the seasons and the different forms of energy that emerge with the arrival of each shift in the weather. They discovered that good health, success and happiness could all be achieved by obtaining the correct balance of these energies—via the right food and exercise, correct timing, auspicious architecture and even the right kind of interior design.

It sounds far-fetched but nowadays more and more strands of ancient Chinese culture are becoming accepted all over the world. Western orthodox doctors are investigating the incredible power of acupuncture and Chinese herbalism. Massage therapists are learning techniques such as acupressure and tuina and finding that their clients respond with amazing results. Feng shui, the Chinese art of placement in architecture and interior design, is becoming ardently accepted by businesses keen for greater success and higher profits, while ordinary people are busy shifting furniture and hanging up crystals and silver balls in the hope of greater luck, better love and, of course, more money. And even the complex oracle, the *I Ching,* one of the most ancient books in the world, is being used more and more as a tool for greater happiness and success, teaching people the best and most auspicious time and way to proceed in important life choices.

To the Chinese it all seems very obvious. All of life is energy and energy is constantly changing, constantly flowing. The energy that abounds with the bright morning sun is quite different from that of the glowing sunset; the vigorous thrusting energy of spring cannot be compared to the apparent emptiness of winter. A forest feels quite different to a mountain top; a cluttered apartment has a completely different atmosphere from a soaring cathedral. In order to pass through life smoothly, healthily and successfully you need to get into the flow, to move seamlessly in harmony with the vital energies of the earth and cosmos, rather than fighting against them. It's like swimming easily and effortlessly with a gentle current rather than trying to fight your way up a series of rapids.

The underlying philosophy is that good health (in body, mind and spirit) revolves around the correct flow of *chi,* the subtle energy of the body. *Chi* flows around the body in channels called meridians, and along the meridians lie hundreds of points which link the various organs and functions of the body.

If we look after ourselves, eat the right kinds of food, do the right kinds of exercise, keep our bodies and minds balanced, the *chi* in our bodies will flow smoothly and correcting. If we fall into bad ways, our levels of *chi* drop or are blocked and the consequence is lack of vital energy, or even disease. In a similar way, *chi* flows through houses and landscapes and can be blocked or allowed to rush through in a completely undisciplined manner. The art of feng shui looks at how to harmonize our environment to keep this external flow of *chi* beneficial to us. Then there is the oracle of the *I Ching,* which teaches us the art of good timing: how to get in step with the elemental energies of the year; when to act and when not to act for the best results.

The whole Chinese lifeview is immensely complex and, some might say, almost obsessive. *Chi* can be depleted or lost through too much, too little or the wrong kind of food, drink, exercise, work and even sex. Your emotions can become out of balance and affect your health. And, of course, not taking notice of the shifts in seasons can lay you low as well.

According to TCM, the world is also divided into two forces—*yin* and *yang*. *Yin* is considered to be dark, cold, negative, passive and feminine, while *yang* is light, active, warm, positive, and male. Disturb the balance of *yin* and *yang* and, once again, the result is disharmony, possibly ill health. In addition, there are the five elements to consider: each of us contains within us the elements of fire, earth, metal (or air), water and wood. When TCM practitioners diagnose, they don't just check for the flow of *chi,* they also look to see how much of each element is within the body and what kind of energy is being transmitted. Then they can stimulate or quieten unbalanced organs or body systems by food, exercise, massage, herbs or acupuncture.

Interestingly, the Chinese divide the four seasons once again to produce the four mid-season points—in all, the year is divided up into eight slices (just as in the ancient Celtic calendar). While Western science is just beginning to accept the idea of biorhythms, natural shifts in human energy, the Chinese have known about it for thousands of years. They divide each day into different phases according to the kind of energy that prevails: *yang* rules from midnight until noon, while *yin* moves in to govern noon until midnight. Recognizing that human energy shifts accordingly, early morning has always been associated for the Chinese with high energy, while mid-afternoon (high *yin* time) is yawning siesta time. Orthodox physiologists are now discovering what the Chinese have always known: each organ receives energy at different times of the day or year. Asthma attacks don't occur more frequently at dawn from chance but because 3 A.M. is the time when the lungs are at the height of their energetic activity. High noon is the most likely time to have a heart attack because this is the hour of the heart's maximum activity. Why do most people have their major bowel movement first thing in the morning? You could put it down to potty training, but more likely it's because the largest intestine receives the largest amount of energy at that time.

Yin and *yang* work in larger cycles too. Each month has its *yin* and *yang* phases—*yin* rules from the full moon until the new moon while *yang* takes over from the new moon until the moon is full once again. And the whole year shifts to the *yin/yang* rhythm—fresh new *yang* rises with bounding energy and vitality in spring and reaches its full, abundant maturity in the height of summer. Then *yin* begins to rise and takes us down through the quiet of autumn into the depths of winter. For a Taoist or follower of Chinese medicine it would be sheer madness not to adapt their lifestyle to fit the seasons—diet, daily activities, exercise, herbs and even sex are changed and adapted according to the shifting seasonal energies.

We all carry all the various elements within us and, in an ideal world, they would all be in balance. When this happens, we enjoy perfect health and abundant vitality. A person who is balanced adjusts naturally to the cycle of changing seasons and is in perfect harmony with the world around. However, given the stress, strain and pollution of modern life, few of us are naturally in balance. Bad food, insufficient exercise and the numerous environmental pollutants in the world take their toll. The result is that our bodies don't adapt naturally to the shifts in energy that occur with each season, and so we fall ill or feel generally under par. The Chinese would say that we have fallen prey to an "evil" energy, which upsets the delicate internal balance between *yin* and *yang* and causes all kinds of problems.

THE FIVE ENERGIES

Wood The element associated with spring, wood is the fresh *yang* stage of the seasonal cycle—young, expansive, energetic, thrusting and explosive. It provides creative energy, increased sexuality, vigor and growth. Wood energy within the body nourishes the muscles and the tissues. It governs the gall bladder and the liver. Within the psyche it calls for free expression, for the freedom and space to explore new ideas, to try new things. If wood is blocked it will cause feelings of frustration, stagnation, jealousy and anger.

Fire The element of summer arises when the creative power of wood grows and matures into the full *yang* of fire. This is the creative power at its height—everything is expansive, fully grown, satisfied. Fire, quite naturally, warms the heart and human emotions. It pulses the blood round the body and keeps our own vital energy, or *chi,* moving and also controls the small intestine. Fire is open and generous, abundant, joyous and brave. If fire is blocked, it can cause heart problems, hypertension or disorders of the nervous system, making people nervous, hysterical or neurotic.

Earth Although the Chinese divide the year neatly into four seasons they also recognize a fifth—a period between high summer and autumn in which everything is in perfect balance. It is a mellow time during which neither *yin* nor *yang* rule. This is the fulcrum of the year when everything is poised, everything is full and ripe, providing a feeling of ease and well being, comfort and completeness. Earth is the embodiment of nourishment and vitality and governs the stomach. So, if earth becomes unbalanced or is deficient in your system you will find you have problems with digestion.

Metal Energy is shifting into its *yin* phase as autumn arrives, contracting, condensing, beginning to store and save itself for the lean months ahead, just as in the fields the harvest has been brought in to feed humans and animals through the winter. It is a time for jettisoning the old and unnecessary, keeping only the healthy and vital to see us through the dark days ahead. In the body, metal (or air) controls the lungs and the large intestine. Blocked metal energy will produce chest infections, skin problems, flu, colds and respiratory problems. On a psychological level it will cause feelings of grief and sadness, melancholy and anxiety.

Water In winter *yin* has moved into its most extreme state. Everything is still and cold, waiting and resting. Energy is being condensed, conserved, held in storage until the thrusting *yang* energy rises again. To the Chinese, water is considered a highly concentrated element whose power is awaiting release, like a cat bunched and poised to spring. In our bodies, water rules over the fluids in our systems—the hormones, the mysterious lymph, the slow bone marrow, the essential enzymes. This is a time to store and to keep warm, a time to conserve vital energy and go deep within. If water becomes unbalanced it can cause chills and fevers, headaches and a variety of other bodily aches and pains. It can even cause sexual impotence.

The best ways to calm and balance your energies will be discussed throughout the book, in the relevant seasons. However, if you have a chronic problem it would be worth consulting a practitioner of TCM so he or she could work out precisely how to balance your energies. TCM is a highly complex system of health care which can produce remarkable results. In the hands of a skilled practitioner it is powerful medicine and you should always inform your GP or consultant if you do decide to try it.

Balancing the Doshas: Ayurveda and the Year

The other great seasonal adviser is Ayurveda, arguably the oldest form of medicine on earth. Its principles were said to have been passed down to humankind from a chain of gods leading back to Brahma, the father of all gods. Ayurveda has been called "the mother of medicine" and is generally accepted to be the forerunner of all the other great world healing systems: the Tibetan, the Greek, the Arabic, even the Chinese (although they might argue about which came first). Written texts show that the ayurvedic medicine practiced from about 1500 B.C. to A.D. 500 was incredibly advanced. Students studied six philosophical systems: the study of logic, of evolution and causality, of the discipline of body and spirit (yoga), of moral behavior, of pure esoteric knowledge and even the theory of the atom. Historians of the ancient world wrote of the great universities which taught Ayurveda, but when India started to suffer invasions in the Middle Ages the system began to fall apart and the universities were broken up.

The British were the final nail in the coffin of Ayurveda: they brought their own brand of modern Western medicine with them and established their own universities. Ayurveda was in danger of dying out altogether. Fortunately the Indians realized what they were losing and the Indian Congress affirmed support for Ayurveda; in 1921 Mahatma Gandhi opened the first new college for ayurvedic medicine. Now Ayurveda is being practiced alongside Western medicine in India and is becoming popular in the West as well.

The ayurvedic philosophy is remarkably similar to that of the Chinese. Ayurveda is basically a preventative discipline which teaches that, if you can bring your body, mind and soul into perfect balance then you will live in good health and emotional happiness. Not only will you live well, say the ayurvedic texts, but you will also live long. Like the Chinese, the ayurvedic sages saw longevity, even immortality, as their ultimate goal. The ancient texts say that the human lifespan should be around 100 years and that all those years should be lived in total health, both physical and mental.

So the ayurvedic practitioner is looking to balance the body and mind, to ferret out health problems before they occur or to nip them in the bud before they do any real harm. Unfortunately, the texts say, the causes of illness (and the shortening of life) are caused by virtually every ill of modern life: constant stress; irregular meals; eating the wrong kind of food; taking the wrong medication; having bad posture; breathing in polluted air; allowing microorganisms to enter the body; becoming injured; not digesting food properly, and living out of balance with the natural rhythm of the seasons.

As with Chinese philosophy, Ayurveda sees the world and everything in it consisting of five elements—earth, water, fire (as with the Chinese) and air and ether (instead of metal and wood). They even understood the concept of the atom and used this tiny block of matter to demonstrate the action of the elements teaching that the weight of the atom comes from earth, its cohesion from water, its energy from fire, its motion from air and the spaces between its particles are made of ether. So the whole human body is made up of the five elements, and Indian philosophy says that an excess of one or more elements can be the cause of imbalance and so lead to illness.

Over the centuries, Ayurveda came up with a kind of shorthand for the elements—it combined the five elements into three bio-energies or *"tridoshas"*: *vata, pitta* and *kapha*. *Vata* comes from a combination of ether and air; *pitta* from the fire with a little water; and *kapha* from water and earth. In an ideal state, we would have all three *doshas* in perfect balance, but this is rare. Most of us have one or perhaps two which overbalance the others. The whole of ayurvedic medicine aims to balance the *doshas* in order to restore health.

As with the Chinese system, the *doshas* are responsible for different parts and functions in the body. *Vata* produces movement in the body; *pitta* produces heat and so is responsible for the metabolism, while *kapha* produces growth and structure. All three are essential for life: without *vata* we couldn't breathe, our blood wouldn't pump around the body, food wouldn't move through our guts, nor would any chemical impulses fly to and from the brain. Without *pitta* we would not be able to process the air, water and food that runs through our system. And without *kapha* we simply wouldn't hold together: it keeps our cells bonded together and fuses bone, muscle, fat and connective tissue.

The *dosha* that dominates within our bodies gives rise to our *prakruti,* or body type—the basic predominating psychophysiological force which affects everything about us—from our shape and our weight to our predisposition to different illnesses; to the forms of exercise that suit us; the kinds of food we should eat; how we think; how we react to situations, to how we perceive the whole world. Above all, Ayurveda teaches that we should follow a seasonal routine to keep ourselves in balance as the seasons and prevailing energies change. They even have a name for the process—*ritucharya. Ritucharya* doesn't involve overturning your lifestyle every few months, rather simply being aware of the shifts in the seasons and moving the emphasis of your diet and activities.

Although there are general guidelines for how to cope with the seasonal changes, Ayurveda believes that we should further adapt our lifestyle in each season according to our own individual *prakruti.* It is especially important to watch the season that matches your body type: *pitta* corresponds to summer, which can be a tricky time for *pitta* types; *vatas* should take care in winter, while spring is the time to watch for *kaphas.* For a complete understanding of your *prakruti* and how to adapt it perfectly to the year you should seek out a good ayurvedic physician.

WORKING OUT YOUR <u>PRAKRUTI</u>

Few people have just one *dosha* predominating—most of us are a combination of two. If you are truly balanced already, you will be a perfect balance among all three but, as you might imagine, that is quite rare. The following questionnaire should help you gain a general understanding of the *doshas* that govern you.

Read through the following questions and tick off those apply to you.

Your Physical Body

1. What were you like at birth and as a child?
   a) Small at birth, and a thin child.
   b) Average size at birth, and a medium-sized child.
   c) A large baby, and plump child.
2. What is your build now?
   a) Thin with light bones and prominent joints and tendons. Perhaps either very tall or very short, you hardly ever put on weight.
   b) Of medium build and bone structure. You can easily gain and lose weight.
   c) Large boned and quite heavy or dense in build, with broad shoulders or wide hips. You find it hard to lose weight.
3. What is your skin like?
   a) Dry, delicate skin that is easily affected by the weather.
   b) Soft skin. A ruddy or freckled complexion.
   c) A pale complexion with thick skin. Skin can be oily but will usually be cool to the touch.
4. What kind of hair do you have?
   a) Normal to dry, dark, wiry or kinky.
   b) Normal to fine hair, blond, red or prematurely gray.
   c) Normal to oily, thick wavy hair.
5. What are your eyes like?
   a) Small, dark and constantly moving.
   b) Quite penetrating in their stare, light green, gray or hazel.
   c) Large beautiful eyes with lustrous, brown eyelashes.
6. What kind of appetite do you have?

a) Irregular: sometimes you feel ravenous, sometimes you can't be bothered. You like to snack or nibble and often have eyes bigger than your stomach when it comes to larger meals.

b) Good: you hate to skip meals and feel irritable, even ill, if forced to do so. You like high-protein foods such as meat and fish, eggs and pulses.

c) Healthy: you enjoy food and don't like skipping meals but if forced to do so, you suffer no ill effects. You love starchy, fatty foods such as bread, sweets, cakes.

7. How are your bowel movements?
   a) Irregular, often hard or constipated.
   b) Regular, tending to soft, loose and profuse.
   c) Regular, steady, thick and heavy.

8. How do you sleep?
   a) A light sleeper, with sleep often short and interrupted. You might find it hard to get to sleep or be liable to insomnia.
   b) A regular and sound sleeper, rarely any problems.
   c) A heavy, long sleeper. Can be liable to oversleep or feel drowsy during the day.

9. What are your hands and nails like?
   a) Cold hands with little perspiration; nails are often brittle.
   b) Hands often perspire, nails are flexible but quite strong.
   c) Hands sometimes perspire, nails are thick and strong.

10. How do you walk?
    a) Quickly, lightly, always seem in a hurry.
    b) Medium pace but in a determined, purposeful fashion.
    c) Slowly and steadily, calm.

11. What kind of illnesses are you prone to?
    a) Sharp pains, headaches, nervous disorders, gas or constipation, eczema or dry rashes.
    b) Rashes and allergies, inflammation, heartburn, ulcers, acidity, feverish complaints.
    c) Fluid retention and excess mucus, bronchitis, sinus problems, asthma, congestion.

Your Mind and Emotions

12. What is your basic personality?
    a) Enthusiastic, outgoing, talkative but with changeable moods and ideas.
    b) Strong-minded and purposeful. You thrive on challenges and tend to be quite forceful in expressing your opinions.
    c) Calm, placid and good-natured; easy-going, reliable and steady.

13. What are you like at work?
    a) Quick, imaginative and alert. An active and creative thinker with an endless fund of ideas. You become bored with rigid routine or discipline.
    b) A natural leader with a keen intellect. Efficient, you like well-planned routine and tend to be a perfectionist.
    c) You keep projects running smoothly and calmly. You enjoy a regular routine.

14. How do you react to stress?
    a) Tendency to become anxious or nervous.
    b) Become angry or irritable.
    c) Try to avoid it at all costs.

15. How do you dream?
    a) Frequently, but often you can't remember your dreams on waking.
    b) Vividly, often in color. You find it easy to remember your dreams.
    c) You only tend to remember highly significant or clear dreams.

16. What is your memory like?
    a) You're quick to learn but equally quick to forget.
    b) Your memory is generally quite good.
    c) You take a while to learn but your long-term memory is excellent.

17. How is your sex life?
    a) You have an active fantasy but your sexual interest actually tends to fluctuate: sometimes you love sex; at other times you aren't that interested.
    b) You have a pretty average sex drive.

c) You love sex and, although you might take a while to "warm up," you have intense sex and great stamina.
18. Do you spend or save money?
   a) Money is there to spend. You tend to be an impulse-buyer and have large credit card bills.
   b) You are a sensible spender, buying useful and classic items.
   c) You are a great saver and always have enough money.
19. How would you describe your lifestyle?
   a) Erratic, always changing.
   b) Busy with plenty of plans. You achieve a lot.
   c) Steady and regular. You may feel a bit stuck in a rut.

Assessing Your Score

There are no trick questions here—simply add up how many a's, b's and c's you ticked. A predominance of a's signifies that you are most likely a *vata* type; b's indicate *pitta,* and c's indicate *kapha.* Few people ever have just one *dosha,* so don't be surprised if you have two scores quite close. Most of us are a combination of two *doshas*—some people even have all three.

Mainly a's

Vata Speed and movement are the keys to *vata,* so it's not surprising to find that *vata* is the *dosha* of wind and air. *Vata* is always on the go, both physically and mentally. *Vatas* are ideas people, full of imagination and often artistic. They are quick, creative and flexible, reveling in new things, new ideas, new sights. However, it is hard to pin them down to one task or one idea; they are changeable and tend to flit from one thing to another. *Vatas* pick up new subjects very quickly and easily but often forget them just as quickly.

Vata as an energy is most active in the late afternoon and early evening (from 2 P.M. to 6 P.M.) and just before dawn (2 A.M. to 6 A.M.). Its season is autumn and winter. When *vata* is imbalanced, it can cause constipation, bloating and wind, aching joints, dry skin and hair, brittle nails, failing memory or confusion.

Mainly b's

Pitta Fire and water are the elements of *pitta. Pitta* people have initiative and good energy; they are determined and force-

ful, confident in their abilities, courageous, intelligent and generally happy. *Pittas* grasp information quickly and easily and can
put their knowledge into practice. They are great organizers in
whatever field they find themselves—either as highly organized
parents or the leaders of giant corporations.

Pitta as an element is strongest between 10 A.M. and 2 P.M.
and from 10 P.M. to 2 A.M. Its season is, not surprisingly, high
summer and this is when *pitta* people need to be especially
careful. If *pitta* becomes imbalanced, you can fall prey to sun-
burn, rashes and irritability in the sun. Sore throats, inflammations
and fevers and intense feelings of anger, frustration, or jealousy
are all signs of imbalanced *pitta*.

Mainly c's

Kapha Solidity is the key word for *kapha,* the *dosha* of
earth and water. *Kapha* is solid, strong and enduring, and *kapha*
people often have great stamina. They are also wonderfully calm,
grounded, honest and trustworthy people who prefer to shun the
limelight and quietly work on the task in hand. *Kapha* people
crave security—they enjoy routines and the comforts of regularity.
They most definitely like their food and are susceptible to comfort eating and putting on weight.

Kapha times are 6 A.M. to 10 A.M. and 6 P.M. and 10 P.M. The
kapha season is spring. When *kapha* falls into imbalance, you
will find excess weight and mucus building in the body; sinuses
will become blocked and colds will become common. Depression is the bane of imbalanced *kapha*.

FINDING AND BALANCING YOUR DOSHAS

Finding and balancing your *doshas* can be a truly liberating experience. People who have never been able to lose weight easily
can find the excess simply vanishing as they rid their body of
the foods that increase *kapha*. Equally, those who never seem
able to put on weight however much they eat can find a *vata*-
soothing diet will bring them down to earth. The benefits aren't
just physical: soothing imbalanced *doshas* can help your memory
and concentration, allow you to sleep better, help you deal with

stress and depression, make you less irritable and even improve your sex life.

Where Ayurveda can become confusing is when you find that, although you are predominantly, say, *kapha,* you also seem to have several strong characteristics of another *dosha* that seem to contradict your main *dosha*—for example, you are having trouble sleeping, your hands and feet are cold, and you are having bad constipation. In this case you are a *kapha* person who is suffering from a *vata* imbalance and would need to soothe *vata* as well as keep your own constitutional *dosha* in balance.

Finding Imbalances

The following should give you an idea whether you have an imbalance in any *dosha*. Once again, simply tick the questions that you can answer "yes" to. If you have several ticks in any one category it is quite likely that you have an imbalance in that *dosha*. Ideally, you should see a specialist in Ayurveda for an individualized program.

Vata imbalance
1. Are you seriously underweight?
2. Do you have eczema or dry, rough, chapped skin?
3. Do you suffer from constipation or bad wind?
4. Are you finding it hard to concentrate, difficult to relax? Do you constantly jump up to do things?
5. Is your sleep very disturbed? Do you find it hard to get to sleep or have bad insomnia?
6. Are your hands and feet often cold? Do you have bad circulation?
7. Do you often have headaches or migraine?
8. Are you constantly overexerting yourself?

Pitta imbalance
1. Do you suffer from heartburn, ulcers or acidity?
2. Are you frequently irritable, impatient or critical?
3. Are you over-ambitious, too demanding and stubborn?
4. If you are stressed do you tend to overreact, by getting angry or frustrated?
5. Do you break out in rashes easily? Are you very susceptible to bad food or environmental pollution?

6. Do you often have diarrhea?
7. Do you often get feverish colds and flu?
8. Do you react badly to the heat and sun?

Kapha imbalance
1. Is your skin dull and congested with enlarged pores?
2. Are you very overweight and finding the excess weight impossible to shift?
3. Do you become possessive and overattached to people and things?
4. Do you feel uncomfortable in cool, damp weather?
5. Do you have a lot of mucus, sinus problems, asthma, bronchitis or phlegm?
6. Are you very lethargic and over-complacent? Do you lack the energy to change?
7. Do you often oversleep or find yourself dozing off during the day?
8. Are you greedy?

If you do have an imbalance, try the following guidelines to soothe the *dosha*. Sometimes you will find that the *dosha*-calming activity might contradict the general seasonal guidelines. This is quite likely as the guidelines are just that, guidelines. I can't emphasize enough how individual we all are and how much we all require slightly different things at different times. That is why this book is *not* a precise, point-by-point regime. Try to listen to your body, get an intuition of what *feels* right, what your body really needs at a deep level and try following that course.

Balancing Vata
Follow these guidelines if you are predominantly a *vata* type or have a *vata* imbalance.
• You need regularity in your life above all else, which isn't an easy thing for *vata* types to achieve. But do try, because regularity will give *vatas* a far more steady and balanced output of energy and you will find you can keep going for far longer rather than expending masses of energy in short bursts followed by periods of complete collapse. Make yourself eat your meals at regular times, at the same time each day. Always sit down for your food—eating on the run or snatching snacks will aggravate

vata very quickly. Try to get to bed at the same time each night and get up at the same time each morning. If you can get to bed early (around 10 p.m. is ideal) you will find less anxious and agitated.

• When you find yourself in overdrive, recognize it and purposefully slow down. Learning meditation, yoga, chi kung (an exercise and meditation system that combines breathing techniques with precise movements and mental concentration) or autogenic training (mental exercises that combat stress) could really help here.

• You love fast, high-energy sports and activities, but to balance your *dosha* you should try something more calming and lower in impact. Again, yoga is great, so is t'ai-chi. If you always go running or do high-impact aerobics, take down the pace and try hill-walking or low-impact aerobics. And rather than doing nothing all week and then exhausting yourself in a two-hour squash marathon at the weekend, try to take a regular amount of steady exercise throughout the week.

• As a *vata* you will naturally be drawn like a wasp to jam to fast-action sports and exciting new experiences. You revel in sensory overload but it can be the worst thing for anyone with a *vata* imbalance. Try to avoid very loud music, flashing lights and swift-action computer games. Calm, gentle, creative pursuits might sound boring but taking up painting or tapestry could be very beneficial. Cultivate the fine art of doing nothing. If you're going on holiday, resist the urge to book the safari or the "learn a different sport a day" adventure break. Pick a beautiful spot and stay there; give yourself sun and warmth and simply revel in the relaxation.

• The ideal *vata*-calming diet should include warm, even slightly heavy, foods and sweet fruits. Above all, you should avoid cold and iced foods, chilled drinks and raw food—raw apples and greens are not a good idea. Make sure your food is easy to digest—soups are great, and dry foods like rice or pasta need only a little oil or butter to lubricate them. Go easy on beans as they won't help the *vata* wind—the best choices are split mung beans, yellow dhal or black lentils (known as urud dhal). Never eat very dry food, frozen foods or leftovers.

• Keep warm. *Vata* needs warmth in all senses—not just physical warmth but spiritual warmth as well. Try to put yourself in a safe, warm, caring environment. Saunas and steam rooms are wonderful environments for *vata*, so relax in one whenever you can.

• Learn how to express your feelings. *Vata* types often find it hard to speak their mind, and suppressing feelings will only aggravate *vata*. If you feel this is a problem, try assertion training or counseling.

• Get enough sleep. *Vata* types should avoid late nights, working late, particularly jobs that involve night shifts.

Balancing Pitta

Follow these guidelines if you are predominantly *pitta* or have a *pitta* imbalance.

• Keep cool. Avoid the physical heat, stay out of the hot sun, keep clear of steam rooms and saunas (although you probably love them) which combine heat and humidity, the two things you need to shun. If you have a warm bath or shower, finish off with a cool rinse. Get out in the open air as much as you can but, if it's hot, keep cool in the shade.

• *Pitta* types are normally highly organized, so maybe you need to introduce just a touch of spontaneity into your life. Be careful that you don't become too goal-orientated, too focused on objectives and nothing else. Try taking a walk "for the hell of it" or just sitting in the garden or gazing out of the window—not doing anything in particular, just musing, which is very therapeutic for *pittas*.

• If you're a typical *pitta* you thrive on challenge, hate being bored and love a little competition in life. Obviously you shouldn't get bored, but don't take on too much or challenge yourself too far. Be careful that you don't end up sacrificing everything just to win.

• *Pittas* are naturals in competitive sports. They adore tennis and squash, and even an innocent game of ping-pong brings out the killer serve. They can easily take sport far too seriously, and if you know you're a *pitta* type you should avoid anything too competitive. Water sports are wonderfully calming and soothing for *pitta,* and of course winter sports in the snow and ice will cool that *pitta* fire.

• *Pittas* love hot spicy foods, meat and alcohol—the curry and beer or steak and red wine-drinking business-type is a typical *pitta,* but these foods are there absolute bane. Avoid or at the very least cut right down on oily or greasy foods, caffeine, salt, red meat, alcohol and any highly spiced foods. Foods that tend to cool and calm *pitta* include fresh fruit and vegetables, milk, soft cheeses (not hard cheese), cottage cheese, ice cream. Whole-grains are fine for *pitta,* and greens provide the bitter taste that can balance *pitta* so well.

Balancing Kapha

Follow these guidelines if you are predominantly *kapha* or have a *kapha* imbalance.

• Let go. *Kaphas* are great hoarders, they hold on to things— be it weight, people, or emotions. It can be very beneficial to loosen up, to trust a little, to release.

• Allow change, unpredictability and excitement into your life. *Kaphas* love routine and feel safe and secure when everything stays the same, but taking the odd chance or allowing the pulse rate to speed up a little from time to time will give any sluggish *kapha* energy a good boost. Even little things can help—vary your route to work; shift the furniture around in your office or home; if you always have a drink at 6 P.M. go for a walk instead.

• *Kaphas* love to sit doing nothing in particular. Leisure and relaxation are favorite words. To balance *kapha* you need to get your system moving, give it a bit of a shake-up. You need to take on new activities and challenges that will stimulate you both physically and mentally, so try a new sport, a night class or go and see a different kind of film from the type you normally watch. Keep your activities varied; if you do aerobics, try switching your routine or doing step or slide aerobics or boxercise. *Kaphas* need plenty of physical exercise, so try to incorporate some activity into every day. On holiday, *kaphas* are the ones whose idea of fun is flopping into a sun-lounger in the morning and having to be pried off it in the evening. To stimulate *kapha,* choose a touring holiday or, horror of horrors, try an activity holiday where you will have constant stimulation.

• Avoid iced foods and drinks, cut right down on sweets and don't eat too much bread. Dairy produce will aggravate *kapha*— it produces yet more mucus—and wheat can often be a problem too. Heavy, starchy foods are really unsuitable for *kapha.* Instead eat warm, light and dry foods—nothing stodgy or greasy. However, *kapha* does need a certain amount of complex carbohydrate to function well, so try using grains such as millet, barley and rye which are all light and dry. Plenty of fresh vegetables will help, and use herbs and spices liberally.

Naturopathy: Harnessing the Healing Power of the Elements

The system of naturopathy may not have a written tradition that can be traced back thousands of years, but its wisdom is as ancient as the planet itself. Naturopathy is to the West what Ayurveda and traditional Chinese medicine are to the East—a gentle, nature-based, holistic health system that aims to put the whole body in balance. And many of its "cures" involve simple DIY routines that can be incorporated into every regime.

Historically speaking, the roots of naturopathy lie in the darkest antiquity. Hippocrates spoke of *ponos*, the body's incessant labor to restore itself to normal balance, while Aristotle spoke of the life force having a purpose beyond simply existing. Both these viewpoints echo the British Naturopathic and Osteopathic Association's description of naturopathy as "a system of treatment which recognizes the vital curative force within the body."

In its current standardized form, naturopathy has been around for over 100 years. One of the early pioneers of naturopathy, Dr. Henry Lindlahr, defined disease as an "abnormal or inharmonious vibration of the elements and forces composing the human entity on one or more planes of being." Again, we're back to the Indian and Chinese concepts of energy and elements within the body responsible for health and ill health. These disturbances, he believed, are due to lowered vitality; an abnormal composition of blood and lymph; an accumulation of morbid materials and poisons within the body.

What brings on such disturbances? Partly hereditary factors and partly early environment (both before and after birth) but, most importantly, the lifestyle we lead. Most toxic of all is mesotrophy, the slow decline of the cell, which is caused by poor diet. Once again, this is remarkably similar to the Chinese and ayurvedic view.

Naturopathy is the great detoxing therapy. It takes the view that many of our health problems are due to the incomplete elimination of the waste products of our metabolism and the accumulation of toxins. The body tries to live with a growing accumulation of waste, and the result is low-level disease—not a particular illness but a sense of feeling below par. So the aim of all naturopathic processes is to help the elimination of waste by bolstering every one of the body's excretory functions through diet, detox treatments, water therapies and exercise regimes.

Again, if you have a chronic health problem or want a totally individual program you should consult a qualified naturopath. Balance is achieved by using the most natural cures available: fresh air and sunlight, fasting and a fresh clean diet, relaxation and psychological counseling and, very importantly, the healing power of water. In addition, many naturopaths are also trained osteopaths and will treat mechanical problems of the body with a course of manipulation.

Some naturopaths are purists and work only with these most basic tools. They believe that our health is our own responsibility, that we should take strict measures to keep it under control and they consider the use of herbal or homeopathic medicines as taking away the element of personal responsibility. However, many others have incorporated other disciplines, and most naturopaths you will come across are masters of many arts, using herbalism, homeopathy and acupuncture in addition to the traditional methods. They see these systems as important catalysts, pushing the body toward health and helping its self-healing mechanism.

The Transforming Power of Ritual

Alongside ideas for adapting your diet, exercise and lifestyle to the seasons, I have included plenty of information on seasonal rituals and festivities that could be gradually incorporated into your life. I believe that in ignoring or over-commercializing ritual celebrations we are in danger of losing a vital key to our emotional, mental and spiritual health.

In pre-Christian times, rituals marked the ebb and flow of nature. The year spun around, marked with regular seasonal festivals in which all the community participated. In the past, anthropologists and psychologists assumed that these were a means of trying to control nature, to appease the gods and hopefully ensure a good harvest, a gentle winter, peace and plenty. However, some experts are now starting to think differently. Perhaps, they ponder, the great seasonal festivals and all the various rituals of the year were not about controlling or appeasing nature but more a means of coming to terms with the shifting rhythms of the seasons. By following the ups and downs of the year, people could come to grips with the cycles of their own lives, learning that there are times of great energy and joy alongside times of quiet introspection; times of birth and rebirth, but inevitably also times of sadness, loss and death. What worked for our ancestors can work for us, and taking the time to rediscover the great seasonal festivals can provide us with a renewed sense of self and of community.

Unfortunately, nowadays when we think about rituals we tend to envisage boring church services or the tedium of forced family get-togethers. When we think about festivals and seasonal celebrations we imagine the commercialized nightmare of Christmas that starts in September; of children being sick after too many Easter eggs; of card manufacturers cashing in with Valentine's Day, Mother's Day, Father's Day, Grandparents' Day . . . Surely, you might think, we need fewer rituals and festivals, not more.

The key is to make rituals work for you. A good ritual or celebration is not about static, tired customs which you carry out for the sake of it; about routines enshrined in cobwebs. We need to feel free to adapt rituals and festivities to fit in with our lives, our desires and hopes. To be worthwhile and fulfilling, a ritual needs to have the true meaning for all the participants.

A good ritual can become very powerful. Because most rituals rely heavily on symbolic gestures and activities (lighting candles, hunting Easter eggs, sharing certain foods) they speak directly to our subconscious. They help us to come to terms with change, with the passing of time. Incorporating ritual back into your life can seem quite strange at first. When I first began to celebrate festivals like Beltane (May Day) and Lammas (Harvest) I felt like a complete idiot—lighting candles and incense, decking the house with greenery or corn sheaves and so on. But slowly, over the years, it became more and more a part of regular life. When I lived in the city, it turned into a means of reconnecting with the countryside, a world away from tarmac, brick, concrete and cars. Now that I live in the country it helps me become even more subtly attuned to the perpetual change around me. And, if you have children, please please take the time and effort to make rituals and celebrations particularly meaningful and special. Rituals give children a sense of order, of wonder, of being part of something larger and more comforting. They give tender young souls a chance to work out their anxieties and fears in a safe, loving environment. And, apart from anything else, with a little planning, the activities involved in preparing for festivals can keep children happily amused for days on end.

Throughout the book, I have included the major festivals and suggestions for the kinds of rituals that could be carried out at particular times of the year. If you want to know more about the current thinking on the therapeutic use of ritual there are several books available (see the back of this book). However, if you really want to learn about the power of ritual and the beauty of ceremony and festivals, then look at books on paganism. Some psychologists seriously believe that it is a subconscious yearning for our lost or denigrated celebrations that has caused, in part, the rising interest in paganism and other native earth-based religions, with their plethora of satisfying rituals and celebrations. Maybe it's time to reinstate festivals like Beltane (May Day) or Samhain (Halloween) to their proper ritual status. One very important point: please don't equate paganism with satanism or occultism. Paganism is the ancient earth religion which venerates life and seeks always to protect it. It has nothing to do with Satan or devil worship. Rest assured no one will try to convert you (pagans aren't allowed to talk about their beliefs unless you ask them) so suspend age-old prejudices, and you could learn a lot from this ancient faith.

Shan, a working pagan priestess who is also a therapist, taught me so much about the importance of ritual and festivals in the year. "The seasons of the year are less crucial to our modern lives with imported food, heated houses and indoor work," she notes, but adds, "yet our bodies and emotions still go through their important changes which are foolish to ignore." Rituals try to link people and their inner lives with the world outside, with the cycles of the earth, the rhythms of the seasons. They teach us about the nature of change, mark the boundaries between light and darkness; life, death and rebirth. But it's not all serious and psychological. Ritual can, and should, be fun. The pagan calendar celebrates eight major festivals a year, about one every six weeks. And, as Shan puts it, "That gives us about five to six weeks of workaday life, then a break for a holiday or celebration which is an entirely pleasant and very healthy rhythm."

Do try some of the rituals, however small, or think about how meaningful your own rituals (such as Christmas, birthdays, Easter, anniversaries, etc.) are. Small changes or new celebrations can make life far more interesting and could have some surprising knock-on effects.

Where Are You Now? The Self-evaluation Test

Before you start on any of the ideas in this book, give yourself time to fill in the questionnaire that follows. This book is all about your self, the true inner you. So the first place to start is right here and now with how you feel about all areas of your life. Please don't skip over this bit, since this one exercise can make you see your life in much clearer terms. You can only make changes when you're really clear about what you want to change. Often we *think* we know the answer, the one big bugbear in our lives, but there are plenty of other nasties lurking below the surface.

This quiz is designed to make you think about your life—about what is good in it and about what doesn't work so well. There aren't any right or wrong answers, so be as truthful and honest as you can. I would recommend you put your answers in a fresh notebook or journal. Buy one especially for the work you will do throughout this year—it will act as a diary and progress report. Ideally choose a book you really like—something special and beautiful—and keep it solely for your work. In other words, don't use it for scribbling notes to the kids or for the odd shopping list. It should be something very private. You can only be truly honest if you feel no one is going to read what you have written. So tell your family that this is a private zone. If you have nosey children you might consider buying one of those locking diaries!

Answer the following questions in as much depth as you like. The more you start thinking now, the easier the work over the next year will be.

YOUR HEALTH

1. Are you happy with your health? Do you consider yourself a healthy person?
2. Do you like your body? What do you like about it? If you don't like your body, why not? Do you feel comfortable with your body? If not, what parts feel uncomfortable?
3. Are you happy with your weight? If not, why not? What would your ideal weight be?
4. Do you consider yourself to be fit? How fit are you really? Would you like to be fitter?
5. Do you incorporate regular exercise in your life? How much and how often?
6. Is your body flexible? Can you easily bend and stretch, or do you have aches and pains?
7. Do you have good posture? Does your body feel comfortable and easy at all times?
8. Do you suffer from stress and tension in your body? Do you find you hold tension in your shoulders, neck muscles or jaw? Or do you suffer from nervous tension in your stomach? Do you get headaches or migraine when you are tense? What are the physical symptoms of stress you suffer?
9. How do you sleep? Do you suffer from insomnia or interrupted sleep? And what are your dreams like? Any recurring dreams? Nightmares? Perhaps no dreams at all?
10. Think about your diet. What kind of food do you eat? How much of it? Be honest. Write down a typical day's food. Do you eat much chocolate, sweets or cakes? Do you often or occasionally eat convenience food, prepackaged food, junk food or takeaways?

11. What do you drink? How much tea, coffee and fizzy soft drinks do you consume? How much alcohol?
12. Have you had any accidents? Do you suffer pain or discomfort as a result?
13. Do you smoke? How much? Do you take any recreational drugs?
14. Do you live in a very polluted area? Do you spend much time traveling on roads? How is your breathing?
15. Are you on any medication? How much and what for? Do you understand your drugs: what they are for; how they work? Are there any side effects? How long have you been taking medication?
16. Do you feel happy with your GP? Can you talk to him/her about your problems? Or do you feel dissatisfied with your health care?
17. Do you feel in control of your body and your health? Or do you feel it is something quite outside your control?
18. How are your senses? Do you have clear eyesight or do you need glasses/contact lenses? How is your hearing? Your sense of taste? Your sense of smell? Do you ever think about how you feel or touch things? Would you say your senses are acute or dull?
19. Do you worry about your health? Are you scared of becoming ill or of being out of control of your body?
20. List the five things you would like to change about your health.

YOUR PSYCHE: EMOTIONS AND FEELINGS

1. Do you consider yourself a happy person? Or are you more generally unhappy? What is it that makes you feel discontent with your life?
2. Are you fearful? What frightens you?
3. Do you express your feelings? Can you freely express grief, sadness, anger, frustration, love, gratitude, joy, etc.? Are there any emotions you cannot express?
4. Did you have a happy childhood? Were you loved? Did the members of your family get on with each other?
5. How did you cope with adolescence? What were your feelings around puberty?

6. Have there been any major traumas in your life? Any death, divorce, abuse?

7. Are you on good terms with your family—both immediate and extended?

8. Do you have a good relationship with your partner? Is it a partnership of equals or do you feel discontented with it? If you don't have a partner, does that cause you unhappiness?

9. Do you ever suffer from depression? When? Any triggers?

10. Do you have solid friends you can talk to and confide in?

11. Do you ever do things just for the hell of it? Do you take time off to play?

12. Do you have hobbies or interests outside work you really enjoy?

13. If you spend time on your own how do you feel? Do you enjoy it or do you feel slightly uncomfortable or downright unhappy?

14. Do you ever feel trapped by your life?

15. Have you got good self-esteem? Do you believe you are a worthwhile, interesting, valuable person? Or do you feel that you don't really matter that much; that other people are far more exciting and interesting than you are?

16. Can you be assertive if you need to be? Can you stand up for your rights, or do you let people walk all over you?

17. Do you have a good sex life? Are you happy with your sexuality? Is there anything you would like to change?

18. Do you feel in control of your life?

19. Are you scared of your emotions?

20. List five things you would like to change in your emotional life.

YOUR LIFE PATH

1. Do you feel as if you are in the right niche? Are you happy with your career or your life path?

2. Do you feel fulfilled?

3. Is there something you have always yearned to do with your life?

4. Do you have enough money, or is money a constant worry?

5. Do you feel secure?
6. Do you wake up in the morning and feel raring to go, as if each day is a new challenge, or do you wish the world would go away?
7. Do you feel creative in your life? Whether it's in your work, your family and home, artistic pursuits or new ideas and challenges?
8. Can you adapt well to change or does it frighten you?
9. If you could do anything in life what would it be?
10. Do you feel that your outward persona matches your inner self?
11. Do you feel respected in your life work?
12. Do you have good relationships with your fellow workers? Do you get on well with your boss, your colleagues, your employees?
13. Is your work a joy or a battleground?
14. Do you work with people who support one another, or do you work in an environment which thrives on "creative conflict," pitting people against each other? Do you enjoy your work environment?
15. Are you ever bored with your work?
16. Are you doing the best you can, or are you underused and understretched?
17. Does your work environment harm your health in any way?
18. Do you switch off when you leave work, or do you never have a break? Do you take work home with you and work on weekends? How do your family and friends see your work? Does your work compromise your relationships? Are you a workaholic?
19. Does your work give you stress? How do you deal with it?
20. If you could change your work in any way, how would you do it? What career did you want as a child? What is your ideal career? Do you want to work at all?

YOUR SOUL

1. How do you feel about the idea of spirit or soul? Is it an alien concept; something rather embarrassing; something frightening, or is it something you feel quite comfortable with?

2. Do you express your spirituality? Do you have any kind of religion, whether organized or not?

3. Do you fear the unknown?

4. Are you scared of eternity, of death?

5. Do you believe in luck, chance, random events?

6. Do you ever have the feeling that your life is being overseen in any way?

7. Do you blame the misfortunes of life on something beyond your control—on karma, God, fate, past life?

8. Do you give yourself time to dream, to think, to muse?

9. Do you meditate or practice any form of visualization or relaxation techniques?

10. Do you feel as if your life has purpose?

11. Does life fill you with a sense of complete joy sometimes?

12. Do you have time to be on your own?

13. Do you ever escape into nature—whether the local park or countryside? Where do you feel happiest: by the sea, in the mountains, in a forest? Or do you feel happier in the city, surrounded by people, or in a quiet cozy room?

14. Do you feel safe?

15. Do you live in the now, or are you living in the past or projecting into the future?

16. Do you ever stop and just do nothing?

17. Do you feel as if life is just one long trial and that there is nothing you can do to change it?

18. Do you take enough holidays and days off?

19. Do you believe that you deserve good health, great relationships and a wonderful life?

20. If you could do something just for you, what would it be?

As you'll see there are no scores, no summaries. This is a portrait of you at this moment in time, how you feel right now. Keep your answers in a safe place. We will look at them at various points during the year.

SPRING

The Season of the Body

KEY FOCUS
Getting into the body—working on your relationship with your physical self.

SECONDARY FOCUS
Starting to think about your life.

TASKS
Introducing a healthy diet; starting to exercise; detoxification; toning the body; boosting the lymphatic system; increasing flexibility.

QUESTIONS
How might I like to live my life? How do I want to treat my body? Am I willing to take responsibility for my health?

CHALLENGES
Dare to pamper yourself; use dance to discover your emotions; try seemingly irrational exercises!

FESTIVALS AND CELEBRATIONS
Spring equinox, Easter, Beltane.

Everything seems possible in spring. This is the young season, the growing season, the season of buds and blossom, of lambs and all young things. It is, to my mind, the perfect time to turn over a fresh leaf, to start anew. Spring is the season of hope, of fresh life and new beginnings. It's as if each year we get another stab at getting it right or, at least, getting it better.

After the darkness of winter, the days start to get longer and this change in light triggers a deep shift in nature—everything begins to come back to life and vigor. Catkins appear on hazel trees and pussy willow; bluebells cast a hazy sheen through dappled woods; primroses cling to steep mossy banks and larks soar and fall over the plowed fields. Even within towns and cities the onrush of spring can be seen in the bright cheery faces of daffodils and other spring bulbs and the frenzied nest-building of sparrows, pigeons and other city wildlife. You don't even need to *see* visible signs of spring: just stop and sniff the air, there's something fresh about it, a new energy has arrived into the year.

Spring is pure phsyicality—it's the season of the body and the perfect time to start a program to bring you into peak fitness. Take it slowly, one step at a time, and you can transform the way you look and feel. Spring is the time when we need to cleanse and detoxify our bodies, to clear out the debris that has accumulated during the relative inactivity of winter. It's a time to start looking closely at how we feed our bodies; a time to decide on changes that will help our bodies serve us better. You *can* lose weight now, but it's not the best time of year to launch into a fully fledged weight-loss regime. Your body has just come out of its winter hibernation and needs to be cleansed and then fortified, tonified. Far better to spend spring easing yourself into good, honest healthy eating, to cut out toxins and junk food and then launch into weight loss proper (if that is what you truly need) in the summer.

Equally, although spring might seem like the perfect time to change your entire life, it's not a good idea to overturn it right now. Spring is great for deciding upon your focus for the year, but it is not necessarily the best moment to quit your job on whim or to make sweeping life changes. It's the time to start thinking about what you want from life; to consider what you might need to change. But leave the implementation of those changes until that other dynamic season, autumn.

Hopefully, you have already filled in the questionnaire in the introductory chapter. If not, do take time to do it now. Look carefully at the section on your health. Are your answers truthful and accurate or are they wishful thinking? How would you like to see your body? How would you like to feel about your body? Really think about it. Do you know in your heart of hearts, that you eat the wrong food, too much or too little food, too much junk food and not enough fruit, vegetables and fiber? Think about what you're putting in your body. Think about how all your internal organs and bodily systems pounce on the food you put inside you and try to obtain the nutrients they need to make you function properly. Do you give them a fair chance? Or are they scrabbling around trying to keep you going on a pile of empty calories, a sickly wodge of sugar and a dead weight of salt? This spring, the aim is to work on your body, so the least you can do is give it the bare essentials it needs. Try to follow the healthy eating guidelines that are outlined later in this chapter.

And what about exercise? Think about the muscles of your body—not just your pecs and biceps but also your heart and your lungs. Exercise on a regular basis can strengthen the whole body. Go through the whole questionnaire and really delve deep into your answers. What changes could you make to your body right now? What changes do you want to make over the following year? Make a list of everything you would like to improve or change and give yourself a timescale. Also write down how you would do it. For example, if you want to start exercising your list might read:

Goal: improve physical fitness. Be able to run for the bus without gasping. Be able to play netball and go jogging again.

Right now: walk up escalator every day on way to work. Look up gyms and sports centers in Yellow Pages and check out membership details and facilities.

Over the next month: join gym and start regular workouts.

When the weather improves: fix bike and start cycling to work. Get outside in lunch hour—maybe start walking or jogging.

In three months time/when fitness levels improve: join netball team.

Again, don't try to do it all at once. But just do it.

The Season of Wood and the Evil Wind

In the Chinese system, spring is the season of the element wood and it is filled with the expansive, explosive energy of young *yang*. Young *yang* is boundless energy, but it can be reckless, impulsive, impatient. It is like an adolescent, straining at the bit, wanting to race out and make a mark in the world but not quite sure of his or her own limits. Wood is the element that makes us feel that we need free expression to find our own way, to try new things and meet new people. It is open and energetic and can lead to great enthusiasm and new endeavors. However, it can also become out of control and can lead to the feeling of "spring fever," obsessive, undisciplined mania. It's unpredictable—think of *mad March hares,* April showers, sudden heatwaves that vanish equally suddenly in squalls and sleeting rain, or the sneaky frost that can devastate your garden overnight.

Spring is also, quite naturally, the season of sex and sexuality. It is the season of procreation in the natural world and, just because we humans can mate at any time of the year does not mean that we are not moved by the primal seasonal urges. Lust rises in spring—it is the time for starting relationships or recommitting to old ones.

The color associated with wood is green. The direction that governs the spring is east, which also rules the beginning of the day, the morning. The secondary element that the Chinese associate with spring is wind. Wind is the fresh air of spring, that whisks away the old and sweeps in the new. But too much wind can be harmful, and the Chinese say that the great danger of spring comes from the wind "evil." If we are balanced and healthy, then the wind can do us no harm. However, if our energy is low or stagnant then we might not be able to cope with the fluctuation in the external energies of wind and wood. The troublesome wind can invade the body and throw *yin* and *yang* into even more imbalance. The result is that we go down with colds and flu, coughs and snuffles, hot sweats or even more serious ailments.

Some practitioners of TCM say that the wind evil is allowed free rein in our modern world through central heating and air conditioning which shock our bodies and don't allow them to adapt to the outside conditions. Microwaves and radiation equally come under attack, but then no one would suggest that radiation is particularly healthy. Avoiding any of these evils is pretty difficult nowadays, unless you live in a cave up an isolated hill. But there *are* ways to minimize the damage:

• Fortify your body with good, clean food. Avoid sweets, soft drinks and snacks made from refined sugar, and steer clear of junk food, deep-fried food and over-processed foods.
• Take a daily good quality multi-vitamin and mineral supplement.
• Try to avoid shocking your body by plunging from extreme heat to extreme cold. Wear a sweater or a vest rather than turning the heat up high.
• Install an ionizer in your home and office, particularly if you live in a large town or city.
• Keep a window open, especially at night. If you can avoid sleeping with the air-conditioning or central heating switched on, do so. Try using a fan to generate cool air. Program your central

heating timer so that the heating comes on an hour before you get up rather than being on all night.

• Practice the techniques of good breathing. The Chinese recommend that chi kung breathing exercises be carried out every day and that twenty minutes of chi kung will re-establish your energy levels, enrich your blood, soothe the nervous system and the endocrine system and put your autonomous nervous system into the calming, restful parasympathetic mode. Practitioners of yoga say the same for their practice of *pranayama,* which teaches the art of good breathing. There are exercises for simple breathing exercises in my previous book, *Supertherapies,* or, for best results, join a yoga or chi kung class and learn the correct technique.

Food Guidelines for Spring: Easing Yourself into Healthy Natural Eating

We have just come out of winter, the season of thick, warming, sustaining stews and comforting stodge. Most of us have probably put on a few pounds over the winter season. By now you may well have already tried to lose weight after Christmas or as one of your New Year resolutions yet found yourself constantly digging into the biscuit tin or having a second dollop of pudding. Don't beat yourself up over it; you are just doing what virtually every creature does—storing extra fat in case of a lean winter and to keep you warm through the cold. Now spring has come, it's time to gradually shed the excess and to get the body moving.

Whatever you do, don't leap in with a draconian diet. It may be spring, but your body needs nourishing, not starving. And anyway, as you should know by now, diets simply don't work. All you're doing on a strict diet is starving your body into a panic in which it sends out alarm signals to the cells screaming "hang on to every bit you can!" Your metabolism naturally slows down to preserve your stores of fat and, after a while, it becomes harder and harder to lose weight.

What I would suggest at this time of year is that you commit yourself to introducing healthy eating habits into your life. You may find that a few simple adjustments alone will bring about quite surprising changes: your weight should begin to balance itself; you should certainly experience an increase in energy and alertness and, quite probably, you will find your mood improving.

Do remember that food is fuel for your body. If you want a high-performance car to run smoothly and speedily, you fill it with the right fuel and lubricate its engine with the right oil. Put a low-grade or unsuitable fuel in a car and it will run poorly or not at all. Racehorses are fed a carefully balanced diet which is designed to help them stay in peak condition. In both cases there is an obvious link between what goes in as food and what comes out as performance. So why should we think we can get a supercharged performance out of our bodies when we are shoveling in poor-grade food?

There are any number of eating regimes. Some people swear by veganism or macrobiotics; others believe we were born to eat steak. Many people swear by food combining—not eating protein and carbohydrate in the same meal—yet some scientists say our stomachs don't care whether we put in protein and carbohydrate at the same time. I don't believe there is any one "perfect" diet for everyone. We are all different and we all need slightly different regimes. This is where most nutritional programs or diets fall down. Finding the optimum diet for you can take time and effort, and if you really want a tailor-made nutritional plan, then I suggest you consult a well-qualified naturopath or nutritionist. Practitioners of Ayurveda and TCM can also offer you a diet to balance your body type.

However, the majority of people can make vast changes for the better in their health and vitality by following these general good health guidelines. I'm not asking you to take them all on board at once—or even at all—but, if you want to follow some of the suggestions further on in this book, you will really benefit by gently easing your body into a good, basic healthfood regime. I'm not suggesting you eat brown rice and lentils every day of the week. Good food needn't be boring food.

THE GOLDEN RULES

• Buy your food as fresh and natural as possible. In other words, you need to look for food that has been tampered with as little as possible. The ideal would be to choose organic vegetables, freshly picked, and free-range organic meat. Unfortunately, the ideal can be hard to sustain. Organic produce is very expensive, and many supermarkets and stores simply don't stock it. If you can't find organic produce, try to buy fresh, local produce, if that's possible. Much of our food is transported halfway across the world—quite unnecessarily.

• Buy food in season when you can. It's no accident that certain foods grow well at particular times of year. Spring greens and young spring vegetables are perfect spring food; solid turnips and swedes are fine winter fare. Buy food in season, and it will be at its peak, full of essential vitamins and minerals.

• The bedrock of your diet should be complex carbohydrates (starchy foods like bread, pasta, potatoes, rice and cereals). About half your daily intake of calories should come from these prime foodstuffs. This may come as a surprise to many people who think such foods are fattening. The truth is they're not, providing you go for a jacket potato rather than a plate of chips, and eat your spaghetti with a roasted vegetable sauce rather than dousing it with a sauce containing half a pint of double cream. There are endless delicious options with this type of food—risottos and pilaffs, pasta in all its guises, baked potatoes stuffed with all kinds of interesting fillings, sandwiches made with thick wholemeal bread. Experiment also with the more unusual grains that are arriving in the shops such as wild rice, millet and couscous.

• Boost your intake of fresh fruit and vegetables. Aim for at least three pieces of fruit a day, plus around 600 grams of vegetables. It may sound like a lot but your body will love it. Fresh vegetables are packed with vitamins and minerals and are generally very low in calories and fat. They will help protect your body from pollution and boost your immune system to deal with infections. They really are your bodyguards, so eat them any way you can. If the thought of vegetables sends you to sleep, try cooking them in different ways. Delia Smith swears by roasting vegetables—just pop them in the oven with a drizzle of olive oil. She's spot-on—they taste delicious and make a great base for a pasta or rice sauce. Or try barbecuing vegetables—a small amount of meat boosted with plenty of barbecued onions, peppers, mushrooms and tomatoes makes a substantial and highly nutritious meal. Add some pitta bread, and you've got the perfect balance. Other ways of cooking vegetables include stir-frying with plenty of garlic and herbs, or you could experiment with oriental flavorings like ginger, galingale, lemongrass and coriander. And if the vegetables are really fresh, just lightly steam them, perhaps adding a little lemongrass to the steaming water—delicious!

• Eat sufficient protein but don't overdo it. Whether you eat meat or not is totally up to you. I know plenty of super-healthy meat-eaters and plenty of very unhealthy vegetarians, and vice versa. But if you do choose to eat meat, please try to get hold of organic, free-range meat. I know it's more expensive than mass-produced meat, but not only is it a more ethical choice, it is also much better for your health. The added bonus is that you really can taste the difference. After that, the key factor is to choose lean cuts with as little fat as possible. It's not the meat itself that's bad for you, it's the saturated fat that comes with it. That's why chicken is a good option, as it contains less fat than red meat. Fish is also an ideal source of protein, and some of the fats in fish are positively health-giving. Perhaps surprisingly, game is a relatively healthy option as well. Venison, for example, is very low in cholesterol.

Vegetarianism can be a very healthy way of eating, but vegetarians often fall into the trap of eating far too much dairy produce. Cheese and eggs are fine in moderation but, as they are high in fat and cholesterol and also encourage the body to create mucus they should not be eaten in large quantities. Vegetarians (and meat-eaters too) should experiment with the huge range of pulses now available and also try products like tofu (the smoked version is lovely) and Quorn which, although utterly tasteless on its own, will pick up the flavor of whatever it is cooked with.

We need to get away from the idea that all meals should be based around protein. In fact, we need only around 70-80 grams of protein a day. So take protein off center-stage and just use it to add flavor and interest. Some of the healthiest cuisine in the world is poor peasant food—thick vegetable stews flavored with a little meat, beans or lentils and a handful of herbs and spices.

THINGS TO WATCH OUT FOR

• Steer clear of additives and preservatives. Sadly, most foods nowadays come coated or treated with insecticides, pesticides or fungicides. Vegetables are sprayed, injected and coated with chemicals to kill anything that might eat them—and then *we* eat them. Animals are pumped full of antibiotics, steroids and all manner of hormones and, as we eat the animal, so we ingest these in turn.

Always wash fruit and vegetables very thoroughly, and take extra care if they aren't organic. There are now special washes on the market that help clear pesticide residues (check with your local healthfood shop). There's not much you can do about non-organic meat, except to buy it as fresh as you can and from a reputable butcher, and campaign for free-range organic meat, at reasonable prices.

• Avoid over-processed and junk food. It's so easy to eat out of tins and packets; to stock up the freezer with ready-meals; to pop into a burger bar instead of cooking a meal from scratch. Life's often too busy to shop, cook and prepare fresh food. But please try—at least for part of the week. Slowly wean yourself off convenience food and try eating "real" food. It needn't take hours or be haute cuisine: a bowl of pasta with a fresh tomato sauce takes under half an hour; so does lemon-grilled chicken and Greek salad; or blackened fish and couscous. The list is endless. It might take a little more thought and forward planning than plopping a ready-meal in the microwave but your body (and mind) will thank you for it.

• Cut out sweets and snacks as much as possible. A bag of potato chips might taste nice but provides little nourishment. A chocolate brownie might cheer up the afternoon (at least for the two minutes it takes to eat it), but your mind and mood won't thank you for it. These are empty foods, dead foods, so try to limit your intake. I'm not going to say you should always opt for raw vegetables instead of a Mars bar because there's no way a bunch of carrots has a hope in hell of measuring up to a Mars bar in all its sticky, sickly glory. But just be aware of how depen-dent you are on snack foods. Do you eat them every day? At particular times of the day? When you hit a particular kind of mood? If they're for comfort, try a warm drink instead. If they're for instant energy, you'd be better off with a banana or a cup of hot water with honey.

• Watch out for fat. To listen to some "experts" you'd think fat was a dirty word. It isn't, but you need to know the good fats from the bad guys. Some fat is necessary as it provides essential vitamins and fatty acids, but you don't need too much. In fact, you don't need that much at all. A few teaspoons of olive oil a day is more than enough, given that many of our foods already contain fat. To cut down on your fat consumption try alternative ways of cooking such as grilling, steaming, stir-frying rather than frying. Watch out for "hidden" fat in dairy produce, mayonnaise, crisps and snacks, pastry, sausages and burgers.

• Cut down on your salt intake. We almost all eat too much salt. Bear in mind that loads of foods already contain salt, so you need to keep an eye on the ingredients lists of packaged foods as well as watching what you sprinkle on your plate or add to the pan while you're cooking.

The reason we're advised to keep salt intake low is because high levels of salt can cause high blood pressure which in turn can lead to heart disease and strokes. A high salt intake also increases the risk of osteoporosis as it causes calcium loss from the bones. It can be a contributory factor to kidney disease. Cut down gradually, and avoid adding extra salt where you can. Check food labels and choose foods marked "low salt" where possible. If you're buying canned food, choose ones canned in water rather than brine. Adding celery when you cook can help add flavor, or try squeezing lemon on meat, fish and vegetables for a tart, tangy taste.

YOUR DAILY PLAN

Try to eat three meals a day using the above-mentioned foods as your guide.

• Breakfast really does set you up for the day—choose something like cereal or toast with a piece of fruit and perhaps some live yogurt.

• Lunch is important too, but in the middle of a busy day it's all too easy to stick a ready-meal in the microwave or grab a sandwich and a doughnut from the trolley at work. Five minutes' preparation in the morning could set you up with a super-healthy sandwich of thick wholemeal bread with a little meat and tons of salad; or try pita breads with hummus (it only takes five minutes to make in a blender) and tomato, a salad in a pot and some fruit. If you have to buy lunch out, try to find a sandwich shop that makes fresh sandwiches and ask them to boost the salad or vegetable content and go easy on the cheese or meat. Or, for a change, you could try the vegetarian options in your local restaurant.

• In the evening, try not to eat too late. Ayurvedic physicians say we should eat no later than 6 P.M., which in my book is pretty unrealistic. However, it makes sense to eat as early as possible in the evening to allow sufficient time for you to digest your food before you go to bed. Many experts recommend you have a light meal in the evening and that you eat your main meal at lunchtime. Again, this can be tricky for most people, but do be careful not to overload your system at night.

EXTRA HELP FOR YOUR BODY

What else can you do to help your body? Plenty of things.

• If you smoke, please please start thinking about cutting down and, hopefully, stopping altogether. You don't have to do it right now. Just become aware of how smoking affects your body and your nerves. Concentrate on how your *body* actually feels when you smoke and how you feel afterward. Start to think about whether you want to give up and what emotions and thoughts this raises in you.

• How much alcohol do you drink? All the evidence shows that a reasonable amount of alcohol is fine and that the occasional glass of wine might even help your heart. But do you rely too much on alcohol? If you drink too much, you will be damaging your health. Think about keeping some days alcohol-free. Add sparkling water to white wine to make a spritzer so that you halve the amount of alcohol you drink. If you feel you rely on alcohol, start to think about when and why you drink. Again, you don't have to cut it out right now or even at all; just be aware of how you use alcohol.

• How much water do you drink? Many of us actually spend most of the day dehydrated and, often, when we feel hungry, we are in fact thirsty. Aim to drink around two liters of water a day. Not only will this make you feel better in general but your skin will undoubtedly improve as well. If you don't like the idea of drinking water straight from the tap, buy a water filter, or keep a bottle or two of mineral water on your desk and drink it through the day.

• How much caffeine do you take? If you feel edgy or irritable, you could be overdosing on caffeine—not just from coffee but also from tea, soft drinks and supplements like guarana. Drinking five cups of espresso in the morning is not the best way to kick-start your day, nor is coffee the best afternoon pick-me-up. A good breakfast containing complex carbohydrates such as cereal or bread will give you a good level of energy for the morning. If you feel dozy around teatime, don't automatically reach for a coffee and a doughnut, try hot water and honey, and a banana.

I'm not saying you have to cut out coffee and tea altogether— I'm a complete tea addict myself. But do try to cut down, or try interspersing your caffeine fix with a cup of herbal tea or a long drink of water. Peppermint tea is a good pick-me-up; so are some of the citrus fruit blends, rosehip and hibiscus. And one last point, if you do drink tea, try to have your cuppa in-between meals—the tannin in tea reduces the absorption of essential minerals like calcium and iron—otherwise you'll be reducing the nutritional quality of your food.

• Do you need supplements? If you are following my eating guidelines and, in particular, munching through plenty of fresh, seasonal fruit and vegetables then, in theory, you should be obtaining all the vitamins and minerals you need. However, sadly, many of us may still lack or be low in certain essential micro-nutrients. The fact is that by the time the food reaches our tables, many of the nutrients have vanished, either processed away or leached away by long journeys, long shelf-lives and overcooking. To be on the safe side, I don't think it does any harm to take a precautionary multi-vitamin and mineral supplement once a day. A good-quality one won't be cheap, but it will ensure you are getting the optimum amounts of micronutrients in the right balance. I really wouldn't advise anyone to try to work out their own deficiencies and to treat themselves with a little bit of this and a little bit of that. The way minerals and vitamins work with each other and with your body is very complex and best left to the experts. If you do feel you are seriously deficient in a particular vitamin or mineral, then consult your doctor or a fully trained nutritional therapist.

• Take it one step at a time. Try to switch your diet onto healthy guidelines over the next few weeks and months. Don't try to do it all at once, otherwise you will find you get bored or rebellious. For example, cutting out your daily doughnut *and* all coffee *and* your glass of wine *and* crisps and peanuts all in one go is just too much. Try cutting down on the coffee first of all—have three cups instead of six. Have wine at the weekend, not every night. Try substituting a banana and a herbal tea with honey for that coffee and doughnut.

Exercise: Getting Your Body into Gear

We weren't meant to be couch potatoes. Evolution hasn't designed us to sit for ten hours a day behind a computer screen and then slump for the rest of the day in front of a television. Our bodies are designed to move, to work, to be fit and active. In the past, most of us would have relied on the earth for our livelihood—we would have spent our days in the open, working physically very hard. Nowadays, our daily bread tends to come from the supermarket, and so we need to find other ways to keep active and fit.

Do you really need to exercise? Yes, I'm afraid you do. If you want to live longer and more healthily, the single most important thing you can do is incorporate regular exercise into your life. Exercising regularly reduces your risk of early death by an impressive seventy percent. It keeps your lungs and heart working at their optimum level and helps prevent heart disease. Stress levels drop when you exercise, and your mood naturally elevates. Regular exercise can even help you sleep better as well as perk up your sex life! On a more prosaic note, it can regulate your blood pressure and boost your immune system. Some physiologists reckon it can even increase your creativity. On the other hand, if you don't exercise you are asking for trouble—you will be putting yourself at risk of heart and artery disease; your muscles and bones could develop problems; you could find yourself prone to gastrointestinal problems and you will be more likely to suffer nervous or emotional upsets and illnesses.

The good news is that you don't have to live in the gym or run for hours every day—in fact too *much* exercise can also be bad for you. But you do need to do some form of exercise regularly.

So why is exercise such a bugbear? The main problem is that many people take up forms of exercise that they don't enjoy, or that they aren't naturally good at. The result is they get bored, disillusioned and give up. The key to making exercise work for you is to find something you actually enjoy—not what you feel you *should* do but what you would really *like* to do. So you don't have to race out and buy on-line skates because it's trendy, when you have absolutely no sense of balance and are terrified of speed. And you don't have to do acrobics because all your friends do, or play squash because your husband wants some practice. I know so many people who have forked out a small fortune on a gym membership only to find that they hate pumping iron and they loathe step aerobics. Before you join a club, test it out for a while. Any club worth its salt will offer a trial membership for a month or so.

Throughout this book are ideas on how to incorporate exercise into your life and some suggestions on different things to try. For the time being I simply ask that you start to try out some form of exercise.

Take a look at your local sports center—pick up a brochure or take a wander around and I'll bet you'll be surprised at the variety of different sports and programs on offer. My local center offers everything from trampolining to five-a-side football, from boxercise to table tennis (and it's only a small rural center).

Think about the sports you enjoyed in school—are there any you'd like to take up again? Netball can be brilliant fun, or volleyball or softball, if you like team games. Or get back into badminton, squash or tennis. Many adults take up gymnastics and love it, or learn something new like golf. It's worth remembering that the key issue here is fun. You don't have to be brilliant or the best; you just need to do it and enjoy it. A friend of mine has started belly-dancing and adores it. She reckons she's the worst belly-dancer ever but doesn't give a hoot.

KEEPING MOTIVATION HIGH

In order to keep exercising you have to stay motivated. There are several key points to remember here:

• Be realistic about your size and body shape. Hoards of exercisers lose heart because however hard they work they don't end up looking like Cindy Crawford or Elle McPherson. Dump unrealistic role models—these people spend hours, and a small fortune in personal trainer bills, to look that way.

• Start slowly. You shouldn't try to change your exercise habits overnight or you will become demotivated because you don't see changes happening immediately. Make gradual changes to your lifestyle and they will become a permanent way of life without any special effort.

• Break through the one-week barrier. Sports psychologists promise that if you can get past the first week, you've passed the period in which half the dropouts occur. If you manage to work out regularly for six months, you're likely to have created a long-lasting habit.

• Try to get a friend involved. Exercising with someone else is the supreme motivator. Sportsmen and women have coaches; most super-fit actresses and models have their own personal trainers and, if you've got the funds, a personal trainer will undoubtedly get you moving. However, a good mate will often do as well. It is much easier to stick to a regular exercise schedule if you know that someone else is waiting for you in the park, the gym or the pool. Choose someone who is of a similar ability to yourself, and make a commitment to your health and each other, then stick to it.

USE THE WISDOM OF AYURVEDA TO PICK
YOUR IDEAL SPORT

John Douillard, author of *Body, Mind and Sport,* outlines an entire new system for choosing the ideal sport to keep you motivated, year after year. First and foremost, he insists, fitness must be fun. The key, apparently, is to get back to the mindset we had as children, when sport and exercise was, above all, a game. He's quite right. As a kid I used to climb mountains for the sheer hell of it; now I find myself thinking more about how many calories I'm burning. On a recent holiday I staggered up a peak almost chanting, "100 calories, 200 calories . . ." and not even taking in the scenery.

Rob Parr, a trainer who has toned superbodies like Demi Moore, Christy Turlington and Maria Shriver, agrees. He insists the only way to stick with fitness for life is to make it fun and make it part of your lifestyle. "With each client I try to design a routine that incorporates activities they already enjoy." Hence his plan for Bruce Willis and Demi Moore incorporated the outdoor activities they loved, like kayaking and skiing.

According to Ayurveda, there are two ways of looking at the exercise equation. You work out your body type (see page 16) and choose a sport that suits your *prakruti,* or you can pick something that will balance your basic nature. To begin with, you will probably be drawn to something that matches your predominant *dosha* but, as you become more aware of your body throughout the coming year, you may find yourself feeling you need something else—a form of exercise that actually balances your mind-body type. Refer back to the introductory chapter for a complete rundown on the *doshas.* What follows is a brief summary of which kinds of exercise suit which people.

Vata

Description People with a predominance of *vata* in their constitution tend to be small-framed with active minds and restless bodies. They talk a lot, ask a lot of questions and can't seem to sit still. Quick, light and agile, they are not very muscular and don't have a lot of endurance.

Natural Inclinations Running, sprinting, any kind of track sports.

Sports to Balance Anything that will soothe and calm their restless natures. Low-impact jogging or aerobics, walking, hiking, cycling and swimming.

Pitta

Description *Pittas* tend to be fiery, aggressive, competitive and vocal people who often assume the leadership role. They are usually strong, medium-framed and well-coordinated.

Natural Inclinations The more competitive the sport, the better.

Sports to Balance Anything that isn't intensely competitive. Cycling, swimming, skiing or golf.

Kapha

Description *Kapha* types usually have heavier frames than *vatas* or *pittas,* with strong bodies and high endurance levels. They are often slower moving and slower speaking, easy-going by nature.

Natural Inclinations Sports requiring endurance and power. Any shot-putter is likely to be a *kapha*. They do well with team sports and thrive under the motivation of others.

Sports to Balance They need speeding up, enlivening, so any fast sports that require endurance, such as tennis, rowing, running and high-intensity aerobics, are all excellent for *kapha* types.

WORK WITH YOUR RHYTHMS

Exercise guru Kathy Smith says that many people drop out of fitness programs because they push themselves too hard at the wrong time. She claims the key to successful, long-term fitness is to find your personal rhythms and exercise within them. "Keep a notepad or calendar handy and every morning and night jot down four or five words to describe your energy level, your frame of mind, your physical condition and what you have done workwise," she says. "After a period of time you can review and identify patterns—when certain parts of your body are tired; when exercise makes you feel great; when you're tired; when you're raring to go. Then make adjustments."

Also remember that it is not written in stone that your workout should stay exactly the same, month in, month out. Most good gyms and clubs will alter your program every few months to keep you interested. They will also test your fitness levels and assess your progress so that you stay motivated. Cross-training— in other words, varying your activities—will stop you from getting bored and demoralized and has the added advantage of enabling you to exercise different muscle groups. If you always train with weights, try a body-conditioning class for a change. If you have a solid diet of step and low-impact aerobics, try something different like slide aerobics or boxercise. Balance high-intensity workouts with quieter, more precise forms like yoga or chi kung.

WALK YOUR WAY INTO SPRING

I am a great fan of walking and I encourage other people to do it whenever I can. It really is a great way to start easing yourself into exercise and, if you are pretty fit already, you can always set yourself new challenges.

Why walking? Because you don't need fancy equipment or expensive gyms—you simply need your legs, a pair of shoes and somewhere to walk. Also, it is pretty well a perfect form of exercise—effective and safe. Performed properly, walking provides all the benefits of running (and more), without any of the dangers. Brisk walking will raise your heartbeat and help improve your cardiovascular system; you will pump fresh oxygen and nutrients into every cell of your body and you will burn calories quite effectively.

Walking tones plenty of muscles too—the buttocks, thighs and calves—so your legs will soon look firmer and trimmer. And if you swing your arms as you go, you will give your upper body a slight workout too. Slot in a few hills and you will really notice a difference in your body shape. Walking briskly for forty-five minutes four times a week could enable you to lose between ten and fifteen pounds (around four to seven kilograms) in a year without your making any changes to your diet. And, even more importantly, you won't be doing yourself any damage while you walk. Running, on the other hand, can jar the whole skeleton and puts great pressure on the joints. However, when you walk you are only putting one or, at the most, one and a half times your weight on your feet. The action is smooth so there's no danger to your knees or hips. Walking is so safe that it can be done by anyone—pregnant women, the very overweight, the elderly—and is ideal for everyone who wants to avoid injury.

I have outlined many more benefits of walking in my previous book, *Supertherapies,* but here are the main points on how to start up a walking regime.

1. Set a manageable target. Start off gently and gradually build up your pace and distance.
2. The aim is to build up to a regular three times a week, with each session lasting a minimum of half an hour.
3. You should be aiming to work at a level at which you perspire and your heart rate is raised. The simplest way of gauging how you're doing is to take the "talk test." You should be able to pass the odd word with a friend as you walk. If you can't even breathe a word, you're doing too much; if you can gossip merrily, you're not working hard enough.

Preparation

1. As with all exercise, avoid eating for about an hour before you set off.
2. Drink plenty of water before, during and after your walk. If you're thirsty, it means you're becoming dehydrated.
3. Warm up. Walk gently for the first five minutes to get your muscles warm before you pick up the pace.
4. A few gentle stretches after your warm-up will ease your body into the exercise.

The Technique

1. Keep your weight centered: imagine a straight line stretching from between your feet and ahead of you down the road. Keep your legs parallel to this line and your toes pointing directly ahead.
2. Take the longest stride that is comfortable and let your arms swing naturally at the same speed. Relax your shoulders.
3. The heel of your leading foot should touch the ground just before the ball of the foot and toes. As your heel reaches the ground, lock your ankle and shift your weight forward with the knee bent. Rock onto your toes and use the movement to push you on to the next step.
4. Breathe from your abdomen, not from your chest. Inhale and exhale rhythmically and easily through the nose.

It sounds strange giving instructions for something so mundane as walking, but using the correct technique turns it into a serious workout. Once you feel happy with walking this way and have built up a fair level of fitness, you might try extending your walk into a whole outdoor workout. Try doing push-ups against the back of a park bench or triceps dips on the edge of the seat; a branch of a tree would be handy for pull-ups, but do check that it's secure first.

If you're walking with a friend, try incorporating some backward walking. This uses the muscles in a slightly different way and can be slightly harder on your muscles.

Walk Safely

Walking may be the safest form of exercise, but there are still a couple of points to watch:

• Don't be tempted to add handweights to your walk. The shoulder is an unstable joint and could be prone to injury if you walked with weights.
• Don't drink coffee just before your walk—or before any kind of workout. Caffeine gets the heart pumping, and so you may feel as though you are warmed up for exercise when you're not. Caffeine will dilate the arteries in the central part of your body but it won't reach your arms and legs, so you could leave yourself prone to strains.
• Watch out for pollution on hot inner-city days. When the air quality is bad you'd be better off avoiding the streets.
• Be seen and be safe. If you walk at night, wear fluorescent strips. And, if you can, walk with a friend for security. If you do walk on your own, make sure someone knows when you are expected back and where you are walking.

APPLY A LITTLE PSYCHOLOGY

Here are a few final tips on exercise to keep you motivated:

• Be practical. Make sure you choose an activity that fits in with your lifestyle. If you enroll in a gym that's miles away, you're unlikely to use it often enough.

• Put out your exercise kit the night before so that the next day there will be no excuses about not having time to pack.

• If you see exercise as a real chore and a hopeless bore, then standard aerobics simply won't suit. Instead, try sports that don't seem like exercise such as dancing (ballroom, square, tap, belly), hiking, trampolining, horse-riding, rollerblading.

• It's hard to motivate yourself to go to a gym or join a team if you're feeling overweight and undertoned. Start the process at home with exercise videos, stair climbing, or regular walking or cycling, and wait until you've hit your initial target before you join up.

• Once you've reached that stage, you'll probably do better in a class or gym unless you're highly motivated. Having an instructor egging you on makes you get far more out of your workout and gives you a greater sense of achievement.

• If you like to compete and exercise with other people then consider joining a league or a club for your chosen sport. Then, you know that if you don't turn up, you'll be letting the other members down.

• Being part of a team can really foster motivation. You'll share the same goals and, again, if you don't show, the team will miss you.

Above all, remember that exercise, in whatever form, will make a huge difference to how you look and feel. If you follow the eating and exercise advice given in this chapter I can promise you that, by the end of the spring, you will be feeling completely differently about your body. There is no doubt that eating sensibly will make your body feel stronger and healthier. Your mind should feel clearer and your mood should be more balanced. Add exercise, and your muscles will start to feel toned. Your aerobic fitness will steadily improve and you won't be gasping if you have to walk up an escalator or run for a bus. It doesn't happen overnight but it can happen quite quickly. Most people notice a distinct difference after six weeks. And, once you start to notice and enjoy the benefits, you'll be hooked. Why live life half-heartedly when you can enjoy it to the full?

March

It may seem cold outside, perhaps even bleak, but the new life of the year is starting to push up and into the world. March is the herald of spring, a month of promises and new beginnings. The Native Americans call March the Welcoming Back, the advent of the new year. Traditionally it is the month of blustery winds, of "mad March hares," a clean fresh open time. In the garden the crocuses are shining through the grass like bright little beacons and the grape hyacinth are scattered in a blue haze. The magnolia trees are heavy with swollen waxy buds while the delicate catkins dangle in country lanes and city parks.

March looks forward to the 21st, the spring equinox, which is a joyous festival of spring, a welcoming celebration of the return of energy and life after the long cold hibernation of winter. This is the time of spring-cleaning—not just physically, but emotionally as well. It's a time to get rid of things you have outgrown and to end projects you don't really want to complete in order to make room for the new. March is the beginning. The start of a fresh new life.

Hopefully, already you will be starting to move your body gently into a more healthy way of being. Making some adjustments to your diet and taking up exercise are two huge steps which will certainly bring you boundless rewards. Remember, you should not try to be too radical at this point. If you want to make any changes stick, you have to alter your lifestyle gradually and carefully. And you have to really want to change deep inside. If you don't have that inner desire, nothing and nobody will be able to push you into lasting change.

Spring-cleaning: Space Clearing

Something that will pave the way is to have a really thorough spring-clean. If you seriously want to make changes in your life you need to start from a position of clarity. You need space in your life and a clear mind before you can begin to decide what you need and what you can live without. So the first task of March is to provide yourself with a clear space in which to work.

When things go wrong in life we tend to look inside ourselves for the reasons. Psychotherapists talk of clearing our minds, while holistic practitioners exhort us to purify our bodies and cleanse our emotions. But a new theory states that to affect your inner being, you need to take a good hard look at your external surroundings. Before you can make changes in your life you need to make changes in the physical world around you. The process is called space clearing, and one of the acknowledged world experts in this new technique is Karen Kingston.

In fact, technically, the concept is not new. As Kingston points out, many traditional cultures, such as the Zulus, the Native Americans, the Maoris and the Balinese, have some form of cleansing ritual. We even retain elements of it here in the West, although often we have long forgotten the true purpose behind certain rituals and ceremonies. The incense wafted around a church is cleansing the atmosphere; the bottle of champagne crashed against a ship is a form of consecrating ritual, and the bells that ring out on Sunday morning were not originally just intended to call worshippers to prayer but also to cleanse the parish through sound.

Kingston has been "clearing spaces" for twenty years now. But why bother? If we have lived all these hundreds of years without space clearing in Britain, why should we start now? "Suppose a room hadn't physically been cleaned for ten years," she suggests, "you can imagine what it would look like. Well, I'm talking about clearing a room on an energetic level; clearing it of all the emotional and mental traffic of the people who have been in the place since it was last cleared. In the case of most buildings, that has never been done." So most of us are probably living in the psychic equivalent of a rubbish dump. But how would we know?

"The symptoms are clear," says Kingston. "Your life doesn't seem to move; you want it to go in a particular direction but nothing seems to happen. You might feel low in energy or find you have the same problems recurring. You might even get more colds or be more constipated than other people."

It all sounds very airy-fairy and, frankly, unbelievable, but Kingston insists that the whole procedure is very down-to-earth. In Bali, where she spends about half the year studying with healers, space clearing is taken very seriously as a way of life. No one would envisage moving into a new house without thoroughly cleansing the psychic aura as well as the floors.

DIY SPACE CLEARING

The first step to space clearing is none other than good old-fashioned housework, a solid dose of spring-cleaning which leaves every corner sparkling and every old pile of papers sorted and, preferably, thrown away. Don't throw away all your magazines just yet—you will need these for the next step (the treasure map) and then they can be put in the bin.

If you want to change your life you have to sort out your clutter and get rid of whatever you can. If you haven't used an item in the last year and you don't absolutely love it, give it away, let it go. The reasoning is that by clearing the space, you are creating room for something new, something better, to appear in your life. If you have a pile of papers in your room, your energy automatically dips because you know it needs attention, argues Kingston. Every time you walk into your home and there are objects that need repairing, letters that need answering, junk that needs clearing, your energy can't flow internally because of what is happening externally.

If your house and workplace are both clear and tidy, you will find it much easier to think. But don't just tidy things away—pushing a pile of papers into a cupboard won't solve the problem. Sort things out: decide what needs to be kept and what can go. It's not just papers. Are you holding on to old clothes that you know you will never wear again? Be ruthless. Weed out anything that doesn't fit, that is stained or that you haven't worn in two years, and give it all to charity. Check your food cupboards for tins and packets that are past their expiration dates. And check medicine cabinets for old medicines and prescriptions, ancient vitamins and supplements which are well past their dates. Clear them out.

Having had your huge turn-out, the house should look clearer and more spacious. You might feel slightly different already. Now take the time to really clean it, from top to bottom. Don't skimp, but as you are cleaning the outside aspect of your environment, imagine that you are also preparing yourself on the inside for the new. I often use essential oils in cleaning. Adding a few drops of lavender oil to furniture polish or popping a couple of drops of grapefruit, lemon, or lavender oil into the vacuum cleaner bag gives the whole house a fresh scent that is much nicer than the synthetic smell of most household cleaners. If you want further ideas on how to use essential oils around the home, check out Valerie Ann Worwood's book *The Fragrant Pharmacy* which is packed full of tips and hints.

Cleaning your house thoroughly will help enormously, but there are further, more esoteric, steps you can take. Experts in space clearing say you need to "clap out" the corners of the room which is where stagnant energy is most likely to gather. To do this, move to the first corner and, holding your arms up high, start to clap in a regular fashion, moving your hands down the wall as if you were sending the clap from the ceiling down into the floor. Imagine the noise is clearing away any debris. It may feel silly, but try to concentrate. Carry out the same procedure in each corner of the room.

"Clapping pulls the energy down and disperses it," explains Karen Kingston. "As you go round each corner in the room, and when you are about three-quarters of your way round the room, the sound of your clapping will suddenly change from being dull to being sharper and crisper. It means the job is almost done."

The Japanese apparently have a variation of this ritual whereby they attack the trapped energy in the corners with swords. The effect, says Kingston, is the same.

Next Karen uses a bell to "put a circle of sound around the room." She uses a beautiful golden Balinese bell with a note of shimmering purity. It sends shivers down the spine and, by moving the bell in a circular movement, the sound reverberates round and round in the air. Kingston explains that she is putting a circle of sound around the room: every time the sound is about to die, she rings the bell again, taking it right around the room and ending with a figure eight movement. "This is the symbol of eternity," she says. "It tells the energy to go on and on." You could use any bell you like providing it has a clear, pure sound that appeals to you.

Some people also burn incense to clear spaces although many experts say that the effects don't last as long.

It may sound like crazy mumbo-jumbo but, apparently, when spaces are cleared, people experience quite remarkable results. In one instance, while Karen was space clearing a woman's house she found very thick, heavy energy in the back extension. When questioned, the woman admitted that it had been the scene of terrible rows with an ex-boyfriend and that she avoided the room whenever possible. When the space had been cleared, she immediately felt better about it and now it has become her favorite room.

Likewise, a young man inherited a house from his grandmother after her death. He constantly felt sad in the house and all his attempts to find flatmates were unsuccessful. Once the space had been cleared, however, he suddenly found his phone ringing virtually nonstop with potential tenants.

Frankly, when I first came across space clearing I found the principle rather charming but could not rationally cope with the idea that clapping and ringing bells could alter my life. However, I did try out one technique that Karen had shown me. I was living in London at the time and my house had been burgled twice in the last few years, so I was certainly willing to try out a "shielding" technique which is supposed to protect your home. You stand at each corner of your home and imagine yourself bringing down a force field with a sweep of the arm. Ultimately the four fields will merge and create a safe haven. I performed the ritual and then promptly forgot all about it until later that evening when I suddenly realized my sister was about an hour late for supper. When she finally arrived, she bore a puzzled expression on her face. "I don't know what's going on," she said, "but I've driven round and round the street and, although I know fully well where your house is, I kept seeming to miss it. It's as if it had become invisible." Pure coincidence? Perhaps, but now I always do a space clearing when things seem stuck in life.

The Treasure Map

Having done all that cleaning and clearing, you're probably feeling physically shattered. So the next exercise is a pleasant change and involves nothing more taxing than browsing through a pile of old magazines. Give yourself a few free hours, preferably a whole evening and start to think about your life, about your dreams, your ambitions, your plans. Consider the following:

• If you could have anything you wanted in life, what would it be?
• In your ideal world, where would you live? How would you live? Who would you live with? What would you do for a living?

Be honest and really think about what you want. Would you *really* want to be married to an egocentric film star? If you won the lottery, how would it make your life better? Would you feel comfortable living in a huge mansion in the country or would you really prefer a comfortable cozy town house? Don't worry about realism on the other hand. This is about dreams, about wishes and fantasies. It's about building a treasure map.

Now start to flip through the magazines and pick out images that sum up your dreams. It might be pictures of the kind of places you'd love to visit, a picture of your ideal house, of your perfect figure, of your dream career, or it could be more abstract images that sum up the kind of lifestyle you would love. Pick out any words that seem suitable as well, if you like.

Now take a large sheet of paper or a couple of sheets of

newspaper stuck together so that they're firm. Find a recent photograph of yourself, put it in the middle of the sheet and arrange your images around it. Now pin the "map" up where you will see it every day.

The idea of the treasure map is that it speaks to your subconscious mind in the powerful language of symbols. First, it gives you a chance to think about what you truly want. When you see the map on the wall, an image might start to jar or not seem right in some way. If it feels wrong, take it off and add something else. Your map does not have to stay static. But sometimes the images on the map have a curious way of becoming reality. People who use treasure maps regularly believe that the subconscious sees the images and tries to make them happen. Sometimes it succeeds or at least comes close.

I like using treasure maps because they serve to focus the mind on what I really want in my life. But I have found them coming true in the most peculiar ways. While I was still living in the heart of London I made a map which expressed my deep desire to move out into the country. It had lots of images of fields, a picture of a robin, a shot of a crazy-looking dog, dreamy photos of picnics under trees by a tranquil pond, and loads of seriously large, ridiculously grand houses I'd snipped from the property section of *Country Life*. Now I knew that in my wildest dreams I couldn't afford a Georgian stately home, but the pictures appealed and so up they went.

Six months passed and I actually did it. I moved away from London where I'd lived for most of my life and out to deepest Somerset. A short while ago, I found the old treasure map again and was stunned to find how accurate it was. I now live in a rather grand Georgian rectory, just like the ones in the pictures. It's not the whole rectory, I hasten to add, but just one half of it that has been stripped of its surrounding land. What I found so interesting was that it seemed as if my subconscious had looked for a way to get as close as possible to the map—and had done pretty well, given the budget! Other details fitted too: when friends come to visit we have tea under the trees by a small pond while the robin watches with beady eyes. A friend bought me a ridiculous puppy with a crazy look in his eyes, and the house is surrounded by fields. You could argue that these were all quite possible goals and that I simply went out and got them but, to be truthful, when I put together that map I honestly didn't think I'd ever manage to make the move, let alone live in a lovely old house and have a daft dog. My current map has lots of pictures of people relaxing on sun-kissed beaches and a fair few immaculately toned models. Hopefully, I'll end up walking along a Caribbean beach with a supermodel figure. I'm handing the details over to my subconscious and hope it comes up with the goods!

Pampering: Exploring the Joys of Massage

Spring may be the season of the body but it doesn't have to consist of whipping your body into shape. Getting started on a healthy eating plan and introducing sensible exercise may seem tough at first, but after a while it will stop feeling like torture and become something you actually enjoy. However, I'd also like you to think about getting in touch with your body in a really pleasant way. Massage is about the most gorgeous therapy you can do, not just for your body but for your entire being—your mind, emotions, and soul as well. It eases the aches and pains of everyday life; it can soothe away stress and tension and have highly therapeutic effects if you have any health problems.

On quite another level, massage will help your mind—not only by relaxing it but also by boosting your self-esteem. That may sound strange but, by allowing yourself to have a massage, to give yourself up to something so utterly blissful, you are sending a very strong message to your mind and body. Effectively, you are telling your body that you value it, that it deserves nurturing. You are also telling your mind that you can have time for yourself, that you are worth pampering. And on another level altogether, you will possibly find that as your body relaxes, it will let go of its deepest held tensions. And when age-old tension goes, often so do the negative emotions, the ancient hurts, that accompany it. We will talk more about this aspect of bodywork in the summer.

For now I would love you to think about treating yourself to regular massage sessions. I can guarantee that once you have started, you will find the habit hard to kick. But this is one addiction that won't do you any harm. And yet I'm willing to bet that most people reading this are already making excuses. "Oh, I don't have the time," "I couldn't possibly afford it," "It might be a bit dodgy, mightn't it?" "I'll have to take off all my clothes and I'm so fat/thin/bony/ugly/veined." Why, oh why, do we put off pleasure so much and so often? Massage is one of the greatest gifts you can give yourself. More than anything it allows you to experience the healing power of touch. We simply don't have enough touch in our lives nowadays—we are almost scared of being touched. We hardly even kiss one another any more—we "air kiss" or briskly pat a shoulder. There are now so many different kinds of massage that you will easily find one that suits you—from the very deep to the light and soothing; from the highly chaste (all swathed in fluffy towels) to the almost brazen (naked as the day you were born). Some take a luxurious two hours; others can be squeezed into a short half hour—although I always think you really need at least an hour to relax truly.

Equally it doesn't need to cost the earth. If you can afford to have professional massages, then do so—once a week is wonderful but even once a month will help a lot. When I was really hard-up I still used to have massages; I found a training school for beauty therapists and offered myself as a guinea pig! Quite a few colleges will be grateful for spare bodies to practice on. Some might ask for a nominal charge; others will pound and press you for free. Of course, you won't be getting a true expert touch but it's better than nothing. Another option is to teach yourself the rudiments of massage. Plenty of specialist colleges and even local education authority night classes offer short courses in DIY massage to practice on family and friends. There are also videos, but I would recommend you take a course if you can manage it—it can be quite tricky to get it just right from a video. Persuade your partner or a friend (even better, a whole bunch of friends) to learn with you and then you can trade massages.

Rest assured that massage is no longer synonymous with massage parlors and "added extras." Sex certainly won't be on the menu unless, of course, you answer an ad that reads "busty maiden offers massage" or "man to man deep sensual massage" or something of that ilk. Far better to go to a local gym, a health club or a natural health center. While most beauty salons and sports clubs will offer traditional massages such as Swedish or therapeutic massage, there are now a host of specialist massage techniques available. They are all quite different and offer varying results. They also require various levels of undress. Here's a brief lowdown:

AROMATHERAPY

This is the ultimate feel-good massage, and if you are new to massage, I would suggest you start here. Aromatherapy massage is now readily available, although, for the best results, you will need to find a well-qualified aromatherapist who will select oils that not only smell delicious but that also can help any particular health problems you may have.

A good aromatherapist will always take your case history and ask quite detailed questions about your health—past and present. If you have sensitive skin, problems with blood pressure or epilepsy, your aromatherapist will need to know. In particular, it is very important to inform the therapist if you are pregnant: certain oils are not used during pregnancy because they can induce miscarriage.

The aromatherapist will then choose the oils. If you have no specific health problems, general relaxing oils are usually selected. Some aromatherapists work on the more esoteric theory that your body will know precisely what it needs and will ask you to smell a selection of oils and pick out the ones you like. However, many will look at your symptoms and problems and choose oils on a strictly therapeutic basis.

Aromatherapy is a discreet form of massage: you won't be expected to lie stark naked on the floor or couch. The therapist will usually leave the room for a few minutes while you get undressed and put yourself on the couch, with a towel to cover yourself. Some people strip right off: I personally like to keep my knickers on for modesty's sake!

Each aromatherapist has a different way of working, but a full-body massage usually includes plenty of time devoted to that key stress-holding area, the shoulders and neck. Most will include a hand and foot massage, and often your face will be included—oils can be wonderful for cosmetic purposes, and most beauty salons now offer an aromatherapy facial.

Many aromatherapists have also learned massage techniques which are therapeutic in their own right. It's far from uncommon to have acupressure or shiatsu techniques incorporated into the massage. Some practitioners have studied TCM practices and will choose particular oils because of their *yin* or *yang* properties—they may go very deeply into the underlying causes of your illness or stress.

ACUPRESSURE/SHIATSU

Acupressure and shiatsu work in much the same way as acupuncture, by stimulating the pressure points (the acupoints) and the meridians (the energy channels) and so allowing the correct flow of *chi* (vital energy) throughout the body. Acupressure generally tends to be incorporated in other forms of massage—such as tuina, aromatherapy, and Tibetan massage—rather than practiced on its own. Shiatsu also incorporates large amounts of acupressure. It is always performed on the floor, on a mat, rather than on a couch, and you will not be asked to remove any clothes (apart from shoes and jewelry)—make sure you wear loose comfortable clothing though.

First you will be asked for a full case history. Then your pulses will probably be taken and you will be asked to lie down on a mat. Here the therapist will palpate (diagnose by touch) your back and abdomen. *Hara* diagnosis is a fundamental part of shiatsu—the *hara* is the abdominal area which can be read almost like a map. Just as a reflexologist can tell about your health by touching your feet, so a shiatsu practitioner can gain vital information by the feel of your *hara*. This, together with the case history, gives him or her the information needed to decide on your treatment.

The shiatsu practitioner's aim is to free the meridians so that your *chi* (energy) flows smoothly and clearly. Pressure is applied to individual points, and intense stretches are used to stimulate or soothe the whole length of the meridian. Expect to find yourself being moved and held in various positions, not just with the therapist's hands but also with their elbows and arms, feet and knees. Every so often you get a wonderful sense of "that's it" when a muscle or joint frees up. Sometimes it's subtle; other times your whole body seems to be creaking, cracking, and groaning. Your entire body will be worked on. After the large body stretches, the therapist will often use long, slow pressure on points along individual meridians. It's not uncommon for old thoughts and memories to be released during a session although, personally, I find this happens less with shiatsu than with other forms of bodywork.

TUINA

Tuina or tui-na (pronounced twee-nah) is one of the great remaining secrets of Chinese medicine. While acupuncture and Chinese herbal medicine have become well-known and respected in the UK, few people have heard of tuina. And yet in Chinese hospitals it is practiced equally alongside acupuncture and herbalism as a profound healing therapy.

Tuina is thought to predate acupuncture, and has been used by the Chinese in healing for over four thousand years. Fundamentally, it is an intense, deep massage that uses a positive barrage of techniques to work on the soft tissue and the joints. It is superlative for treating neck, shoulder, and back pain, sciatica, frozen shoulder, tennis elbow, and migraine.

Before a session the therapist will ask a few questions about your health; whether you have any injuries, any serious illnesses or are pregnant. Tuina is not suitable for people with fragile bones or osteoporosis, and practitioners need to be very careful when treating people with cancer and heart problems. Certain points are avoided in pregnancy because they could induce labor. As with shiatsu, you do not need to remove your clothes. You will probably be asked to move around during the session— you'll perhaps sit on a chair for some work, or on the couch for other parts of the body.

Tuina is a deep, therapeutic massage, and its primary aim is to get you physically well, not to send you to sleep. So this isn't the best choice if you simply want pampering. I would also suggest you try something like shiatsu before launching into tuina. However, if you are a bit of an old hand at massage and want something new, or if you like the idea of deep, powerful massage, then give it a go—it's wonderful stuff.

TIBETAN MASSAGE

This massage is really only a part of the whole Tibetan treatment, but it is well worth discovering in its own right if you can find a practitioner.

The session starts with careful questioning and pulse-taking to gauge health. Expect far more diagnosis than is usual with many other forms of massage. You might even be asked to provide a sample of urine for diagnosis. The therapist is looking to find out which of the three "humors"—very like the ayurvedic *doshas*—are out of balance. This will help him or her decide which oils to use in massage or even whether you need a massage at all.

Pray you do require massage because it is quite lovely. You are generally asked to strip down to your pants, but you will be well covered with towels at all times and should never feel uncomfortable. Practitioners often use oils such as ginger and cardamom and focus on freeing energy blockages via acupressure points. One difference from many other forms of massage is that Tibetan practitioners will wake you up if you start to doze off—you apparently need to be aware to gain the most benefit.

THAI HEALING MASSAGE

Traditional Thai healing massage helps you stretch yourself to the limit. Often called "lazy man's yoga" or "passive yoga," it reaps the benefits of stringent yoga postures without all the hard work—the masseur flexes you into positions you would never dream of reaching on your own. In a one and a half hour session your body will be bent and pulled, stretched and soothed. You walk out feeling taller and looser, more open and expansive, as if every part of your body had been unlocked allowing you to move and breathe more easily, more freely. Like many Eastern massage systems, the Thai method works not just on the physical body, on unleashing tension in muscles and soft tissue, but also on the energy lines of the body—the meridians. As an acupuncturist works with needles, so the Thai masseur works with his or her hands, feet, and elbows to release blockages in the energy flow and to allow vital life force, *chi,* to run smoothly around the body once again. The result, they say, is improved flexibility, better circulation of blood and lymph, and an exhilarating dose of vitality.

Thai massage, like shiatsu and chavutti thirumal, is performed, not on a couch but on a mat on the floor. Although Thai massage is generally suitable for most people, practitioners will check to find out whether a client is pregnant, has a severe back problem, or has high blood pressure: if so, they will adapt the massage. Thai massage is usually performed, like shiatsu and tuina, in loose comfortable clothing. The stretches are very deep and can be quite uncomfortable. As with tuina, I would not recommend this for newcomers to massage as it is quite intense.

No part of the body is ignored in Thai massage—it really is a head-to-toe affair. Hands, arms, and shoulders get the stretching treatment, and tension is soothed away from face and head as the masseur gently but firmly presses on the pressure points.

CHAVUTTI THIRUMAL

Chavutti thirumal is a curiously named massage which is practiced in a decidedly bizarre fashion, using the feet rather than the hands. But while the idea of someone's toes probing your body might sound rather unpleasant, devotees of massage by foot pressure simply adore being trodden upon. Not only does it feel quite delicious but its benefits are enormous: it soothes and relaxes; stimulates the circulation, immune, and lymphatic systems and can ease arthritis. Regular sessions will apparently rejuvenate the body, liberate the mind, and could even help you lose weight.

Although, as yet, there are few practitioners outside India, this is quite certain to become one of the massage techniques for the future. If you are wary of baring your body, this one isn't for you. There is no massage couch, just rush beach mats laid on the floor with a large white towel in the middle. A thick rope is suspended above head height for the practitioner to balance on. There are no discreet swathings of towels: you are left lying on the floor naked. The practitioner will ask a few questions before starting on the massage: have you ever broken any bones, any back problems, any asthma or epilepsy? The only contra-indications are cancer and heart disease, but it's good for the practitioner to be aware of any problems.

Massage by foot sounds clumsy but it is actually very precise and very deep. A trained pair of feet can do all that hands can do—and more. And, if you *can* face the total nudity you will soon find that your inhibitions fall away under the absolutely exquisite sensations. The massage kneads, probes, stretches, and soothes every muscle and ligament in the body—starting with the shoulders and working right down to the fingers and toes. Nothing is missed: even your face and head receive attention.

It is one of the most satisfying massages you could ask for. It isn't all uninterrupted bliss, though: some parts of your body may feel sore or tender as they are probed and pressed. However, the net effect after an hour and a half is that your body feels like singing.

KAHUNA BODYWORK

Kahuna, or Hawaiian massage, is a system of bodywork that has been practiced in the Polynesian islands for centuries. Unlike normal massages, which simply aim to relax, the Hawaiian method has a much more profound purpose. Its practitioners believe they can put you back in touch with your body, teaching you to accept and love yourself, whatever your shape or size. And once you accept the beauty within, they say, you will start to recognize the beauty that surrounds you.

Aside from deeply relaxing the physical structure of the body, Hawaiian massage also affects the body on a vibrational level. It is said to accelerate the vibrational rate of the cells and the energy fields of both the physical and subtle bodies. However, the deepest difference between this and other forms of massage is its ability to make you feel your body as a whole. The smooth, repetitive movements which cover the whole body induce the body into almost a hypnotic state. Meanwhile, the practitioner's heart is concentrating on smothering you with unconditional love, acceptance, and joy. The idea is that your body, cocooned in all this love and acceptance, will begin to believe that it is, indeed, lovable and beautiful. The length of the massage (often up to three hours) allows the message to be reinforced. This is not a quick pick-me-up but a lesson in love for the body, a chance to remember its worth.

As with chavutti thirumal, kahuna massage is performed nearly nude—save for a brief loincloth—and so the treatment room is always very hot. You feel very exposed and, initially, the experience can be uncomfortable. Using light scented oils, the practitioner starts by massaging the back, sweeping down from the head right through to the legs in long fluid movements. The movement is rhythmic and repetitive and, after a few minutes, it becomes hard to remember where one stroke ends and the next begins. Performers don't just use their hands but also the whole length of their forearms for some moves. Kahuna massage uses techniques from a variety of massages but the whole is far more than the sum of its parts.

Again, not an ideal massage unless you feel you can cope with the nakedness and the almost "intimate" nature of the massage. Not everyone feels comfortable being showered with unconditional love!

Celebrating the Spring Equinox

The major festival of March is the spring equinox, a celebration of joy, energy, and life. By space clearing and making a treasure map you have already fulfilled two of its tasks—the clearing out of the old and the welcoming in of the new. Now you just need to celebrate.

This is an ideal time of the year for short breaks, for weekends away—spend some time walking in the countryside in the bracing weather. If you can't get away and there isn't any countryside to hand, spend time in parks or even in the garden. Bring spring flowers into your home— cheery bunches of daffodils, the sweet scent of hyacinth. These are such simple things to do but they are as much rituals as the swinging incense and chanting of High Church ceremonies. You are connecting yourself to the land, to the upsurge of the year. Be aware of the changes in nature—see how the days are beginning to grow longer. As the clocks go forward, the evenings become lighter. Everything is alive and you are part of the celebration. Enjoy the elements—the wild winds, the sharp air. Dress up warmly and take a kite out to play.

The fourth Sunday in Lent is Mothering Sunday. In the past it was the day when children would return home to their mothers for a visit, carrying with them small gifts—often money if they had been working away from home, or a posy of spring flowers or an item of clothing. The day had its own cake too—simnel cake—a rich fruit cake crammed with marzipan in the middle and marzipan on top, often decorated with almond paste, eggs, or balls as well.

Nowadays, of course, Mothering Sunday has become commercialized. We call it Mother's Day and we generally send a card and, if we remember, a bunch of Interflora flowers. When I was a child we made cards and were given posies in church to hand to our mothers. It all seemed purer, sweeter somehow. Even now, I cannot quite bring myself to buy the gaudy bouquets and cards. I normally pick wild flowers or a posy from the garden and choose a simple card. Obviously, what you do is up to you, but if you have children why not encourage them to make their own cards and pick their own flowers? And remember that, first and foremost, this is a festival that celebrates motherhood. Take some time to appreciate your mother—she gave you birth, she took you through childhood, and without her you wouldn't be here. If you are not on good terms, then make a special effort at this time of year to get your relationship back on track. Make the first move—what will it cost but your pride? And if you have deep-seated problems with your mother, if you feel she has done something unforgivable to you in the past, maybe this is the time to forgive. Forgiving is a powerful tool. It can liberate you quite as much as the person you forgive. This, however, may be hard at this stage. If so, leave it for now—we will deal with these sorts of issues later on in the year.

April

April is fresh, bright, light, and cheery. While March may hark back to the chill of winter, by April there is no doubt that the new year is here to stay. The daffodils are still brightening the garden with their cheery yellow, but now they have been joined by bold tulips and splashes of purple aubretia. On the riverbanks, the primroses shyly turn their faces to the sun while the forget-me-nots give a shimmer of blue. There is a fresh green glimmer over the whole land. Weeds appear overnight, the fields are plowed and lambs are everywhere. To the Native Americans, April is the Awakening Time and it's not hard to see why: April simply shouts "Wake up! Get out there! Live!"

By now your body should be becoming used to a good, clean, healthy diet and be positively enjoying it. Your exercise program should be showing effects too. Now is the time to add some more powerful medicine in the shape of tonics.

It's also time to think about introducing flexibility into your body. You may be getting fit, you might be able to run up stairs and your muscles should be toning up nicely, but a truly healthy body is also a flexible body, supple and easy in itself.

Boosting Your Health with Tonics

In days gone by, our ancestors adapted to the new season by wearing different clothes, eating different foods, and taking different herbs. They would enliven their diet with the fresh spring greens, making zesty soups from the young nettles and herbs growing all around, tasting the sharp piquancy with delight after the heavy root vegetable stews of the winter months. Nowadays, of course, we rarely bother to adapt our diet to the seasons. However, in cultures like China, where the tradition of herbal medicine has continued uninterrupted for thousands of years, it's still common practice to prepare your body for the new season by taking a tonic. There are tonics for the blood, tonics for the immune system, tonics for regulating and balancing the entire body. As Kenneth Wingrove-Gibbons of the CHI Center for Traditional Chinese Medicine in London explains: "Chinese medicine works on the principle that everything is in balance. So you should really change everything to suit the season you are in. When you come out of one season and move into the next you sometimes need a boost to help you through the changeover period."

Some of the Chinese arsenal of tonic herbs have become quite familiar: ginseng, bee pollen, and royal jelly are well-established on the supplement counters of chemists and health-food stores. Some, like licorice, we use without any idea of their medicinal importance. But there are countless other plants of which we have no knowledge whatsoever. Benny Mei of The AcuMedic Center in London points out, as an example, the incredible effects of *Dong Chong Hia Cao*—the preparation that lay at the center of the controversy surrounding Chinese athletes a few years back. The Chinese athletes were performing so very well that Westerners thought they had to be taking steroids or other powerful pharmaceutical drugs. They weren't: they were simply supplementing with *Dong Chong Hia Cao*. "It is a tonic which builds up your body's strength," Mei explains, "and it is also a great aphrodisiac." Sadly, it is also very expensive. As a child, Mei grew up with tonics: "In the Far East you go to the grocers and ask for a cooling tea for summer, or your mother will give you something when your body is toxified after winter."

"A good tonic," says Kenneth Wingrove-Gibbons, "will permeate right down through the system, balancing and strengthening each and every organ, allowing them to 'talk to each other' in harmony. It's like an upright pinball machine. The medicine runs through all the little gates and attaches itself to each ball, or organ, and tunes it as it passes. When it gets to the bottom it takes away all the toxins and waste you don't need and leaves everything cleaner. It's as if someone went in and polished everything. Your whole system can communicate because there is nothing in the way."

Keen to encourage some meaningful dialogue within my body, my first stop was my local health-food shop where I was offered Korean ginseng extract. At around £20 for a small jar it wasn't cheap but, I was assured, it was good quality. You drink it like a tea, mixing a tiny spoonful in hot water and adding honey if you like. Surprisingly, the taste wasn't that bad—earthy and sharp. And the effects were quite distinct: I felt brighter, more alert and clearer-headed. It was like drinking strong coffee without the side effects.

Next stop was East-West Herbs in Neal's Yard, London, where I discovered the wonderfully named Move Mountains, a combination of ginseng plus equally celebrated tonic herbs astragalus, schizandra, lichi, and dendrobium. The label promised that it "increases endurance, stamina and cheerfulness, helping one jump out of bed in the morning . . ." Around fifteen drops added to carbonated spring water was definitely an acquired taste but, again, not unpleasant. Once again, I was impressed. The little bottle was a firm friend while undergoing the horrors of moving, keeping energy levels high and spirits more or less up.

However, Kenneth Wingrove-Gibbons warns against this kind of self-diagnosis and treatment. "In China, people know what to buy and how to use it," he admonishes. "Take ginseng for example: first there is red or white ginseng. Then you choose between Chinese, Korean, or American ginseng. The capsules generally won't do anything, but the real root is very potent. They say you can bring a man back from death's door with a sliver of raw ginseng." Sounds wonderful. However, ginseng is not suitable for everyone and the unaware could easily take too much. "You could increase your heart rate and your blood pressure," he warns. "You're putting in something to stimulate the system and, if you put it in wrong, you can overstimulate the body. It's like driving a car too fast—you take off."

He recommends that you either take your chosen product to a qualified herbalist to check out or, better still, you have a tonic tailor-made for your system. To demonstrate, he took me to meet Dr. Li at his clinic. Initially, it felt very strange admitting to a doctor that there was nothing technically wrong with me, that all I wanted was something to make me feel *even* better. But Dr. Li didn't bat an eyelid—she simply looked at my tongue, took my pulses, and observed me very closely, as if trying to see what made me tick. Did I sleep well? How were my periods? How were my bowels? Did I have a good appetite? Nothing is sacred to a practitioner of traditional Chinese medicine. I was prescribed an herbal tea comprising eleven different herbs and instructed to drink it twice a day for a week.

In the pharmacy, they threw handfuls of herbs onto seven large platters: bits of bark, bundles of leaves, sliced dried mush-rooms, corn-type husks, and something that looked suspiciously like pearl barley. Throwing each day's supply into a paper bag I was presented with a large carrier bag of herbs to take home. Then started the arduous process of brewing the "tea." The herbs need to be boiled twice with one dose taken in the morning and one in the evening. The first day I didn't notice much of a differ-ence. The second day I felt as if I had a bad cold with a runny nose and congested head. But by day three I felt like a six-year-old, running up the stairs two at a time and attacking my garden like a human tornado. By the end of the week I was feeling distinctly different: clear and calm, with abundant but more con-trolled energy.

The following are the most widely used Chinese tonics.

Astragalus **(Huang Qi)** One of the most widely used en-ergy tonics in China, astragalus is a great immune enhancer. It boosts the production of white and red blood cells, interferon (a protein that inhibits viral growth), immunoglobulins (a protein that acts as an antibody) and the function of the adrenal cortex. In the USA it is being investigated for use with cancer and AIDS patients.

Lichi **(Gou Qi Zi))** This is a gentle tonic for the kidneys and the liver that helps poor eyesight and even benefits the com-plexion. Modern research shows that the fruit promotes regeneration of liver cells and lowers blood cholesterol levels. It can prevent the formation of atherosclerosis (hardening of the arteries) and tends to reduce blood sugar.

Codonopsis (Dang Shen) As famous as ginseng in China, codonopsis tonifies the life energy and, in particular, strengthens the lungs, spleen, and stomach.

Schizandra (Wu Wei Zi) A famous sex tonic for both men and women, schizandra has the added benefit of softening and beautifying the skin. Modern researchers have found it balances the nervous system, increases endurance, and reduces fatigue. It can help lower blood pressure and is a useful expectorant.

Chinese Liquorice Root(Gan Cao) This is a remarkable root which can detoxify the ill effects of drugs, balance blood sugar levels and relieve pains and spasms in the digestive system. Liquorice also stimulates the action of other herbs. Japanese research shows that the glycyrrhetic acid contained in liquorice can inhibit tumors.

Chinese Angelica (Dang Gui) The most famous blood tonic in Chinese medicine, *Dang Gui* is particularly important in treating menstrual disorders. However, it should be avoided before and during pregnancy. It is often used to help combat exhaustion and debility.

Ginseng Renshen is the Chinese ginseng, useful for tonifying a system weakened by disease, overwork, or old age. It is an adaptogen (both stimulant and sedative according to the body's needs) and very useful in stress. *San Qi* or *Tian Qi* is another form of ginseng which has been shown to give pain relief, lower blood pressure and cholesterol levels, and to reduce swelling. *Xi Yang Shen* is American ginseng, a mild and gentle tonic which has been used for treating tuberculosis. Modern research shows it has a sedative action on the brain while exciting the central nervous system.

Try the following casserole as a way of introducing several of these powerful tonics into your life.

CHICKEN QI TONIC CASSEROLE
SERVES 4–6
As recommended by the East West herb shop, this is an energizing and tonifying main course ideal for exhaustion, debility, as a general pick-me-up and energy booster. East West advise you to

eat the roots as well, although as astragalus is somewhat indigest-
ible you can give that one a miss! The tonics can be found in
Chinese pharmacies or ordered by mail (see Further Information
at the back of this book).

1 medium free-range chicken
2 sticks astragalus root
1 stick American ginseng
2 sticks cadonopsis root or *Panax* ginseng
10 shitake mushrooms (fresh or dry)
1 cm (½ inch) slice fresh ginger root
2 tsp. French or English mustard (prepared)
3 sticks celery, chopped
3 carrots, chopped
1 tbsp soy sauce
bunch of watercress, roughly chopped
salt and pepper to taste

Place the chicken and all the ingredients except the soy sauce
and watercress into a large saucepan and cover with water. Bring
to the boil and simmer for one and a half to two hours, then
remove from the heat.

Add the soy sauce and watercress. Test for seasoning and add
salt and pepper if necessary.

Serve with fresh brown bread or on a bed of rice.

OTHER TONICS

The Chinese don't have a monopoly on tonics. If you see a
practitioner of medical herbalism, Ayurveda, Tibb (the Arabic
form of natural medicine also known as *Unani* medicine, Greco-
Arabic medicine, or *Sufi* medicine) or Tibetan medicine they will
also provide you with tonics to suit your needs and constitution.
However, there are plenty of tonics nearer to home (sometimes
as close as the back garden), some of which we can all use with
perfect safety.

Dandelion The humble dandelion is a superb cleanser and
tonic. The young leaves (providing they're totally clean) are very
nourishing for the body. Make tea from the fresh leaves or, better
still, put them straight into salads or soups. The dandelion root
is a blood, liver, and kidney cleanser as well as being a tonic.

Just one warning—dandelion is also a master diuretic. Not for nothing do the French call it *pis-en-lit* (wet-the-bed).

Sassafras This herb is not well known but deserves to be. It purifies the blood and acts as a mild stimulant to the system. Sassafras is also excellent for the skin and joints, the bladder, the kidneys, and the chest. It will ease rheumatism and arthritis and can soothe and tonify the stomach and the whole digestive system and relieve trapped wind (remember the dangers of excess wind in spring according to the Chinese system?). As if that weren't enough, sassafras can ward off colds and sore throats. It is also stuffed full of essential minerals. So no wonder that many naturopaths recommend you start spring with a dose of sassafras. Don't overdo it— like all herbs, sassafras is powerful and too much could be harmful. Take a cup of sassafras tea every day for a few weeks throughout April to cleanse your system: simply add a couple of teaspoons of the root or bark to a mug of boiling water and allow to steep for about a quarter of an hour. Strain the brew and drink—you may find you need to sweeten it with a little honey.

Nettles Take a healthy green leaf out of our ancestors' book and eat young nettle leaves. I'm always being told that the young ones don't sting and that you can put them straight in salads or chopped over potatoes. But, to be frank, I've always been a little too nervous to try. Instead, I wear a wimpish pair of gloves when I pick them, and then pop them into soup. Don't overcook them—they're a wonderful source of calcium phosphate, iron, and other minerals and vitamins.

The Big Stretch: Gaining Flexibility in Your Body

Hopefully, by now you'll be well into your exercise routine and starting to feel the benefits. If you have joined a gym or are taking aerobics classes, no doubt you have been advised to follow a stringent stretching routine as part of your workout. And ten to one, you probably won't bother with it. Think again. A truly healthy body is one with complete freedom of movement—total flexibility. We think we're flexible but often the truth is that we're painfully distorted. Even if you can touch your toes without effort or put one leg behind your head it doesn't necessarily mean you have perfect flexibility. I can do a perfect lotus position, but I'm far from flexible.

My legs will quite happily bend because, for some inexplicable reason, my big brother taught me how to do the posture when I was very young. I kept practicing, and my muscles adapted to the routine. Even the most fluid dancers and the most contortionist gymnasts don't always have complete balance in their bodies.

As April is such an expansive month, it is the natural time to begin a program of coaxing your body into greater flexibility. It's a time to stretch and move, to discover new possibilities, to extend far beyond your former limits. I'm not asking you to become an elastic being which can bend every which way but simply to pay some attention to flexibility within your body. It's something we often ignore. I watch loads of people at the gym hurl themselves around, doing aerobic exercise on the machines or in classes, lifting weights for muscle tone and yet, at the end of their workout, they race off without a single stretch. Yet every fitness instructor you'll meet will tell you of the importance of stretching. Not only does it improve your flexibility, it also prevents your muscles from becoming sore; it lessens the risk of injury and takes your body down from the arousal of intense activity to a more relaxed state.

And there is another, more subtle benefit. As we've already discussed, your body affects your mind and vice versa. So imagine the effect of a rigid, stiff, inflexible body on your mind? It really does seem to be the case that, if you can introduce flexibility into your body, your mind will follow suit. You will find it easier to come up with novel solutions, you will become more adaptable, you will become far less scared of change. On a practical level your body will hold less tension—there will be fewer places for it to hide. You will develop better coordination and balance and find you have fewer aches and pains. Quite simply, your body will work more easily—it's like oiling the hinges.

So how do you start? Begin quite gently by introducing simple stretches into your day. Watch any animal on waking and notice the first thing it does. It stretches—slowly, luxuriously. Learn from the animals. When you wake up, don't leap straight out of your bed but spend some few minutes simply becoming aware of your body. How does it feel? As you lie in bed, start to stretch your body, slowly flexing it. Make yourself long, as long as you can by stretching out over your head and as far down as your toes. Then take your knees up to your chest and let them gently fall to one side of your body. Slowly turn your head and arms to face the opposite direction. Hold

the stretch and then take it the opposite way. It should feel good—
you might find (as I do) that a vertebra or two clicks back into
position. Next, gently take yourself to a sitting and then to a standing
position and continue stretching. Let your head *gently* stretch from
side to side. Now roll it softly round—first clockwise, then counterclockwise. All these exercises should be done very slowly and very
smoothly—the object is to softly nudge your body into the day, not
give it a rude awakening.

Next, I would recommend you try a series of postures known
as the Sun Salute. These come from yoga and are the perfect
way to start the day, as they stretch virtually every muscle in
your body and massage the internal organs as well. In ancient
India they were part of daily spiritual practice and were performed in the very early morning facing the sun, the deity for
health and long life. Practice this sequence regularly, and the
benefits are legion. You will become far more flexible, particularly in your spine. It also increases your breathing capacity and
can tone the abdomen. There are twelve spinal positions, and
each stretches different ligaments and moves the spine in different ways. At first, this series of postures will seem jerky and
uncoordinated. But if you persevere, as you begin to learn them
by heart you will find you can move fluidly and smoothly from
one stance to another. Start off with just one whole set and
gradually build it up to the optimum twelve. Please be aware,
however, that although this is one of the most familiar and safe
yoga routines, it is not suitable for people with hypertension,
hernia, low back pain, and venous blood clots.

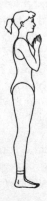

POSTURE ONE:
Standing upright, bring your feet together so that your big toes are
touching. Your arms are by your
sides. Relax your shoulders and tuck
your chin in slightly—look straight
ahead, not down at your feet. Bring
your hands together in front of your
chest with palms together as if you
were praying. Exhale deeply.

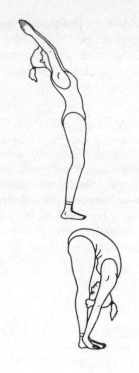

POSTURE TWO:
Inhale slowly and deeply while you bring your arms straight up over your head, keeping your palms together as you finish inhaling. Softly look backward toward your thumbs. Lift the knees by tightening your thighs. Reach up as far as possible, lengthening your whole body. If you feel comfortable, you can take the posture back slightly further into a bend.

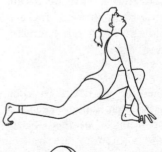

POSTURE THREE:
Exhale as you bend forward so that your hands are in line with your feet. Aim to touch your head to your knees. To begin with, you might find you have to bend your knees in order to reach. Eventually you should be able to straighten your knees into the full posture.

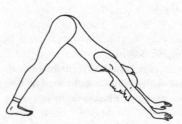

POSTURE FOUR:
Inhale deeply and move your left leg away from your body in a big backward sweep so that you end up in an extended lunge position. Keep your hands and right foot firmly on the ground. Your right knee should be between your hands. Reach your head upward, stretching out your back.

POSTURE FIVE:
Exhaling deeply, bring your right foot back, in line with the left, so that your body is in an arched position (known as the dog). Your arms are in front of your head, palms facing directly in front, arms shoulder-width apart. Your

back should be in a straight line with your head and arms. Keep your feet and heels flat on the floor.

POSTURE SIX:
Exhale and lower your body onto the floor. This is a curious posture known as *sastanga namaskar* or the eight-curved prostration because only eight parts of your body should be in contact with the floor: your feet, your knees, your hands, your chest, and your forehead. Try to keep your abdomen raised and, if you can possibly manage it, keep your nose off the floor so only your forehead makes contact. Don't worry if it's an impossibility at this point—just keep the idea in mind.

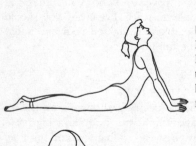

POSTURE SEVEN:
Inhale and bend up into the position known as the cobra. With hands on the floor in front of you, arms straight, bend backward as far as feels comfortable. Look upward.

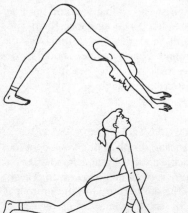

POSTURE EIGHT:
Exhale and lift your back back into posture five. Remember to keep your feet and heels (if you can) flat on the floor.

POSTURE NINE:
Inhale and return to posture four, this time with the opposite leg forward, so your left foot is in line with your hands while your right leg is stretched back.

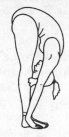

POSTURE TEN:
Exhale and return to posture three.

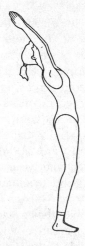

POSTURE ELEVEN:
Inhale, raising the arms overhead and back backward into posture two.

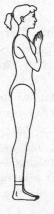

POSTURE TWELVE:
Return to a comfortable standing position, feet together, arms by your sides. Look straight ahead and exhale. To close, bring your hands back together in a position of prayer.

The Ultimate Stretch

Introduce simple stretches into your life, and you will notice a considerable difference. However, if you really want to change the way you look and feel, experiment with one of the superlative super-stretchers. Many forms of exercise and bodywork will help your flexibility, but some stand out way in front.

YOGA

If you enjoyed the Sun Salute, you may find yoga the perfect way to extend your stretching. If you look at anyone who practices yoga seriously and over a long period of time, you will see that their bodies are usually beautiful—supple and flexible with long lean muscles. Frankly, I cannot recommend yoga highly enough. It will tone your whole body, give you wonderful levels of flexibility, help you control your weight, assist your circulation (both of the blood and the lymph) and generally make you feel brighter and more cheerful. The wonderful thing about yoga is that absolutely anyone can do it—no matter what your age, size, or level of fitness. Providing you find a good teacher, there is nothing to stop you.

Recently I have been going to a class which has a wide cross-section of people. One woman had a Cesarean not long ago; another had a hip replacement and finds this is the only form of exercise she can safely take; others have bad backs, stiff necks, weak knees. The teacher simply adapts each posture for each individual, adding supports and props where necessary. Sometimes it looks like a torture chamber with a couple of us helping someone else get into a posture with the aid of straps and cushions.

What I love about it is that yoga is (or certainly should be) totally noncompetitive and nonjudgmental. Nobody mocks or stares—everyone just gets on with their own thing. And you usually find that everyone has their good bits and their bad bits. I can do a perfect lotus and bend my legs round my head, but I've got absolutely no balance and couldn't do a headstand to save my life. Do give it a go. And if you're quite fit and think yoga is a bit static and boring, check out some of the more dynamic forms of yoga that are becoming popular. There's nothing namby-pamby about *these* classes—they are just as tough as a circuit training routine.

How deeply you get into yoga depends on you. Nowadays we tend to think of yoga as purely a form of exercise, but in reality it is a complete system of self-discipline designed to harmonize, strengthen, and purify not just your body but also your mind and soul. When practiced deeply, the yogic path consists of far more than just correct exercise. You learn proper breathing, proper diet, proper ways of relaxation, proper meditation and correct ways of thinking (studying the philosophy of yoga). Taken like this, it offers a complete system of health.

THE FELDENKRAIS METHOD

When you see a cat walk across a room, it's like watching perfect fluidity in motion: supple and flexible, perfectly balanced, perfectly poised. The Feldenkrais method has been described as a way to "find the cat in you" by teaching effortless movement through improved mind and body coordination. It's the secret behind the poise and control of countless actors and dancers; the magic ingredient that gives sportspeople the edge in improving their performance or fine-tuning their game. In Germany it is so highly regarded as a tool for rehabilitation that it can be claimed on health insurance. And yet, in the U.K., hardly anyone has heard about this gentle exercise system that coaxes bodies back into ease and comfort, that can banish pain and give back freedom of movement.

The Feldenkrais method was developed by Moshe Feldenkrais, a Russian Jew with a Ph.D. in engineering and physics. A keen sportsman, he introduced judo to prewar Paris and then, when the Second World War broke out, escaped to Britain, and worked in a submarine base in northern Scotland. Still sports mad, he damaged his knee through playing football and was told by his doctor that the only treatment was (possibly ineffectual) surgery. Feldenkrais decided to take his health into his own hands and applied his knowledge of structure and motion, combined with his martial arts training, to tackle the problem. Through long and detailed observation of his body, he concluded that stiffness and pain are often not caused by physical defects, disease, and degeneration, but by limitations in movement. By reeducating his body to move more freely and easily, he cured his knee and began a quest to help other people find the same release.

He noted that most people are quite unaware of how they hold their bodies, which parts move easily and which are stilted or lacking in mobility. By gently moving a person's body in unfamiliar ways, Feldenkrais found people could become more aware of how their bodies moved and that, by repeating the movements, he could actually alter the neuromuscular patterns that organize and control movement. The result was freedom from pain, increased flexibility, and a wonderful feeling of truly being in the body.

The Feldenkrais method is taught in two distinct ways. One-to-one sessions are known as Functional Integration and comprise gentle manipulation, generally carried out on a low couch. Alternatively, you can learn the method by attending Awareness Through Movement classes and workshops in which small groups carry out gentle exercises guided by a teacher. Some people come for just a few individual sessions or the odd workshop; others take up the classes on a regular basis.

Like yoga, the whole philosophy of Feldenkrais is kind. Whether you choose to work alone, with a teacher, or as part of a class, the entire process is noncompetitive and nonjudgmental. "Feldenkrais accepts people at any stage," says Barbara McCrea, who teaches the technique in London. "You are never pushed beyond your limits, you are never forced into anything. You use comfort as your guide and simply work at your own pace."

Feldenkrais is often compared to the Alexander technique and certainly the two systems share the same emphasis of educating the body into freedom of posture and movement. However, to be honest, Feldenkrais is a lot more fun than the Alexander technique. Many of the movements taught in Awareness Through Movement classes are drawn directly from babyhood and childhood, so you're quite likely to find yourself rolling or twisting on the floor just like a toddler. "As we grow up we learn to edit out natural movements," explains Barbara McCrea. "Our sedentary lifestyle is partly to blame but also social constraints. It is no longer seemly to sit on the floor or to run freely and easily. We limit our range of movements."

Feldenkrais can give back the joy of movement. The freedom and joy of a child can coax the adult back to poise.

THE MEZIERES METHOD

The Mezieres method is little-known outside its native France but, with any luck, it will become more widely available. It's a powerful bodywork technique that will not only give you better flexibility but, if you are really committed, it can imbue your body with perfect harmony. I became convinced when I met U.K. practitioner Joel Carbonnel.

Carbonnel believes in perfection. He firmly states that within us all is "hidden a Greek god or goddess with harmonious physical proportions." No saddlebag thighs, no bulging bottoms, no rounded shoulders, no flabby waists. It's an impressive claim and surely overly optimistic? Yet however much I pushed Carbonnel he refused to budge. "A beautiful body is not only our birthright," he says, "it is also a prerequisite to health and well-being." So his patients report not only an often radical reshaping of their bodies but also freedom from aches and pains, from arthritis and sciatica. The Mezieres method can correct long-term distortions of the body, from kyphosis (Dowager's hump) and scoliosis (spinal curvature) to flat feet, knock-knees and bow-legs.

In its native France the Mezieres method has been quietly revolutionizing bodywork for the last forty years. Its originator was Francoise Mezieres, a teacher of physiotherapy and anatomy. Like all physiotherapists, she had been taught that the muscles in the back are generally too weak and need to be strengthened. But one day while she was examining a patient it suddenly occurred to her that in fact the very opposite was true: the muscles in the back were actually too *strong*. Their strength caused them to become shortened and to lose their elasticity, creating tension and eventually pain. This imbalance of strength was occurring all over the body, but it was particularly pronounced in the back because the muscles in the back overlapped to form a chain running the entire length of the body. There was, she realized, absolutely no point in relieving stiffness or shortening in just one

muscle or muscle group as it would simply cause compensatory
shortening in another area: the whole chain needed to be
stretched and readjusted at the same time.

Mezieres could hardly believe what she was formulating. The
idea directly contradicted everything she believed in, everything
she taught her students, so she set out to disprove her theory.
Two years later, after endless observation, she admitted defeat
and began to reshape entirely her way of working.

The Mezieres method is no easy ride. It involves intense, pains-
taking work by both practitioner and patient. Joel Carbonnel sees
patients once or twice a week and frankly admits it may take
several months to reshape a body. "Often you can get rid of pain
in one session," he says, "but it will never be long-lasting unless
you work hard to correct the cause of that pain."

Correcting the cause involves literally unraveling the distortions
of the body—it's a little like slowly and patiently taking the kinks
and knots out of a badly twisted rope and stretching it so that it
lies smooth and flat once again. And, like a rope that has been
wound for a long time, the body fights against being straightened
and stretched. Put one part in place and another bounces out
of line.

I found it one of the most difficult—yet most rewarding—methods
I have tried. First Joel asked me to strip down to underwear and
to simply stand with my feet together, ankles, knees, and toes
touching. Easier said than done—my knees turned inwards, preventing my feet from coming together. Then he asked me to
slowly bend forward as if to touch my toes. I can happily put
both hands on the floor and expected instant praise. Wrong:
"Your hamstrings are relatively supple but your legs are too far
back in relation to your ankles." He paced around, observing me
from all angles and concluded that I'm in a bad way.

So to work. I lay down on my back on the floor and Carbonnel
began to put my body into a precise position. He moved my
head slightly to the right and instructed me to gently bring my
shoulders down and pull my chin in. "Keep your pelvis on the
floor, bring your whole lower back onto the floor," he instructed,
and my knees shot up. He laughed: "Every time we correct one
part, another leaps out of line." I could see what he meant. Next
I had to bring my ankles together and keep my feet from turning
out. It sounds simple but within seconds I was begging for mercy.

"Now breathe out deeply from your abdomen," instructed Carbonnel. I failed dismally.

More movements followed—all involving tiny adjustments, all held for several minutes, all unbelievably difficult. I felt like an overstuffed packing case: you press down one side and something pops out the other; you stuff a sweater back in and your washbag flops out. However, I didn't have to do all the work. Sometimes Carbonnel used his body weight to add to the stretch; sometimes he kneaded tense stiff muscles to help them yield. At the end of an hour I was exhausted. My feet had pins and needles and my legs felt numb—a common reaction to Mezieres in the early stages.

As I walked down the street afterward I felt as if I had been given a different body—I ached in places I have never ached; my legs seemed to walk in a different way. The next day I felt as if I had been in the gym for three hours. Obviously my flab had not vanished overnight: that would take time (and quite possibly a change of eating habits, lectured Carbonnel), nor had my knock-knees miraculously straightened out. However, I could clearly see how the system could work, given application and patience.

"It is not a quick fix by any means," says Carbonnel. "You worked for years to make your body what it is today and you cannot change it back overnight." He insists that anyone who sticks the course can and will see profound changes. Obviously you cannot alter your height (although people often find they "grow" an inch or so) and nothing will change large bones. But with determination almost anything else can, and will, change. "The method gives us the means whereby we can mold and reshape the body so that the beauty, strength, suppleness, and smooth functioning we deserve are ours," insists Carbonnel.

As yet, Carbonnel is the only practitioner of the technique in the U.K. He combines it with the Alexander technique which is, to his mind, the only other form of bodywork that really gets to grips with our problems. In the future, he hopes, more practitioners will learn and teach this revolutionary form of bodywork. Then, he smiles, we could all transform our bodies into those of the gods.

Celebrating Easter

Easter may sometimes fall in March but generally we celebrate it in April—so here it is. We think of Easter as the great Christian festival and, certainly, it celebrates the triumph of Christ over the cross, the great mystery behind the Christian faith. Yet, Easter is not all Christian. The name Easter actually derives from Oestre or Eostre, who was a very un-Christian Saxon goddess of the Dawn of the Year. Our cuddly Easter bunny was originally a fleet-footed and highly fecund Easter hare—an ancient symbol of fertility and regeneration. Our Easter eggs are again quite obvious symbols of birth and continuation. In the old days you would have painted them with symbols and pictures of whatever you desired from the year. The eggs would then be buried in the ground so that the Earth mother could be told your hopes and dreams.

So Easter is about regeneration on a large scale—not just the rebirth of Christ but the regeneration of all of nature. Even the hot-cross buns of Good Friday have a much more ancient history than you might imagine. Such cakes were originally eaten in honor of the Goddess of the Spring. The equal-armed cross was an ancient symbol of the goddess, demonstrating her power over the four seasons. Some people say that hot-cross buns have healing properties and will last indefinitely if stored in a dry place. In fact I can testify to the latter—I have a hot-cross bun that apparently dates back to the 1930s. My grandmother put it in a marble pot and there it stayed. It's quite blackened and dried to a crisp, and I certainly wouldn't eat it, but it is clearly a hot-cross bun. Whether it has healing properties or not I couldn't say. Please don't think I'm in any way denigrating Christianity by explaining the pagan past of many of its celebrations. It's merely that the earlier origins of festivals often show their original purpose—the celebration of the cyclical nature of the year, the joyful passing of the seasons.

Don't ruin all that healthy eating by munching your way through loads of chocolate eggs. Instead go back to the old customs and decorate the real thing. Eggs make wonderful minicanvases. You can paint them as they are (but be careful) or boil them first. Onion skins in the boiling water will turn the shells a golden-brown color, or you can use food dyes. If you draw on the eggs with a wax crayon and then boil them in colored water you will get an interesting effect. Why not use the old custom and paint on your egg whatever you want for this year—something symbolic of your aims and aspirations.

There's a tradition that says that sowing parsley on Good Friday will help the seeds sprout early. The reasoning was that the devil stopped the seeds from germinating, but by sowing them on a holy day you were effectively tying his hands. I'm not so sure about that but it's not a bad idea to think about herbs now. Plant up pots of dill, basil, thyme, chervil, and chives indoors, ready to go on the window ledge when the warmer weather comes.

Another interesting aside is that if you want to encourage your hair to grow this is the time to have it cut. As everything around you grows and shoots and sprouts, why should your hair be any different? Cut it now and it will grow even faster.

May

The Native Americans call May the Growing Time. May thrusts upward and outward in a glorious upsurge of energy, freedom, and growth. May doesn't hold anything back, in fact it simply doesn't seem to care. It's like a beautiful, wayward adolescent who wants to get out there and do it all, see it all, feel it all, be it all. It shows nature in its full early beauty: everything is fresh and green and lush; a gentle haze softens the countryside. In the woods the bluebells shimmer like a magical carpet. There are daisies splattered jauntily over lawns and thick peony buds promising riches to come. The lambs are getting bigger, and plump pheasants wander innocently over roads. As the promise of summer comes tantalizingly close, animals start to molt, dog hairs everywhere.

Exercise should be easy now. As the days get warmer, the clear spring sun should tempt you out of doors. Gardens need all the hours you can give them—and gardening is great exercise too (but mind your back).

Beltane: The Wild and Wonderful Festival of May

The lessons of May are about freedom, about energy and about determination. It's a dynamic time—not just of growth but of destruction too. As Shan, pagan priestess and therapist, says: "Freedom is stressful. It means making decisions, balancing opportunities, it means the freedom to break." She points out that many marriages and partnerships cannot take the sheer scrutiny of May and break up around this time. It's also a season when many people choose to die. "It's a natural time to end things," she says. "It's like new energy being put into an old vessel. If the vessel isn't strong enough to take the energy, it will break."

Of course, this all ties in with the principal festival of May, which is May Day or, in the ancient calendar, Beltane. No point in being coy about it, Beltane is the great sex festival of the pagan year. The maypole is a blatant phallic symbol plunging down into the fertile (female) earth. It is said that the pole also stands for the movement of energy between heaven and earth, the vital energy of the sky coming down to combine with the growing earth which brings about the fresh new upsurge of spring. As an interesting aside, it appears dowsers can detect spiral energy patterns in the places where maypoles used to stand.

All kinds of greenery were used to celebrate this vibrant festival. Houses were decked with the fresh branches and leaves of spring. Why not revive the custom and decorate the house with garlands and wreaths or, if that seems a bit embarrassing to explain to the neighbors, make sure you have plenty of flower arrangements using masses of greenery and leaves in place of stiff carnations. You could even follow the old custom of going "a-Maying," bringing in armfuls of the freshly flowering hawthorn. However, be sure to obey the old rule that the blossoms only stay in the house for the one day. Branches of rowan can be picked too and placed over your front door as a protection. Or twist a wreath from birch twigs and give it to your beloved— a traditional gift at this time.

In the old days Beltane was also a great fire festival—like Hallowe'en. Our ancestors had a practical use for the fire: they burned magical and medicinal herbs in it and drove their livestock through the smoke to fumigate them against illness. But fire is exciting as well as purifying and, above all, Beltane is an exciting time, almost a dangerous time. People jumped through the fire—not necessarily a custom I would advise you reinstate unless you are pretty agile. If you don't have access to anywhere to enjoy a large bonfire, then light a festive fire in your grate, if you have one. Traditionally the Beltane fire was lit with a bundle containing three pieces each of nine different types of wood: birch (for fertility and the goddess); oak (for the male principle or god); rowan (for life and protection against evil); willow (to represent death); hawthorn (for purity and purification); hazel (for wisdom); applewood (for love); vine (for joy); and fir (for rebirth, the symbol of immortality). While you watch the fire burn, toast the fresh new year with a May bowl—simply place a few flowering sprigs of woodruff in a bowl and pour over a bottle of white wine and a wineglass of strawberry wine or strawberry liqueur. Mix and sweeten if necessary.

A Time for Cleansing

If you have followed the advice of April you should be well equipped to deal with much of the wild energy of May. You will have started to learn about flexibility and so are more able to bend, to withstand the powerful energy. And you will have fortified your body with tonics so that it won't fall prey to the potential imbalance of the May energy. After that, who knows what will happen? Be aware of the shift in energy this month; feel how it affects you, become aware.

This month we undertake the first real cleanse of the year. Your body should be well prepared—you have been following a good clean wholesome diet for almost two months now and have given your system a goodly tonic dose as well. Now, as the warmth of summer approaches, it is time to shed off the accumulated stodge of winter and the toxins that have built up over the years.

It's also the time to explore other forms of exercise—more creative forms that don't just stimulate the physical body but also bring emotional issues to the fore. We're beginning to ease into summer, the Season of the Emotions, so inevitably emotional topics will begin to come to prominence. May is still very much about the body, about the physical, but already we are seeing the focus shift—other people are coming into the picture. We're starting to think about relationships. Sex rears its head as naturally as the buds burst out of the trees. Our lives start to move into a more sociable phase.

Detoxing

Detoxification is a thorny subject and one which I discussed at greater length in *Supertherapies*. I am still slightly wary of all the wonder treatments and supplements that claim to detox you overnight or at least over the weekend. I think that the whole detox lark is a rich source of revenue for a great many people and as long as there is money to be made there will be a never-ending supply of amazing products and treatments to whisk away our toxins. I'm not saying they are all worthless, but I recommend you be circumspect when parting with your money.

Having said that, I do accept that we live in a rather nasty toxic world, assaulted on all sides by pollution in the air, in our homes, in the foods we eat, and the clothes we wear. We are polluting the earth with scarcely a thought; our livestock are pumped full of drugs and dunked in chemical baths; our crops are sprayed with powerful pesticides and fungicides, many of which have side effects no one is quite sure about. Some scientists predict that we will see a vast increase in neurological disorders, in cases of Alzheimers, a proliferation in the cases of cancer as a horrific by-product of all this pollution. They warn that we will find old diseases rearing their heads once more and new ones appearing as well. It can be quite terrifying. But there are things we can do.

First and foremost, we can campaign for cleaner food, cleaner air, and a better environment. Badger your congressman about environmental issues. I never understand why the environment comes so low in our political concerns. If we turn this planet into a toxic wasteland, where are we going to go? Let's try to preserve what we've got.

You can create a market for cheap organic food by demanding it and, if you can possibly afford it, buying it whenever you can. The more land that is given over to organic farming, the fewer chemicals we will have polluting the land. As more is produced, the price should come down so that everyone can enjoy clean uncontaminated food. Do the same with nontoxic paints and chemicals, by choosing environmentally friendly sources. I could go on and on but I don't want to sound like a soap-box preacher so, if you're concerned, check out the facts from groups like the Women's Environmental Network (see the back of the book for details).

To be brutal, for the time being, there really is no practical way we can avoid all these sources of pollution. So we have to find ways to protect ourselves. The key to this is a well-functioning immune system, able to ward off nasties; healthy organs to digest and get rid of toxins—in other words a body in peak health. This is something for which we can all aim (and hopefully achieve). And boosting your immune system and coaxing your body into optimum health is a way of regaining a little power, a little more control over your life in a world in which power is increasingly taken away from us.

I confess I am a wimp and whenever I have undergone a full detox program I have usually run off to somewhere especially geared to the process. It's not a particularly comfortable process—when your body starts to shell off toxins there are plenty of unpleasant side effects. I generally find I develop a screaming headache after a few days. Many other people find they become horribly constipated or unbearably smelly! The good thing about following a detox regime in an establishment is that the people around you will be doing the same thing and suffering in the same way, and the people in charge will be well used to the side effects and can offer reassurance and ways to counteract the worst of the horrors.

If you decide to detox on your own then prepare carefully. Check with your GP or natural health practitioner first and, if they give you the go-ahead, then choose your program. Be careful—for example, fasting is distinctly *not* advised if you are pregnant or breastfeeding, or if you have any medical condition, and particularly if you have any eating disorder. Always ask the advice of a qualified practitioner.

Whichever program you choose, make sure you have no pressing work or family commitments while you're detoxing. You will probably feel quite tired at first and, for the full benefits, you should be detoxing your mind as well as your body. So instead of filling your days with phones, work, and chit-chat you should, ideally, be quietly meditating or just thinking, playing gentle music, practicing yoga perhaps or just lounging around pondering your life. I find detoxing gives an interesting perspective on life—sometimes things slot into place, solutions offer themselves, surprising thoughts come into your head, interesting dreams run past you at night. Don't dismiss any of these—write them down in your journal. They may not make sense now but they might do later.

THE FASTING METHOD

One of the quickest but also the most uncomfortable way of detoxing is a fast. You ease yourself into the fast by having a day on just vegetables and salad, with fresh juice to drink. Then a day on just juice. Then you begin three days of nothing but water.

Amidst healthy skepticism there is evidence backing periodic, sensible fasting. Research has been carried out since 1880 and since then medical journals have carried occasional reports on the use of fasting for the treatment of obesity, eczema, irritable bowel syndrome, bronchial asthma, depression, and even schizophrenia, to name but a few. Most people nowadays, however, use it as preventative medicine. As medical herbalist Kitty Campion says: "Not only does it help the body to maintain peak fitness by periodically unburdening itself of accumulated waste, but, if done properly, it also nips minor health problems in the bud, decelerates the aging process, stabilizes body weight, and helps the body to utilize nutrition far more effectively." Tempting indeed.

She points out that the digestive system uses up to thirty percent of the total energy produced by the body so, by putting the system into a state of rest, the body can concentrate on detoxification and healing. On a health level, she says, fasting can improve your immune function and allow your body a decent chance to deal with its problems; on a beauty level, fasting can make your skin look fresher and more toned, your eyes brighter, and your hair more lush. And, quite obviously, you also lose weight. Six hours after the last meal, the body starts to use glycogen (the carbohydrate stored in the liver and muscles) as its energy source. But after twenty-four hours the body will adapt to obtaining most of its energy from stored fat.

However, don't think about fasting as a weight-loss option; it really isn't your safest or most effective bet if you want to lose weight. As the British Medical Association (BMA) points out, after twenty-four hours your body takes its energy not just from stored fat but also from the breakdown of muscle. If you continue fasting over several days, your metabolism will slow down to conserve energy and, if you fast for too long, the ability to digest food may be impaired or lost entirely because the stomach gradually stops secreting digestive juices. Prolonged fasting also halts the production of sex hormones and your body loses its ability to fight infection. The BMA says that short fasts are fine but that ideally you should only fast under medical supervision.

I think three days on water is fine for most healthy adults, but I wouldn't recommend long periods of fasting. After about seven days, fatty acids can be released into the blood. These are then converted into ketones which make the whole system acidic and can cause a "high." It means we are running our bodies on a different form of fuel.

After your three days, gently rejoin the world of normal eating. Whatever you do, don't plunge straight back in with egg and chips or a vast takeaway. If you can face it, have another day of just juice. Then stick to vegetables for about a week, after which you can ease back into your normal diet. You may find you don't want so much meat or dairy produce; you might not want to put alcohol or coffee into your lovely clean body. Whatever the effects, you should be feeling lighter and brighter—as if you've had a spring-clean from the inside out.

You don't have to fast in order to detox. You can achieve results just as well with less draconian means and, for many people, these modified detoxes will be much more pleasant and manageable.

FRUIT FASTING

Eating just fruit for a few days—no longer than a week—can be a pleasant way to detoxify, especially if the weather is fine and warm. Choose a selection of fruit, but avoid the citrus fruits as they are too acidic. Apples, pears, peaches, apricots, and grapes are all fine. Some people like to stick to one fruit—such as grapes—but I find it easier to have a selection. Eat when you feel hungry, but do not go above one and a half kilograms (three pounds) of fruit a day. If you like, you can juice some of it—it's up to you. Personally, I never find a glass of juice as satisfying as the solid fruit, but that's just my opinion.

THE ALKALINE VEGETABLE AND LIVER FLUSH PROGRAM

This program is loosely based on the theories of polarity therapy—a complete system that aims to balance the body's energy by bodywork, nutrition, exercise, and counseling—with quite a few other influences thrown in. It is similar to the program at Stop the World, a center in Somerset which offered retreats, detoxification breaks, and pampering holidays, where I first learned the gentle art of detoxing. I now often carry it through at home as well and find it ideal because it lets you eat quite large amounts of food and not go hungry while sloughing off the toxins. It's a kind of detox for greedy-guts. It's also a very safe way of detoxing but, again, always check with your doctor or health practitioner before starting it.

For best results follow the program for seven days. This is the plan:

• Ideally, don't follow this program while you're working. Try to make space for a quiet week in which to carry it out. Stock up on all you need for the week and try not to have to go out into the bustle of the world. Your house will hopefully still be clear after all the space clearing—make sure it's clean as well. Choose a selection of music to play which is soothing and uplifting. Try not to watch television or stimulate your system too much. If you can unplug the phone with impunity, do so.
• Allow lovely aromatherapy scents to waft through the house.

Choose oils which are uplifting and purifying—lavender is lovely, so is geranium and, if you can afford them, jasmine and neroli are divine. Avoid peppermint as it will stimulate your appetite.

• Wake up early. Ayurveda tells us to wake up before the dawn if possible. But be awake by 7 A.M. at the latest and spend a few moments just being aware of lying in bed. However tempting, don't fall back to sleep, but do some gentle stretching exercises and perform the Sun Salute (see APRIL).

• Run yourself a bath. Once the water has run, add oils to it. Naturopath and detox expert Leon Chaitow says the following have a profound effect on detoxification—choose the ones you like best: cedarwood promotes elimination through the mucous membranes; chamomile is soothing and antibacterial; juniper and lemon are both tonics and diuretics; rose is a potent antidepressant and stimulates the liver and stomach functions; tea-tree is antifungal and antiseptic. Before you get in, spend a good few minutes brushing your skin with a good bristle brush, always working toward the heart (see page 108 for more information). Now have a good soak in the warm water, imagining all the dead cells and toxins sloughing off and seeping out of your skin into the water.

• Breakfast may take some getting used to. You will be drinking Polarity therapy's famous "liver flush"—a rather pungent mixture of garlic and juice. Mix three to four tablespoons of pure cold-pressed olive or almond oil with twice the amount of fresh lemon juice. Add three to six cloves of garlic plus fresh ginger to taste. Put everything in a food processor or blender and whizz until frothy. Drink immediately. Many people don't find the taste unpleasant at all, but if you're not one of them, try to think of the benefits as you glug it down: it is said to clear the liver, the kidneys, and the intestinal tract and, when combined with a cleansing diet, to restore the chemical balance of your body. You can also have several cups of hot herbal tea made from equal amounts of licorice root, anise, or fennel, peppermint and fenugreek. Add fresh ginger, lemon juice, and honey to taste.

• Mid-morning you can drink 225 ml or more of fresh vegetable juice made from cabbage, lettuce, carrots and beetroot (in any combination). Add radish or onion if you like, plus ginger, lemon, honey, and garlic to taste.

• For lunch and dinner you can choose any variety of alkaline vegetables—either fresh in salads or steamed lightly with some ginger to spice them up. Choose from lettuce (any variety), cabbage, grated carrots, radishes, cucumber, tomato, onions, and sprouts. You may use a little dressing of almond, olive, or sesame oil with lemon, garlic, onion, and ginger. Add a piece of fresh fruit (apples, pears, grapes, melon, pomegranate, papaya) to finish.

• Mid-afternoon have another glass of vegetable juice (as mid-morning).

• For your evening meal, taken ideally around 6 p.m., choose fruit (from the lunchtime list) plus the herb tea (as for breakfast). If you are very hungry you can repeat the lunchtime salad.

• Throughout the day, spend your time quietly thinking and dreaming. Read books, but not horror stories, violent thrillers, or crime stories. Ideally you should pick gentle book with a spiritual message. On my trips to Stop the World I have read many books I would never normally have considered: *Jonathan Livingstone Seagull; The Way of the Peaceful Warrior,* and other books on self-development and mysticism.

• Practice some gentle yoga through the day. Don't choose the rigorous forms here but just some soothing gentle *asanas.*

• If you meditate you might find you can spend longer at your practice. If you don't meditate already, it could be a good time to try. Mindfulness (see WINTER) is an easy, nonspiritual kind of meditation—check it out.

• Get out into nature when you can. Just sit and listen to the sounds around you: the birds singing, the insects buzzing, the wind in the trees. Let your mind wander.

• Go to bed quite early—you'll probably be quite keen to do without all the late-night stimuli of television, going out, or elaborate suppers. Relax and dream.

At the end of the week you should be feeling pretty marvelous—calm, centered, and full of energy. When you taste "normal" food it will be utterly delicious, I promise you. Even simple dishes will seem full of flavor. I find this program gives me back my tastebuds in a quite remarkable way. But, as with all detox programs, don't shock your body by launching straight back into a full diet. Try to stick to a vegetarian regime without too many

dairy or rich foods for at least a week, and don't go straight back
into drinking alcohol and coffee.

Looking After Your Lymph

Detoxing has all kinds of benefits for the whole body, but one
part of your body which will really appreciate all this attention
is your lymphatic system. Our lymphatic system is the Cinderella
of the body. Ignored and systematically abused, we generally
leave it to its own devices. Yet an unhappy lymphatic system
spells an unhealthy body, and we neglect it at our peril. Let's be
honest, most people don't even know what the lymphatic system
does. So here's a potted guide.

A vast, bodywide network of tiny channels, the lymphatic system is primarily a giant waste-disposal system. It helps the body
to get rid of debris: dead cells, bacteria, toxins, and any foreign
waste are all pushed into the lymphatic system to be cleansed
of impurities. Without the continual removal of toxins, we would
die as surely as if we were stabbed in the heart.

Sometimes known as "white blood" the lymph fluid or lymph
is a slow, mysterious substance. While the blood races around
the body, pumped by the heart, lymph moves less dramatically
relying on the force of gravity and the contraction and relaxation
of our muscles to push it through its channels. When it reaches
its destination in the lymph nodes (primarily concentrated in the
groin, behind the knees, in the armpits, and under the chin),
white blood cells get to work to clean out the waste and attack
any dangerous bacteria. A healthy lymphatic system is virtually
synonymous with a good immune system: keeping your lymph
healthy can literally add years to your life.

The cosmetic effects are pretty impressive as well. A fully functioning, healthy lymphatic system has far-reaching effects on the
whole body. Skin appears clear and unblemished, eyes are bright
and shiny, wounds heal quickly and easily, and colds are rare
and easily combated. Even cellulite finds it hard to get a foothold
if the lymph is flowing freely.

Unfortunately modern living is working against our lymph. Increased pollution, toxic waste, and cigarette smoke put a strain on the system, and a sedentary lifestyle and bad diet only exacerbate the problem. In some cases, the lymphatic system becomes overloaded and simply can't keep up. And while mainstream doctors often ignore the lymph, complementary practitioners will often look to poor lymph circulation as a potential reason for anything from fatigue and poor eyesight to rheumatism and constipation. "Our bodies were simply not designed to put up with the amount of pollution which bombards us in this day and age," says naturopath Roberta Stimson Carr of the Kew Naturopathic Practice who specializes in lymph treatments. "Even if the lymph is not actually blocked, it is sluggish in most people nowadays."

Dee Jones is a practitioner of manual lymph drainage (MLD), a gentle but highly effective treatment which is generally held to be one of the best ways of stimulating the lymph pathways. "Clearing the lymph is vital for anyone congested by our Western diet, sedentary lifestyle, and exposure to pollutants," she says. She notices huge changes in her clients, often after just one treatment. "Puffiness disappears, sinuses clear, and colds can vanish. People also feel incredibly relaxed."

The signs of a sluggish lymph, says Dee Jones, can be quite obvious. "Any swollen or puffy areas are the first sign—swollen ankles or knees or puffy eyes all indicate that the system needs a bit of a boost," she says. Frequent colds or slow-healing wounds can also be indications, but swollen glands, perhaps surprisingly, are a good sign. "A swollen lymph node is one that is working," she explains. "It shows that your system is fighting bugs." Iridologists look to the eyes for their diagnosis. "If you have a sluggish lymph, your eyes will seem dull and almost misty," says Sheelagh Colton of the Society of Iridologists. She points out that blue-eyed people are genetically most likely to suffer with their lymph.

The picture is not, however, totally depressing. There are straightforward strategies that can really give the lymph a helping hand, and complementary and alternative health practitioners can offer expert help. With a little more awareness and some general maintenance we can keep the lymph quietly flowing on. After you have completed your detox week, try to continue supporting your lymph with these simple suggestions.

DIY WAYS TO EASE THE LOAD ON YOUR LYMPH

Swim and Rebound Exercise acts as a powerful pump for the lymph, but high-powered aerobics is not necessarily ideal. "If you overuse muscles, they create more waste rather than helping the lymph," says Dee Jones, who recommends swimming, walking, and yoga. Rebounding (bouncing up and down on a small trampoline) is also ideal because it changes the force of gravity in your body which stimulates the lymph. A rebounder doesn't have to be expensive, and it's a form of exercise you can do at any time—when you're listening to the radio, watching the television, whatever.

Carry on with Your Clean-up Diet High-fat diets slow the circulation of lymph and encourage a build-up of waste. Dairy produce and red meats are the main culprits. Continue with the healthy eating plan outlined in Spring, eating plenty of fresh fruits and vegetables. And drink loads of water (at least two liters a day).

Brush Your Skin Simple but effective, regular brushing stimulates the lymph and softens any impacted lymph mucus from the nodes. Herbalist Kitty Campion says: "Five minutes of skin brushing is the equivalent of twenty-five minutes of jogging as far as the lymphatic system goes." Use either a natural-bristle brush or a damp flannel with a bicarbonate and salt mixture and brush smoothly, always moving toward the heart.

Put Rosemary in Your Bath Aromatherapists use a variety of oils to help the lymph. Naturopath Roberta Stimson Carr uses rosemary and combines it with the benefits of cool water. "Put a couple of drops in a warm bath and relax. Then gradually add cool water until the water is quite cold—the change of temperature also stimulates the lymph," she says.

Stand on Your head All yoga positions (not just headstands!), combined with deep breathing, help the lymphatic system to keep pumping, says Swami Saradanada of the Sivananda Yoga Vedanta Center. "If you have no muscular movement, the lymph doesn't drain properly." So keep going with the Sun Salute and try to add more yoga into your life on a daily basis. If you don't have a class nearby, try one of the increasing number of home videos appearing in the shops.

Drink Herbal Infusions "Impacted lymph mucus can be

shifted slowly with herbs," says Kitty Campion, who recommends echinacea as the supreme lymph cleanser. Roberta Stimson Carr swears by fenugreek and suggests either boiling or steeping a tablespoon for around fifteen minutes. "It emulsifies fatty globules in the lymph system, the blood, and the bowel," she explains.

The Mystery of the Moor

At the beginning of this discourse on detoxing, I expressed disquiet over the endless detox products appearing in the marketplace. However, there is one product which seems, without doubt, to have some amazing, and highly detoxifying effects. The Moor system works like a total spring-clean, revitalizing and cleansing the body from both the outside and inside. Its effects can go deeper too: many people swear it can ease rheumatism and arthritis; psoriasis, eczema, and shingles; hormonal and circulatory problems. Some women even say it has cured them of infertility by alleviating inflammation in the fallopian tubes. The Moor works to beautify you too, improving hair and skin condition, promoting weight loss and giving a welcome shot of extra vitality and zest. You can drink it, you can slap it on painful joints, you can pour it in the bath. It appears in various forms: in skin cream, body lotion, mouthwash, shampoo, and hair rinse. There's even an herbal supplement that you can feed to your pets. Surprisingly, this super system does not hail from a high-tech laboratory, nor has it been invented by the wonders of modern science. It is around 30,000 years old and has been created entirely by nature. It's basically herbal sludge.

The sludge comes from the Neydharting Moor in Austria, where it is "harvested," slightly refined and then packaged. Rich in decomposed plantlife, its healing properties have been scrutinized by hundreds of scientists who agree that the sludge extracted from this area of moorland has incredible, almost miraculous, effects. Scientists believe that the remarkable properties of this Austrian moor lie in its geology. The valley in which it lies was formed by retreating glaciers over 30,000 years ago and, as the glaciers left, the valley swiftly became a lake. Flowering herbs, seeds, leaves, flowers, fruits, roots, and grasses were washed into the valley and mingled with the water. Over time the lake silted up and became moorland but, because the basin was made of non-porous rock, the moor never dried out. Over 1,000 different plant deposits are captured in the moor—over 300 are known to have medicinal value and many others are still unnamed or known to be extinct. The unique conditions have produced a substance which has the ability to penetrate directly into the skin and thence into the bloodstream, which proceeds to transport it around the whole body. Its herbal constituents strengthen, cleanse, and balance virtually every organ and every body system. It could well be nature's best preserved health and beauty secret.

Over the past twenty years there have been nine international scientific congresses on Neydharting which have investigated exactly how the Moor works. Scientists have concluded that it has both anti-inflammatory and astringent properties, it absorbs body wastes and balances the hormones. It appears to work holistically, treating the whole body rather than simply pinpointing areas of disease. Although in the UK it is not exactly a household name, in Austria, Germany, and Switzerland the Moor is as well-known as aspirin. The clinic in Neydharting is booked solidly two years ahead and the products are used in hospitals and dispensed by GPs.

The Moor's healing powers are legendary—stretching back into the mists of time. Archeologists have discovered remains of Celtic and Roman spas at the Moor and the sixteenth-century physician Paracelsus believed that the Moor was the very elixir of life itself. Napoleon and Josephine took the Moor cure, and even Hitler saw its value, believing that the healing and rejuvenating properties of the Moor would help keep his "master race" in ultimate health and beauty.

I first came across the Moor at Tyringham, a naturopathic clinic in Buckinghamshire where they give Moor baths to strengthen the immune system, to flush out toxins, to alleviate skin problems, and to promote relaxation. Moor may be good for you but it isn't exactly aesthetic—the bath looked as though it were full of filthy dirty water. Nonetheless I stayed and soaked for about half an hour and then gently toweled myself dry, allowing as much of the Moor as possible to stay on my skin. It was five o'clock in the afternoon and, feeling a little weary, I lay down on my bed for a short nap. I was stunned when I woke up feeling rested and particularly radiant—at eight o'clock the next morning! A pitifully light sleeper, I usually clock in a paltry six hours of interrupted sleep.

Although naturopaths have used Moor for decades, it's not surprising that the products never quite made it on to the bathroom shelf. Its image was distinctly utilitarian and vastly unglamorous—about as sexy as a pot of Vaseline. But all that's changing and now Moor is being taken up by top-class beauticians.

Kiti Hitches is one such convert. A qualified beautician and aromatherapist, she has worked for some of the largest names in cosmetics. But for the past fourteen years she has been using solely Moor products and now trains other therapists in their use. Her utter trust in the Moor comes from personal experience. "It did such miraculous things for me, I was amazed," she says. "I was a bit of a mess really: firstly I was going through a very early menopause at thirty-eight and HRT didn't suit me. I had irritable bowel syndrome and terrible candida. To cap it all, my daughter's horse had trodden on my toe and I had been told the toe was dead and would have to be amputated." Then she stumbled across the Moor and started taking the herbal drink. "It cleared up everything," she says, "even my hormones."

Hitches is now in her fifties but her clear skin and trim figure are those of a woman twenty years younger. "I love it because it is a total complementary healthcare system: it beautifies you, gives you vitality, and sorts out your inner self as well. The Moor detoxifies, strengthens, and heals the whole body. It can balance your endocrine system, the colon, the liver, and kidneys: it totally harmonizes you."

When she treats people, Hitches spends some time working out what a client needs before suggesting a program of treatment. This could include compresses or poultices, massage or facials. She has experimented with novel uses for the various oils and unguents and now offers a bust treatment which she promises "really does give you a lift." Her facials are said to rejuvenate the skin and when she plasters Moor mud on the buttocks and thighs she swears it will help reduce cellulite. A regular dose of the herbal drink will, she says, often take away cravings because it will help balance your blood sugar levels. Hence the weight-loss claims.

Kiti decided my face and feet needed the Moor treatment and she invited me to slip off my sweater and socks and lie on the couch. The facial was lovely: gentle massaging with the light Moor oil followed by a thin coating of lotion and then the Moor mask itself. Despite having been sitting at room temperature for a good hour, the mask was icy cold to the skin. "It always is," says Kiti, "even on the hottest day." While the mask sat on my face, hopefully doing its level best to detoxify, strengthen, and tighten my skin, Kiti moved to my feet which she softly massaged with the oil. I was in seventh heaven: whether it does anything or not for your health and beauty, it's well worth it for the sybaritic experience alone.

After the treatment my face felt very smooth but quite taut. Kiti puts this down to the product's toning properties. "It stimulates cell production and brings new blood into the skin," she says. "It really does give you a face-lift." I found the tautness slightly unpleasant, however, but an extra dose of moisturizer swiftly softened the effect. As I looked in the mirror I had to admit my skin was looking pretty good—clear and glowing, which is unusual for me, as a facial usually leaves me looking like a blotchy adolescent. The downside is that salon treatments with Moor are pretty expensive. However, Kiti points out that once you know how to use the products you can do it all yourself at home. Salons and health shops around the country are starting to stock the products and there is a mail order service available as well.

Initially I was a little skeptical about the large range of products on offer. Surely all the body unguents, foot soaks, hair tonics, and so on are simply cashing in on the Moor's healthful reputation? And the herbal supplement for animals seemed totally over the top. However, after a fortnight of using the moisturizer and body lotion my skin did feel much softer and smoother. And the pet supplement definitely gave my cat and puppy shinier coats and alarming amounts of energy. Most noticeable of all, they appear to have ceased their perpetual hostilities and are now tolerating each other in an almost benign fashion. It's probably coincidence, but if it *is* down to the Moor, then that really is a minor miracle.

Manual Lymph Drainage

Manual lymph drainage (or MLD to give it its more user-friendly acronym) is one of the therapies I find myself recommending over and over again. The reasons are simple: it's highly effective and also totally delicious. Not only is it fantastic for your lymphatic system and quite incredible if you suffer from any kind of edema or puffiness, but it can also help to clear away scar tissue and even help rid you of the dreaded cellulite! Yet, although it has been around since the 1930s, up to a few years ago hardly anyone had heard of MLD.

Dr. Emil Vodder and his wife, Estrid, first developed MLD in France in the 1930s. Vodder noticed how people suffering from chronic catarrhal and sinus infections tended to have swollen lymph glands and, much against medical practice at the time, he started to work with the lymph nodes. The massage he developed had a circular, pumping effect which increases the movement of the lymphatic system of the body. Medical tests have since proven his conviction that when you increase the flow in the lymphatic system, infection is dealt with more effectively.

It's nothing like a normal massage. There is no pounding of muscles, no probing and pulling; an MLD massage feels like having your skin softly stroked by a child's gentle fingers. It's a light, repetitive movement that has an almost hypnotic effect. After my first massage I felt as if I were floating in a deep blue lagoon and I have never been so relaxed. The relaxation comes about because the massage affects the nervous system, instigating a change from the normal stressed "daytime" state of the nervous system to the "nighttime" state we use when we're asleep.

Almost everyone can benefit from MLD because, basically, we all live in a polluted world and we are all laden down with toxins. MLD gives the lymph a helping hand to battle back. MLD practitioner Dee Jones explains: "When your lymph is working well you will not only feel better but you will look better too, as the lymph is the one thing that can absolutely, thoroughly cleanse your system. There are microscopic lymph collectors throughout the body and they pull the debris from both the outside and the inside of your body. Lymph is your body's garbage bin and lymph drainage will clear it all out."

At the very least, MLD will increase your resistance to colds and flu, will firm and improve the look of your skin, and brighten and clear your eyes. Colds disappear in hours or days rather than dragging on for weeks, and sinuses drain as if by magic. Even the medical establishment is beginning to take MLD very seriously. If the massage is given to burn victims soon after the accident, it can rapidly bring the burn down. Scar tissue can be encouraged to build up only where needed, getting rid of unsightly large scars. And now the therapy is even being used following cancer treatment, to reduce the swelling that often occurs. "We have to be very careful with cancer," warns Dee Jones. "We cannot touch live, active cancer with a fifty-foot pole. There are two schools of thought at the moment: one is that MLD could spread the cancer and the other is that MLD could strengthen the immune system and possibly help to cure the cancer. Obviously there aren't many people willing to test the theories, but some doctors are now beginning to think about the second scenario."

More and more people, however, are now visiting MLD therapists for less serious problems. It is an unlikely beauty treatment but one which certainly has longer-lasting effects than a face pack. "Its effects on the skin are pretty spectacular," says Jones. "It draws the skin in and tightens it. When you get the garbage out of the body it gives the skin a chance to regenerate. It won't make you thinner as such but it will certainly make your face *look* thinner. It tightens up all the little saggy baggy bits, all the puffiness. To a degree it's like a face-lift without surgery."

Stretch marks *will* disappear, she promises, but it takes hard work. "If someone came to me after seventeen babies, I'd work on them but I'd also get them to work on themselves at least twenty minutes a day for about six months." And it's the same story with acne and that scourge of modern life—cellulite. MLD *will* help but you have to help yourself. That means learning the technique and clearing your lymph for yourself on a daily basis as well as following a diet program and keeping up a regime of regular swimming. "It's not an instant cure, it takes time and commitment. You have to free the fat and the water that is trapped by proteins, but it will clear."

Jones points out, however, that there is no point in bailing out a boat if you don't plug the leak. Draining your lymph can have miraculous effects, but it can only truly be effective in the long term if you are prepared to make changes in your life. Like most holistic therapists, she will ask you a battery of questions about your whole lifestyle and attitude to life and will make suggestions on how to keep your newly cleansed system in a detoxified manner. As with any system aimed at long-term change, you need regular treatment. "Generally speaking we talk in terms of courses," she says. "A one-off is pleasant and is great for stress; it will make a difference to puffy eyes immediately. If you have a blocked nose you'll notice a swift change as well. But if you want to build up your immune system I would advise treatment three times a week for the first two weeks and then tail off after that. I now only see a lot of my clients every two to three months or if they have a particular problem."

Regrettably, there are some people who are not advised to attempt MLD. Anyone who has suffered from TB needs to avoid it as there is a possibility that TB molecules stored in the lymphatic system could be reawakened. And anyone with heart problems (particularly cardiac edema) is also advised against the treatment.

Living with the Dance

May isn't just about detoxing and purifying. It's not all serious worthy cleansing. May is a fun month, a lively month and, once you're all detoxed, you should be ready to spring into action. One of the most potent symbols for May is the phallic maypole, and the activity that weaves around it is dancing. If the idea of dancing fills you with horror, please don't turn the page just yet. I have a confession: it feels the same way to me. Some people love it, some find it embarrassing. I always fell somewhere in the middle, enjoying a good dance only if I had a fair amount of alcoholic Dutch courage inside me.

As a physical exercise, dancing is wonderful for your body. Don't just think about ballet or ballroom; you could try the rigorous forms of country and square-dancing, the exotic delights of belly-dancing (wonderful for those abdominal muscles), or the clever routines of tap. Some dances are wild and passionate; try any Latin or South American dance classes; some are quiet and meditative—look into the serene circle dancing.

Yet there is more to dancing than pure physical exercise. A good dance can directly engage your emotions and put you in touch with your deepest feelings, your most hidden thoughts. Now, there are forms of dance available that directly seek to tap into this hidden power of dance. They can be quite confrontational and certainly won't be for everyone, but they *are* interesting. Try a session and see what you think.

LIFE DANCE: RIDING THE WAVE

Gabrielle Roth has a twofold mission in life: to create a world of dancers and to give us all a taste of ecstasy. This unorthodox American has designed a system she calls Life Dance, which apparently has quite remarkable qualities: dance the Roth way and you could not only release stress and free the emotions, but you might also give your sex life a boost. And, if that isn't enough, she promises that her dance might even turn you into a true life genius. Most of all, it will show you how to access sheer joy purely through the power of your own body. This, she promises, is "soul" dancing in the truest sense of the word.

Anyone, insists Roth, can dance. "It works for construction workers as well as barristers; for rock stars and the most ordinary person in the street. We are all stressed and there is no exception," she states baldly. She has been teaching Life Dance for close on thirty years since a skiing accident cut short her own career as a dancer. Finding life unbearable without the freedom that uninhibited movement gave her, she looked for a way to make dance accessible for absolutely everyone—dancer or non-dancer, physically able or physically restricted.

The lynchpin of her work is what Roth calls "the wave"—a cycle of five different ways of dancing based on five basic rhythms. She believes that these five rhythms map out the whole human psyche and that by dancing our way through "the wave" we can experience the full extent of our natures. This means not just accessing hidden sources of vitality, creativity, and joy, but also releasing more negative emotions such as grief, anger, frustration, and hate. Her role, she says, is that of an urban shaman,

someone who can move you into a different state of consciousness and alter your perception of life. The aim is to drop the
conventions and strictures of the everyday grind and simply let
go, allowing a release of those emotions that are normally held
in check by our efforts to be polite and "nice." The five rhythms,
she says, are ancient and fundamental; they help us remember
who we really are.

"I don't teach movement," insists Roth, a tall, thin, angular
woman with spiky black hair and spiky black clothes who looks
much younger than her fifty-two years, "because movement can't
be taught. There are no steps, no right or wrong ways to do this.
You simply have to listen to your body, experiment, explore,
and play with space."

Thousands of people hang on her every word. Although there
are several accredited teachers of Roth's work in the UK, devotees
still flock from all around the country to work with the high
priestess of the dance herself. At the workshop I attended there
were several hundred people and, although the evening was
billed as an introduction to Life Dance, ninety percent of the
participants were evidently familiar with "the wave" and most of
them seemed to know each other.

"It's like one big family," gushed one woman who had trekked
down to London from Yorkshire. "We all meet up at workshops."
The minority of newcomers were painfully obvious, huddled
around the edges of the hall while the rest hugged, kissed, and
twirled around while waiting for Roth to begin.

"Begin" is probably the wrong word: quite where her workshops begin and end can be quite bewildering for a novice.
There is no order and very little structure: most of the time you
are left trying to follow your neighbors and I frequently felt con-
fused and slightly irritated by the assumption that we all knew
what we were doing. Roth herself is almost alarming in her inten-
sity: her "teaching" sounds more like a stream of consciousness,
a wild form of poetry, disconcertingly laced with frequent exple-
tives. She paces around, conducting her manic monologue and
then the drums begin to beat and she urges everyone on their
feet for the first rhythm. "This is flowing, fluid, and feminine,"
she instructs. "It is very old and ancient. Relax your face, your
jaw, and go for a very deep breath. Get a dialogue going between
your body parts, get your hands talking to your feet, your elbows

to your knees." Everyone starts to dance, smoothly, softly, volup-
tuously. For a while you are allowed to dance on your own and
then Roth instructs you to find a partner and dance with them,
keeping close eye contact all the time. Some people are naturals,
fluid and sensuous; others are reassuringly flat-footed. One of
the most graceful of all is a woman twirling in a wheelchair with
a beatific smile on her face.

A short pause and then we're back on our feet for the second
rhythm. This is staccato, with a heavier tempo. Roth calls it masculine and aggressive, sharp and spiky, and urges us to accompany it with strong, panted breathing. As the beat gets gradually
faster, people leap around the room, roll on the floor, utter
strange sharp cries. There is clearly some serious cathartic releasing occurring. Movement three launches the room into sheer
chaos—half the participants sit down to allow the others more
room to throw themselves into their own private chaotic worlds.
Then follows the lyrical stage during which we are urged to be
"light as feathers" flitting around the room like fairies at the
school play. Finally, the evening ends with stillness. "Movement
is a way of stopping," says Roth, urging us to find the spaces in
the room, to investigate equally our own empty space.

The five rhythms, says Roth, will free your whole body—your
heart, your blood, your muscles, your sinews. The suggestion is
that by moving your body in these five different ways you can
reprogram your neural pathways, releasing old pent-up emotions
and easing your body into a new, more comfortable way of
being. And once you alter your body, your mind will follow. "If
you live in a body that has never expressed its fear, its anger,
its sadness, then there is no way it can have joy," she opines.
"It is essential that these emotions are released in a positive,
empowering way. It doesn't take ten or fifteen years and it
doesn't take understanding. It takes dance, it takes sweat, it takes
movement." The knock-on effect of all this release is that your
relationships will improve and your creativity will rise. "The goal
is to become a genius," she insists, "to become something
unique. Don't be a McDonalds, be a specialty burger."

It's a tall order but, Roth insists, quite possible if you continue
practicing the dance on a regular basis. As you work through old
emotions you will have the choice to keep the parts of your life
that work and jettison those that don't. On a purely physical

level, Roth is quite certain that the combination of movements has the power to relieve headaches and all the aches and pains caused by modern stress and tension. And, yes, she really does promise that it can improve your sex life. "The rhythms are in a similar sequence to those encountered during sex," she says, "and this helps to enhance your rhythmical sex pattern."

The three-hour workshop left me hot, sweaty, and seriously out of breath. If nothing else, Life Dance is certainly effective as an aerobic exercise and I definitely felt I had stretched and worked every muscle of my body. Grudgingly I will admit that at certain points I felt a touch of the liberation that die-hard fans enthuse about. But then I used to feel the same buzz dancing in a nightclub. Personally I would have appreciated a less daunting approach, a little more explanation, a little less assumption that we all knew how to dance in this liberated fashion. However, the vast majority of my fellow dancers would disagree. As the evening drew to a close Roth giggled quietly: "That was the warm-up," she joked. "Who's ready to go dancing?" The whole room called out for more.

BIODANZA

I must confess I found Biodanza slightly more user-friendly. Groups tend to be smaller and usually begin with everyone introducing themselves. There is also more explanation, which helps beginners. But don't for a minute think this is an easier option than Life Dance. Like Life Dance, Biodanza claims almost miraculous effects—more boosting of creativity, more freedom of expression and, yes, better sex too. It also leaves you with boundless energy. Its fans claim it can take away stress and improve your sleep; it can liberate your creative impulses and even help you replace no-hope relationships with ones that nurture you. After a year of Biodanza, its growing band of aficionados swear, your life will be totally different.

Biodanza is tricky to categorize: it's much more than a dance form but, technically, it's not a therapy, and its practitioners certainly don't like to tout it as a cure. Its creator, Chilean psychologist and anthropologist Rolando Toro, came up with the idea for Biodanza back in 1960. He recognized that tribal societies have always used dance as a way to express deep feelings and to connect both to one another and to society as a whole. However, Western society has gradually, over the centuries, formalized dance to the point where almost all individual expression has vanished. Look into any nightclub and you will quickly see that even the most modern forms of dancing have accepted moves, fashions, and conventions. Toro felt, however, that by dancing in a manner true to our essential "inner" self, we could literally dance ourselves back to wholeness, coming to accept our bodies and learning to feel more comfortable with our fellow human beings and society. Working initially with mentally disturbed patients, he found that certain kinds of music would evoke certain kinds of movements which would, in turn, bring about quite pronounced physiological and emotional changes. Some stimulated the sympathetic nervous system, others the parasympathetic nervous system.

After prolonged observation and study he came to believe that each of us has within us five different modes of living: Vitality (feeling energy, facing the world); Affectivity (feelings of love, tenderness and respect; giving and receiving love from other people); Sexuality (deriving pleasure from our sensuality); Creativity (bringing creative aspects into everyday life); and Transcendence (going beyond ego to find something powerful outside ourselves). Our problems arise, he hypothesized, because we learn to stifle or block out some or all of these living experiences and so fall out of our natural balance. The idea behind Biodanza is to try to bring the whole person back into a childlike sense of wholeness by stimulating underdeveloped areas and bringing all five into balance.

Now well-established in the USA, South America, Switzerland, Italy, and France, the dance is used not just for general well-being but as a specific therapeutic tool in the rehabilitation of people with eating disorders, with the mentally disadvantaged, for children with autism or Down's syndrome, for people suffering from asthma, cardiovascular problems, Parkinson's disease, osteoporosis and gastrointestinal disorders. The very young, the very old, pregnant women—everyone can benefit from Biodanza.

There's absolutely no need to be a good dancer. In this dance class, there is no correct way of doing exercises, the whole point is to find your own dance. As Rolando Toro puts it, "Our proposal is to dance to our own life, to retrieve the condition of being the owners of our body, our emotions, as a whole, a unit." The workshop I joined in London comprised a completely mixed bag of around thirty people: some obviously fancied themselves as potential Dirty Dancers, others clearly belonged to the "shuffle round your handbag" brigade. But at the end of three long, hot, sweaty hours, the funny thing was that I no longer noticed the difference.

Biodanza is only in its fourth year in the UK and, as yet, there are few teachers, mainly because it takes at least three years to master the 2,000 odd exercises and their precise effects. Most UK workshops are taught by Patricia Martello, president of the Argentinean Center for Biodanza. Martello is a tiny intense woman with flowing dark hair and incredible energy. Having asked us all to introduce ourselves, she invited us to join hands in a large circle. As we lightly tripped around the room, we were instructed to be aware of our movements and aware of other people in the group. Eye contact, she insisted, was very important.

Exercises ranged from the simple, marching round the room feeling confident and full of self-esteem, to the complex, discovering our own individual dance within which to express our creativity. Some dancing is done solo, sometimes you are asked to pair up, and sometimes the whole group dances together. Throughout the whole class there is no talking, except by Martello as she explains how to do the exercise. Personally, I found it a mixed experience. I discovered I had hidden depths of energy, and surprising amounts of anger exploded as I did "my" dance. But I did find some of the exercises a bit confrontational, a little too much close body and eye contact for my comfort. However, that, I'm sure, only goes to show how unbalanced and repressed I am. Maybe after a whole course of Biodanza I'd be as relaxed in my body and as peaceful in my mind as the old hands appeared to be. As one woman explained afterward, "Biodanza has given me the freedom to like who I am, the permission to enjoy being in my body and the ability to interact with people with true friendliness and innocent joy." Not bad for a dance class.

HOME DANCE CLASS

In Biodanza every exercise and its accompanying music is carefully planned to have a precise physiological effect. However, you can try the following exercises to experience a taste of Bio-danza in your own home.

1. Walk around the room, or garden, and try to feel connected with your body. Feel your feet connecting firmly with the ground, let your arms swing naturally, and keep your head up high. Gradually let the movement become more fluid, more vital, more exuberant.
2. Put on music with a strong but fluid melody. Dance in any way you choose, but keep aware of your chest and heart area, and dance "into" that area.
3. Change the music for something with a solid, firm rhythm. Dance again, but this time let your movements be governed by your pelvic region.
4. Keep with rhythmic music and play with finding your "own" dance. Forget notions of what dancing *should* look like; don't worry about proper steps or movements. Allow the music to dance you—you might end up jumping in the air, or rolling on the floor: it doesn't matter.
5. Again, pick some music with a firm beat and practice "giving" your dance to someone else. If you are trying these exercises with a friend, one of you should sit on the floor and "receive" the dance while you dance for her/him. If you are doing this alone, imagine you are dancing for someone special and pretend they are sitting in front of you. Again, let the music guide you in your movements and concentrate on really giving the other person what they need. Maintain eye contact all the way through the exercise. Then swap over and receive their dance.

SUMMER

The Season of the Emotions

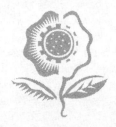

KEY FOCUS
Freeing your emotions.

SECONDARY FOCUS
Learning to listen to your body.

TASKS
Investigate bodywork; improve your posture; regain a healthy relationship with food; boost your self-esteem.

QUESTIONS
What am I hiding from myself? What emotions do I not express in my life? Am I honest in my relationships with others?

CHALLENGES
Rediscover the joy of playing; become passionate; enjoy the natural world; indulge your senses.

FESTIVALS AND CELEBRATIONS
Summer solstice, Lammas.

Summer is sun-time, fun-time, a time for holidays and breaks, for relaxation and play. It's the great season of the outdoors when, in the words of the well-known song, "the living is easy." For our ancestors, summer was a time of relief and relative ease. They no longer had to battle against the cold and damp; instead they were able to spend the long days out in the clear open air. Of course, summer was a time of hard work too: crops were growing and ripening, but so were the weeds that strangled them and the insects that ate them. So there was plenty of work. But it was joyous work, warmed and softened by the regenerative sun.

The Season of Fire and the Evil Heat

Summer is expansive, full, generous. In the Chinese system, summer sees a maturation of the aggressive thrusting energy of spring. The wood energy has burned into the "full *yang*" of fire. Summer is the most obviously energetic phase of the whole yearly cycle; the full heat of the *yang* energy grows and spreads, thanks to the sustaining glow of fire energy. Fire is quite naturally connected to the heart, whose constant pumping keeps blood moving around the body. And, as every ancient system in the world teaches, the heart is the seat of our emotions. It affects all our emotions but primarily those connected with love and joy, compassion and generosity, openness, warmth, and abundance. In the Indian *chakra* system, if your heart center is open, you will usually enjoy all these positive emotions. If it is blocked, on the other hand, the results can be hypertension, hysteria, nervous disorders, and problems with the heart and circulation.

The "evil" of summer is, quite naturally, that of heat—or overheating. We all know the ill effects of too much heat, overexposure to the sun. And obviously the major challenge when the heat rises is to, in all ways, "keep cool." Naturally enough, the color of summer is hot glowing red, the color of fire and blood.

The Native Americans agree. They, too, see summer as the season of the heart, of the emotions, and perceive its color as red. They talk about summer as the season when we should widen our perceptions, become more aware of our feelings, understanding how we give ourselves and how we express love. So this is a natural time to start to look at the whole emotional aspect of our lives. However, that doesn't mean that we can forget about our bodies and one of the quickest ways to rediscover lost or suppressed emotions is through the body. More of that later. For now, there are just a few practical points to recap.

Exercise Revisited

Hopefully now you will be noticing the benefits of regular exercise. You should be feeling fitter, firmer, and with any luck actually looking forward to your exertions. If you *don't* enjoy what you're doing, then maybe you still haven't found the ideal exercise for you. Anything new is difficult for a while, but if you've been sticking to your program, by now it should be easier (though still challenging) and hence much more fun. If not, change your routine. Go back to the guidelines in the SPRING section and think about your choice. Is there anything else you could do? Anything you have always fancied having a go at? Try it—what is there to lose?

Take advantage of the summer and the clement weather. Even if you're quite happy with your routine, try incorporating some forms of exercise that get you out into the open (though don't forget the sunscreen). Swimming obviously comes to mind but there are plenty of other ways to get into the watery element—water polo or volleyball; canoeing; synchronized swimming (don't laugh, it's a tough discipline—great if you like the water and gymnastics); rafting; rowing; scuba-diving. Then there's hiking and hill-walking; tennis; horseback riding; cycling; the list is endless.

Watch the Sun

Enjoy the sun but be very respectful. In recent years we have become more aware of the dangers of overexposure, and yet still we see people walking around looking like lobsters, with bright red skin blistering and flaking from the heat. Overheating yourself in summer can lead to problems in autumn, as I'll explain in a minute, but, even leaving that aside, you need to take care in the sun for the sake of your skin. Skin cancer is a real and growing problem of which everyone needs to be aware. Your best protection is to keep out of the direct heat of the sun. Wear light but protective clothes, a large sunhat or baseball cap, and plenty of sunblock on any exposed bits. If you wear sunglasses, make sure they are a good quality pair with lenses that filter out both UVA and UVB rays. If you're sitting outside, pop yourself under a parasol. If you're playing sports or gardening, make sure your sunscreen is topped up and that you cover as much of your body as is feasibly possible. Wear a baseball cap to shield your face and choose longer-line shorts and tops.

So you won't get an overall tan? So what? Either stick to pale and interesting or buy your tan in a tube—fake tanning creams no longer smell disgusting or leave dirty stains around your knees so, if you like to look bronzed, slap them on. Not only will you protect your health, but your skin will also look much better for it. Look at anyone who spent their formative years sunbathing and you'll be looking at a field of wrinkles. The sun may tint you golden but over the years it is not a friend to your skin, it toughens it and ages it.

Shifting Your Diet into Summer

As you approach summer you need to adapt your diet in order to be able to deal with the hot weather ahead. The Chinese, Indian, and Tibetan systems all agree that this is the time to introduce lighter, cooler foods into your diet, gently shifting your body into the energy of summer while trying to dodge the damage the evil heat could cause. So avoid the mucus-forming foods as far as possible—this is not the season for hearty meat stews or slabs of cheese on thick wedges of bread. Nor should you be overdosing your system with salty or fatty foods. These are bad news at any time of year, but your body will find them particularly difficult to deal with in summer, so cut out the crisps and chips. This is not the time for stodgy comfort food. You need to be thinking about bowls of fresh salads with light interesting dressings (if your constitution does not take cold foods well try warm salads—still light and refreshing); of fresh fish or chicken marinated in light spices and grilled in the open air on a barbecue; of jewel-bright vegetables kebabed next to the meat; of fragrant paella and risottos; of fresh fruit salads and wobbling jellies (homemade ones without all the artificial additives, and stuffed with fresh summer fruits). It's a time to enjoy long glasses of freshly squeezed fruit and vegetable juices.

Now more than ever you should be trying to cut down on your tea and coffee consumption—it's easier at this time of year as you don't need the physical warmth so much. Try cutting out a few more cups and substituting herbal teas—fresh fruity ones are lovely around now and so is mint tea served cool. Simply grab a handful of mint leaves from the garden, wash, and pour boiling water over. Leave to steep for around fifteen minutes then strain and cool. It's lovely and refreshing. Lemon balm is equally refreshing and equally easy to grow. Remember also that you need to keep well hydrated. Often when we fancy a cup of tea or coffee it's because our bodies are actually crying out for water. Keep a bottle of fresh mineral water or filtered water on your desk or in the kitchen and drink at least a liter (preferably two) a day.

A word on icy foods and drinks. In summer when the heat is on, the most natural thing in the world is to shovel ice out of the freezer and transform everything into a chilled or frozen cooler. Unfortunately, ice-cold food and drink is far from ideal for your body. Very cold food shocks the body and can result in throat problems. It also slows or stops the digestion. Ayurvedic practitioners will always ask you not to drink cold water during or after a meal as it will halt your digestion in its tracks. If you like to drink water with your food, leave it out of the fridge to take the freezing edge off it. The key word is *cool*, not cold. I'm not saying don't ever eat ice cream—summer wouldn't be summer without ice cream and sorbets. But if you want a good digestion, eat your sundae or cornet between meals, not directly after. And don't live on the stuff! Most commercial ice cream is stuffed full of additives and preservatives while the more expensive "pure" and natural ice creams are stuffed full of natural cream and natural sugar (not everything natural is good for you)—so you can't really win! A little as a treat is the best option.

Summer is also not a good time to overdose on alcohol. Another tough one, I know, because, think of summer and I (for one) immediately imagine enticing jugs of Pimms, of long gin and tonics, of fragrant white wine and long cool ciders to slake the thirst. However, overdo the alcohol and you will undoubtedly suffer. The combination of alcohol and sun is not a felicitous one. Your hangover will be far worse and you might end up with sunstroke to boot. Also, overindulgence now will set you up for a miserable autumn. What we do in one season will affect our health in the next, and the clear-cut way to autumn ailments is to overdose on the joys of summer. Kate Roddick, who is one of the few Western practitioners of Tibetan medicine, says that most people who complain in autumn of headaches and biliousness have only themselves to blame—for their lifestyle in the hot weather of summer.

Tibetan medicine is not well-known in this country, but it is an equally fascinating, venerable, and effective system of medicine. Like Ayurveda and TCM, it teaches that we should adapt our diet and our behavior to the season, taking particular care when the seasons are about to change. Follow their precise guidelines according to the weather and your own individual constitution and you will enjoy permanent good health and vitality.

In case you have the luck to live near a reputable Tibetan physician (there are several in Scotland), I will briefly summarize the system. Kate Roddick also runs workshops and holidays to introduce people to the Tibetan way of life with a distinct emphasis on seasonal health. They are well worth attending if you would like to learn more.

Tibetan Medicine: A Brief Introduction

Tibetan medicine is very ancient and very venerable. It also appears to work startlingly well. Reports have suggested that Tibetan physicians have cured "incurable" diseases, and many desperate people have flown thousands of miles to ask their opinions and to take their unique herbal preparations known as "precious pills." But the Tibetan tradition of healing has always remained rather arcane and unapproachable simply because few Westerners had the basic tools (a working knowledge of modern and ancient Tibetan) to learn the system or the patience to complete the training (it takes at least ten years).

Kate Roddick explains that the Tibetans classify all of life into five energies which combine to create three "humors"—air, bile, and phlegm. Air controls breathing, speech and muscular activity, the nervous system, thought processes, and your emotional attitude. Bile governs heat in the body, the liver, and the digestive tract, while phlegm controls the amount of mucus in the body and also regulates the immune system. When all the humors are in balance within your body, you will enjoy perfect health. When one or more becomes aggravated or sluggish, problems will occur. The system is very similar to that of Ayurveda and TCM, with which it shares many concepts.

Put like this it all sounds simple, but Tibetan healing is so precise and so complex that it can be mind-boggling; Kate points out that it takes a very experienced physician to bring about the kind of "miracle" cures that occur. However, she is convinced that with just a little knowledge, we could all make ourselves healthier. "Diet is very important," she says. "Sometimes food is the only medicine required to obtain the necessary balance." Her workshops teach people how to work out which humor dominates them and how to soothe any imbalances. "It is people with dominant bile who will suffer most from the heat of summer," she explains, "because they are so prone to overheating." The nightmare situation is for a bile person to be sitting in the sun all day, drinking alcohol, and eating hot, spicy food. "They need cool light food at this time of year," she says, "and to stay in cool shadowy places."

However, Kate points out that the predominant humor in the Western world is actually not fire but air, or wind. "Too much air causes stress which is the common Western condition," she states. Careful questioning and pulse-taking guide Kate toward a clear idea of which humors are out of balance. In addition, the Tibetans use urine diagnosis for precise information on the person. All three conspired to tell Kate that, like many stressed-out Westerners, I had too much air and that, in fact, my system needed gentle heating rather than cooling. Treatment consisted of a wonderful massage using heating oils such as ginger and cardamom, focusing on freeing energy blockages via acupressure points. Then she advised me on diet, suggesting that I heat my sluggish digestion with light but spicy foods and avoiding mucus-forming foods such as dairy produce. I know from experience that the advice was spot-on: in the past when I have eaten to these guidelines I have both lost weight and found myself bouncing with energy. And sure enough, within a couple of days, my digestion was much better and I wasn't screaming at the dog so much.

Kate's hope is that by making Tibetan medicine approachable and understandable, we can all learn how to practice true preventative health care. Simple changes in diet and lifestyle could nip problems in the bud and save us untold misery and suffering. A little Tibetan wisdom a day could keep the doctor away.

WHAT'S YOUR TIBETAN TYPE?

Most people are a combination of types, but the following should give you a rough idea of which humor is dominating you at present.

Air Air causes stress. You might sweat very little and could suffer from insomnia, constipation, back pain, dry skin, and stomach disorders. Your mind might flit from subject to subject. Symptoms include restlessness, dizziness, shivering, sighing, pain in hips and shoulder blades, humming in ears. Air corresponds to the *vata dosha* in Ayurveda.

Diagnosis A clear sign of unbalanced air is watery, almost transparent, urine.

Diet to Balance Paradoxically, you probably need to avoid cold foods such as salads and ice cream, or make sure you have a hot drink beforehand (e.g., ginger tea) or a bowl of warming soup. Base your diet around chicken, onions, carrots, garlic and spices, spinach, and greens.

Bile Bile people often sweat quite a lot. They are precise, analytical people with good mental powers, but can be a little antisocial. They often wake up feeling bright and cheerful, but by midday are feeling irritable. Their weak spot is their liver and they can easily overheat. When bile is out of balance you could feel thirsty, have a bitter taste in your mouth, pains in the upper body, feel feverish, and have diarrhea or vomiting. Bile is governed by fire and so corresponds to the *pitta dosha* in Ayurveda.

Diagnosis Imbalanced bile can be diagnosed if your urine is yellow or brownish in color.

Diet to Balance Choose cool light foods like salads and yogurt, and drink plenty of cool (not ice cold) water. Avoid hot spicy foods, nuts, alcohol, and red meat.

Phlegm The phlegmatic person is generally heavy; they have even, stable and (sometimes) stubborn personalities, and avoid rows. They are prone to oversleeping and like an afternoon siesta. Their problems tend to be bronchial or in the kidneys. If phlegm is out of balance you could feel lethargic and heavy; have frequent indigestion or belching; distention of the stomach, and a feeling of coldness in the feet. You might put on weight or find it hard to lose weight. Obviously phlegm corresponds to the heavy *kapha* of Ayurveda.

Diagnosis Disordered phlegm shows in very pale, foaming urine.

Diet to Balance Keep the digestion warm with spices like ginger, cardamom, nutmeg. Fennel and peppermint will help the digestion too. Avoid dairy produce as it is mucus-forming, and don't eat too much fruit if you are trying to lose weight.

TIBETAN TIPS FOR COMMON HEALTH PROBLEMS

Tibetan lore is full of small interesting tips for health. The following are a brief selection—not necessarily linked to summer, but interesting and worth trying nonetheless.

For insomnia Put two or three drops of ginger essential oil in a base oil (almond is nice and light) and rub into the soles of the feet before bedtime. Children will fall asleep if you massage the sides of their feet.

For chesty/phlegmatic conditions Fill a bowl with hot water and add a few drops of ginger oil. Sit with your feet in it until the water is no longer hot, then massage your feet.

To combat stress and put digestion back into balance Massage the soles of your feet in a circular motion.

For constipation Rub the point between your thumb and forefinger where they meet at the base of the "web" of skin. Regularly drink hot water that has been boiled.

For mid-afternoon tiredness Try taking hot and sweet foods, e.g., honey in hot water.

For anxiety and tension Rub either side of your breastbone.

For hay fever Try taking a spoonful of honey every day for a month before the hay fever season starts.

Losing Weight and the Mind Diet

If you've been champing at the bit ever since starting this program in spring, *now* is the time you can set about to lose weight if indeed you need to. But before you do anything I would seriously ask you to look at yourself—not with the critical eyes of

someone who has spent virtually all their life wanting to be supermodel stick-thin, but as a sane rational human being. How
much do you weigh? How tall are you? How big are your bones?
Are you, hand on heart, *ever* going to look like a beanpole however much you lose?

I'm not going to say that you shouldn't try to lose weight
because that would be wildly hypocritical. I've been battling with
the bulge for as long as I can remember, and a long and bitter
battle it has been. Believe me, I have eaten every diet bar and
drunk every "slim" shake going. I could start a bookshop with
the number of diet regime tomes I've bought over the years. I've
popped every wonder-supplement and smeared on every miracle
cream. None of them worked. One day I worked out, to my utter
horror, that in twenty years of dieting I had managed to put on
over three stones (nineteen kilograms!). Not only that, but I had
blown my metabolism and my digestive systems almost to pieces.
My body was so used to being starved on a regular basis that it
had slowed down to a virtual standstill. My digestion was so
accustomed to subsisting on diet fare that it had lost its tone and
was utterly feeble. However little I ate, I still put on weight.

The key to weight loss is really quite straightforward, very
sensible and very slow.

1. No miracle pill will shed pounds. Maybe in the future (and
   who knows what the side effects will be) but not now.
2. No crash diet will work in the long term. You might lose
   three kilograms (seven pounds) in a week but I can promise you that you will put it all on again—and more—
   within the next few months.
3. The *only* way to lose weight safely and permanently is to
   do it gradually.

I know it's hard to get excited about the idea of losing a measly
pound or two a week (which is what you should be aiming for)
when every magazine and paper on the newsracks is screaming
that you can shed half a stone in a week. But, trust me, the long,
slow way will work. I would also ask you to aim not for a skinny
thin body but for a lean, toned, strong body. Many people really
don't need to diet; they simply need to exercise. If you're not

sure, ask your doctor or the practice nurse—or, alternatively, have an assessment at a good gym or health center.

A thorough assessment should include measuring your height, weight, and blood pressure; testing your quota of body fat and how strong your lungs are; checking your aerobic fitness and your flexibility. You should also be quizzed on your diet and any health problems. Then you will be advised on what you can feasibly do with your body. Sometimes all it takes is exercise. Sometimes you need to modify your food intake as well. But, again, please don't emulate those ridiculous catwalk models. They are not, on the whole, good examples of healthy human beings. Many are unnaturally thin and few of them have good muscle tone. We read that many of them keep their figures by near-starvation diets, heavy smoking, and even drugs or destructive cycles of bulimia or anorexia. They may look "beautiful" now, but I can promise you their health (and beauty) will suffer for fashion in later years.

If you *do* need to lose weight, then read on. Virtually everyone seems to have a theory on the One Successful Way to Lose Weight. Frankly, I don't believe there is one way that works for everyone—it all depends so much on your individual constitution, your individual circumstances, and your individual mindset. However, I do think there are three major factors in successful weight loss which seem to apply to pretty well everyone:

1. Your exercise habits: regular exercise is absolutely essential if you want to control your weight.
2. Your psyche: how you feel in yourself; your self-esteem and your feelings around food.
3. Your food: how much and what kind you eat.

Food comes in at number three for a good reason. You can lose weight by focusing solely on the food aspect of the equation, but it's very unlikely you will keep it off unless you address exercise and your psychological state as well. For really effective, long-term weight loss you need to address all aspects together. This is the reason I wanted you to wait until now to work on weight loss. If you have been following the advice in this book, and have been eating healthy, natural food and taking regular exercise, there is a strong possibility that your weight may have balanced itself already. If that isn't the case, then you probably need to work on the emotional factor as well. To alter your weight permanently, you need to do a lot of work on your self-image, your emotions, your innermost feelings. It's the missing factor in most diet programs. Let's call it the Mind Diet.

"Losing weight is actually not related to the food you put in your body," says Kati Cottrell-Blanc, a psychotherapist who has achieved remarkable success with her clients in the area of weight loss (and indeed the whole range of eating disorders). "You can eat almost anything if your emotional state is good." Vehemently anti-diet, she firmly believes that every diet plan should come with a warning: "Do not attempt if you are feeling low, depressed, tired, or in any negative state of mind." Diets, she insists, are doomed to failure because they simply don't look at the subconscious messages that each individual mind is telling its body. The only true answer to long-term weight loss is to go much further, much deeper than the surface issue of food and to discover the underlying emotional triggers that stop us losing weight. Personally, I do think we need to address the amount of food we eat and the kind of food we eat, but I totally agree with Kati that unless you look at the emotional side of the problem you will not only be unable to lose weight automatically but most likely you will find that you are quite powerless when it comes to sticking to any weight-loss program.

According to Kati there are generally three key negative emotions that scupper our diets: you need to recognize your own hidden enemy.

Fear Are you basically scared of life? Do you worry about everything? Were you frequently frightened as a child? If your deep underlying emotion is fear, then you will find it almost impossible to lose weight, says Kati. "Fear is a holding on emotion, a paralytic emotion," she says. What she means is that your subconscious mind is so terrified that it literally won't let go of anything. It will keep your emotions under wraps and it will hold on to your fat as if a famine were starting tomorrow. This kind of fearfulness often dates back to our early childhood. If you felt unloved or as if you were never quite good enough, you may well be ruled by fear. And, horrible but true, dieters ruled by fear will rarely find their weight budges at all.

Apathy Do you feel as if nothing really matters? As if you simply can't be bothered? That all-embracing sluggish "what's the point of any of it" feeling? When apathy rules, it's not surprising you can't follow a diet. After all, what's the point—surely this diet will only fail like all the rest? Isn't it obvious that it's impossible for you to ever lose weight? Deep-seated apathy is commonly linked to depression and it almost always comes from early traumatic incidents in your life, especially anything that wounded your sense of self-confidence or self-esteem. It also occurs when your body image has been disturbed in some way—perhaps you feel your body is ugly because of early abuse or because you were mocked or ridiculed at an early age. Apathy makes you feel as if you simply don't care—and if you don't care what's to stop you from piling on the weight?

Anger Do you loathe yourself? Hate your body? Feel furious about the way other people make you fat? Do you get in a right state when you see another ad for chocolate being modeled by a skinny stick of a girl? Anger isn't anywhere near as flat a state as fear and apathy, so people whose underlying emotion is anger *can* manage to lose weight but they will often put it back on again—the typical yo-yo dieting. When you are angry you will find your subconscious mind is trying to punish your body—first starving it and then furiously making it binge again. You end up feeling it just isn't fair, breaking open another packet of biscuits—and hating yourself all over again for being so weak.

The underlying causes for these states of mind often hark back to childhood, from the messages we picked up from family and friends. "The problem is that deep down our belief that we are really capable, able people has been damaged," says Kati. "It could come from parents, from the early handing out of nourishment, both physical and emotional. Or it could come from later relationships—whether emotional or work relationships. But always, the common link is a lack of intrinsic self-esteem, of confidence."

So the key is to get yourself back in harmony, into a state of ease in which you can reprogram the negative messages your subconscious is giving to your body. Basically, before you can lose weight, you need to learn how to be happy again. Psychotherapists like Kati insist they never actually treat the weight loss, rather the underlying unhappiness that is inevitably present. But psychotherapy is not necessarily the only, or even the best, way to lose weight for everyone. Kati will often send people off for bodywork, or to see a homeopath. She also suggests psychosynthesis (a form of psychotherapy) and even martial arts and yoga. The key is to find something that suits you, that appeals to you, and that enhances your self-esteem rather than focusing on food.

Kati's own approach is intense and perfectly likely to alter your entire life, not just your eating patterns. She warns that it can be hard work, not just for the client but also for her or his family and friends. Hour-long sessions take place once a week, usually for a minimum of six months. The first time I visited Kati, she asked me to talk not about food but about my childhood. It was quite illuminating. Although there was always food on the table, money was tight and we lived frugally. Like most children at the time, I was encouraged always to finish the food on my plate and to "think of the starving children in Africa." At school we had to sit in front of our slowly congealing lunch until it had been finished—if we wanted to leave anything we had to ask permission, which was rarely granted. By the time I was eight my subconscious had taken on plenty of negative messages including "grab hold of every bit of food you can" and "never leave anything on your plate." It has been frantically obeying ever since! So for my "homework" Kati instructed me to eat whatever I liked. I made my way through the whole sweet shop and takeaway menu—but I felt guilty as hell.

The next week Kati explained that all the while I was feeling guilty about food it would always keep its hold over me. The more guilt you feel, the more inexorable your need for the guilt-inducing food. It's a little like if you're told you can't scratch your head, the first thing you want to do is scratch your head. "Food has to stop being an item," Kati insists. "You have to take the power out of it. Then you can really start to enjoy food again, with wholehearted agreement between your mind and body on a subconscious level. That's when you will start to self-regulate, and lose weight."

Over the following weeks we talked about my relationships, my dreams, my desires, my frustrations in life but hardly ever about food. And every week, she told me to eat whatever I wanted, to stuff myself silly if I wanted. The process was fascinating—and sometimes painful. Not only did I start to see quite clearly how and when I used food as an emotional prop but I also began to look at all areas of my life and question what I really wanted. To begin with, my weight shot up, but after a few weeks it settled and gradually I started to eat good food and enjoy it rather than guiltily bolt "diet" food and feel miserable. Kati agrees that the aim is not to become a stick-like model which is, she says, frankly impossible and unhealthy for most people, but to find the optimum weight for our individual bodies.

"The idea of therapy is to get our body, mind, and spirit into a state of ease," says Kati. "You need to learn how to release emotions. Normally people who are overweight either suppress their emotions (which makes them hold on to weight) or express them (typically in angry outbursts or deep sarcasm caused by anger which, as we've seen, normally causes yo-yo dieting). If, instead, you release them your body is allowed to be in equilibrium." And then, she promises, you can access your own hidden self-confidence. "Once you've done that there is nothing you can't do. And if what you really want is to lose weight, then you will do it."

The whole psychological issues around why we hold on to weight are complex and will vary for each person. What I am trying to do here is simply to start you thinking about the emotional aspects of your weight. Just take a few moments and ask yourself the following questions:

• Can you link your weight gain to any particular event?
• Do you eat more when you are unhappy or anxious?
• Do you binge after a bad or really good day?
• Do you choose different foods when you feel depressed to when you feel good about yourself?
• Does your weight fluctuate? Are you in and out of diets all the time?

If the answers to these questions are predominantly yes, then it is quite likely that you need to address the emotional reasons behind your weight gain.

Over the next few months I will be suggesting numerous ways of fostering self-esteem and getting in touch with your emotions—any of these should help the psychological side of the equation. However, I would not recommend following the "stuff yourself silly" approach on your own (it's pretty scary if you've always had an issue around food). So if you're working on your own, I would suggest you try the plan I outline below to begin with. However, it may be you find that even this plan causes you problems; that you can't stick with it; you're still snacking; you're doing well for a few days and then you just lose it and so on. If so, I really would recommend that you find a therapist or counselor you feel comfortable with and work on this emotional side of the equation.

Equally, there doesn't have to be any deep psychological reason for your weight gain. If you've read through the previous section and it really hasn't struck a chord, then don't be worried. You may simply be eating too much, eating the wrong kind of food, or even eating too little! When I stopped "dieting" and went on a sensible eating plan I was stunned to find how much I could eat—of the right kind of food. If you have dieted for years, it can be alarming to start eating huge amounts of food again but, truly, eating good healthy meals is the best way to lose weight. Once your body begins to trust that you aren't going to starve it, it will relax and start to let go of excess fat. Slowly, slowly, it will shed the stored fat and you will lose weight.

This is not a diet book, nor is it a cookery book so I'm not going to give you long precise plans and menus. But these are the bare bones you need to follow to lose weight safely. Follow the basic guidelines and you shouldn't go far wrong.

The "Eat Masses and Still Lose Weight" Healthy Eating Plan

Let's not talk about calories. You can lose weight by morbidly keeping a calculator by our side and totting up every spoonful of milk in your tea and every smear of margarine on your bread, but it's pretty miserable. It also makes you obsessive about food, which is the last thing you want. Instead, you need to get a rough idea of how much food you should eat to lose weight safely and what kinds of food you need to be careful with.

Essentially, what you're after is a low-fat, low-cholesterol diet that is packed with fresh vegetables and fiber. It's the same kind of diet you have already been following. The only difference is that now we're going to monitor it all a little more precisely.

GENERAL GUIDELINES

1. Make sure you drink plenty of fresh mineral water every day—a good target is a two-liter bottle. Not only will the water help to cleanse your body and ease any constipation you may have as you change eating habits, it will also make you feel full.

2. Try not to skip meals. This eating plan is based on a good old-fashioned three meals a day. If at this point you're saying "but I never eat breakfast" or "if I eat breakfast I carry on eating all day" or "I never have time for lunch," then see a specialist—a nutritionist or an ayurvedic practitioner—as this plan won't work unless you follow it quite precisely. It may be that your ayurvedic constitution will let you miss breakfast but your regime will have to be tailored to suit.

3. Try to stick to a regular daily routine. Aim to eat your meals at roughly the same time each day. If you can make lunch your main meal, then this will undoubtedly help, since from around noon to 1 P.M. your digestion is working at its optimum capacity. If work makes it difficult to do so, then at least ensure that you pay attention to lunch and have something nourishing. If you can make your evening meal the smaller of the two, so much the better. If you can't, then do try to eat earlier in the evening— around six o'clock if you can. Obviously, you will have to do what you can to fit in with your schedules, but if you can move your dinner or supper forward even half an hour it will help.

4. Make an effort over your food. Even if you're just cooking for yourself, take the time to make the food look attractive. And make mealtimes special too: sit down away from your work and concentrate on your food. Try not to eat in front of the television or with a book propped up in front of you. That way you won't notice what you're eating; you might tend to bolt food and you won't feel emotionally satisfied by your food.

5. Don't eat freezing cold food. Allow food to stand at room temperature for a while before eating. And if you're having a cold salad, then preface your meal with a bowl of warm soup—it will heat the digestion and help it cope with the cold of the salad. Equally, as I've said earlier, don't drink freezing water with your meal.

6. To begin with, do weigh out your food just to get an idea of how much you need. I don't think it's a good idea to become obsessive about weighing food, but often you will find that what you thought was a small bowl of breakfast cereal is actually a very large one! Likewise, you will probably find that you can eat far more carbohydrate than you imagined. Once you get used to how much is involved you can stop weighing.

7. Continue with the guidelines for healthy eating: pick food that is fresh, organic (wherever possible), as local as possible, and in season.

YOUR DAILY PLAN

The amounts included in the following meal suggestions are intended as a general guideline. Use the larger amounts if you have a lot of weight to lose or are very big; otherwise try the lesser amount. Only weigh yourself once a week on the same scales and aim for a weight loss of between one and two pounds (half to one kilogram) a week. If you find you're losing more than this, then up the amounts you are eating slightly. If you are not losing weight, then eat the smaller amounts and make sure you are not incorrectly estimating the amount of food you are eating. And don't aim to lose more weight than is recommended for your height and build (check with your doctor, nurse, or gym).

Breakfast
Breakfast doesn't need to be a huge meal, but most people find it helps them to have something in the morning. Keep it light and balanced. Here are some suggestions:

• A small bowl of cereal (around 30–60 g) with skimmed milk. If you think you're allergic to cow's milk, try sheep's, soya, or goat's, although it will be tough to find low-fat versions of these. Or, as an alternative to milk, have a couple of tablespoons of organic live yogurt. Try to wean yourself off sugar and sweeteners by gradually diminishing the amount you have. Although a lot of weight-loss plans suggest you use artificial sweeteners, these contain additives that are slightly worrying. Many scientists feel we don't know enough about the long-term effects of aspartame and the like and how they interact with the body's systems. So, to be safe, try not to use them.

• One slice of wholemeal toast with a teaspoon of butter, soya margarine, or olive oil margarine. Add a teaspoon of honey, marmalade, or a dollop of jam sweetened with fruit juice rather than sugar (utterly delicious and very healthy—all health-food stores stock it). Or top your toast with an egg (but don't fry it in gallons of oil) or 30 g of cheese.

• If you don't have much time, take your breakfast with you. Try a small wholemeal roll with 60 g of low-fat soft cheese or an oatcake with cheese.

• If you feel deprived without a good farmhouse fry-up breakfast try this: have an egg (fried in a teaspoon of olive oil), or a couple of turkey rashers (much leaner than bacon but with most of the taste), or a small vegetarian sausage (normal sausages are generally stuffed with fat and often have all kinds of unpleasant additives). Then grill a mountain of tomatoes and mushrooms. Pile the lot on a slim slice of toast and you've got a healthy but hefty breakfast. Baked beans are also a great start to the day—choose those with reduced salt and no added sugar (again your health-food store can help) and don't have *too* many—about three-quarters of a small tin is about right.

• Whichever option you pick, always add a medium-sized piece of fruit to your meal: half a grapefruit (try the pink ones which are naturally sweeter and won't need sugar), an apple, a small banana, an orange, a fresh fig (more help for recalcitrant bowels). Alternatively, add 30 g of dried fruit to your cereal or, if you prefer, have a small glass of fruit juice. If you always get hungry mid-morning, then keep your piece of fruit to eat when the munchies start. Remember, if you're feeling hungry, keep drinking water.

A note about fruit: fruit is wonderfully healthy and will give you lots of fiber and vitamins, but it is high in natural sugars and, if you eat large amounts, you may put on weight. You should be aiming for three portions of fruit a day of around 120 g a portion.

Lunch

If this can be your largest meal, so much the better for your weight. It's no accident that in many countries the main meal of the day is taken at lunchtime. In the ayurvedic scheme of things, the reason for this is clear: lunchtime is ruled by *pitta,* the fire which stokes the digestion and allows food to be digested and assimilated more quickly. Food eaten at lunchtime will not lay stagnant in the stomach but will be quickly put to work. However, in the UK, for many people this simply is not convenient. Therefore, the quantities that follow are based on lunch being the lighter meal of the day. If, however, you can manage to eat your major meal at lunchtime, then simply switch the information here for that given for dinner, which outlines main meals.

Whether you eat at home or at work, make time for a proper lunch. For an ideal meal you need to balance complex carbohydrates, protein, and vegetables. A good balance of carbohydrate and protein for the lighter meal of the day lies around the following amounts:

Carbohydrate choices: 30–60 g of rice or pasta (uncooked weight); 45–90 g of potato, one to two slices of bread; a muffin or a roll (we're talking about normal dinner rolls here not vast baps).

Protein choices: 60–120 g of white fish, tofu, or Quorn; 30–60 g of oily fish, lean meat, cheese, or offal; 90–180 g of lentils, chick peas or other pulses, one or two eggs.

These can be combined with vegetables, which can be eaten quite freely—the only ones to keep an eye on are peas, sweetcorn and parsnips, which are starchy and count as carbohydrate.

The only other factor to watch carefully is fat—aim for a maximum of one teaspoon of olive oil, vegetable oil spread, or (if you really must) butter.

The choices are pretty endless:

• Stuff a pita bread with hummus. Shop-bought hummus tends to contain lots of oil, so try whizzing up your own in the food processor. Accompany with tomatoes, lettuce, and onions, and sprinkle a little paprika on top.

• Make a hearty omelet in the peasant style with lots of onions, tomatoes, sweet peppers, and herbs (try roasting or grilling vegetables instead of frying).

• Have a jacket potato—without, of course, all the oozing butter. If you make a solid filling based around a little cheese or tuna or grilled turkey rashers boosted with onions and vegetables you shouldn't miss the butter too much.

• Add a side salad to any of the above to ensure you get plenty of those antioxidant vitamins. Pack it full of peppery rocket, young spinach leaves and watercress with spring onions, red peppers, fresh coriander leaves, sweet cherry tomatoes, and add a dash of balsamic vinegar—delicious.

• Have a piece of fruit for lunch, although if you tend to get hungry mid-afternoon, save it for then.

Dinner

Do try to eat this meal as early as you can. Again, ensure you achieve a good balance of carbohydrate, protein, and vegetables. The guidelines here assume this is your main meal of the day.

Carbohydrate choices: 80–90 g of rice or pasta (uncooked weight); 200–300 g of potato; one to two slices of bread, or a roll.
Protein choices: 120–180 g of white fish, tofu, or Quorn; 60–90 g of oily fish, lean meat, cheese, or offal; 180–270 g of lentils, chick peas or other pulses; two to three eggs.

Once again, the above choices should be combined with vegetables which can be eaten quite freely with the same provisos as for lunch. Again, watch your fat intake. This may sound more alarming when it comes to a major meal but, in fact, the options are pretty well endless. Avoid frying as much as possible. Instead, try stir-frying with only a tiny bit of oil, or try grilling, roasting, poaching, steaming, and stewing using spices and herbs to add zest and flavor.

You could, for example, eat a very substantial meal of pasta with roasted vegetable sauce—using lots of onion and garlic and a dash of oregano, marjoram, or basil. Since you only need a drizzle of olive oil over the vegetables to roast them, the dish is wonderfully healthy and totally delicious, and because you can eat vegetables freely you can have a huge pile of food. If you like meat, then use your protein choice to add some lean bacon or turkey rashers or Italian cooked meats. Otherwise, top the dish with parmesan cheese. Or use half of each.

When you first start weighing meat the amounts here look very mean and stingy. The key is to follow the principles of many of the healthiest cuisines in the world and use a little meat to add flavor rather than relying on it to provide all the interest.

An equally robust choice would be a lentil stew, flavored with hearty vegetables and herbs and poured over fragrant couscous (treat as a carbohydrate) or rice.

If you like meat there are endless recipes for grilling and roasting. Choose lean cuts of meat, trim off any fat, and serve with plenty of vegetables. Or whisk up a tangy salsa to liven up plain grilled meats. Or marinade the meat in a teaspoon of olive oil to which you've added balsamic vinegar, a teaspoon of English mustard, a chopped chunk of ginger root, a little honey, and plenty of garlic and freshly ground pepper. Then grill or barbecue.

You don't have to stick to "diet" cookbooks either. I find the vast majority of recipes can be "slimmed down" simply by cutting right down on the fat, boosting up the vegetable content, and cutting down on the amounts of protein and (possibly though less likely) the carbohydrate.

Once again, make sure you have a piece of fruit after your meal, or start the meal with a slice of melon or half a grapefruit.

EXTRA GUIDELINES

• The amounts of protein in this program are quite meager, and you'll notice that you can eat greater quantities of pulses and white fish than you can of cheese or red meat. I would heartily recommend you choose fish, pulses, or vegetable proteins like tofu to provide the majority of your protein needs through the week. Limit the amount of red meat, eggs, and cheese you eat in any one week as they are high in cholesterol.
• Don't, however, scrimp on your vegetables. The key to healthy eating and comfortable weight loss is to pile on the veggies. You can eat almost unlimited quantities of vegetables and not gain weight, and all those vitamins will be wonderful for your health. And remember, you can use vegetables to stave off hunger pangs. Several successful weight-loss programs advocate

vegetable soup as the perfect healthy filler. I couldn't agree more. Simply make up a large stockpot of hearty vegetable soup and eat a bowl before meals or when you feel ravenous and there isn't a meal in sight. Or even after a meal if you're still feeling hungry.

To make the soup, sweat onion and garlic in a large heavy-based saucepan until they're soft and then add a selection of chopped, seasonal vegetables (up to you which you choose, but for the purpose of this soup avoid the starchy vegetables like peas, sweetcorn, parsnip, and potato). I like to add a liberal dose of fresh herbs or, if the weather is cooler, some warming spices. Then simply simmer the whole lot until the vegetables are soft, and either eat it as it is or put it through a blender. Try not to add too much salt—instead, include some celery in your selection and it will add a salty taste.

• Another healthy and filling option is vegetable juice. Few people can wade through mountains of broccoli or carrots, however tastefully steamed and flavored. So, to boost your veggie intake and fend off hunger as well, try juicing. Best, however, to make your own vegetable juice as many of the commercial brands contain added salt and/or sugar (see AUGUST for juicing ideas).

• Ayurvedic and Tibetan practitioners swear by rhubarb as a great diet aid because of its bitter, slightly astringent quality. They say you can eat rhubarb freely on a weight-loss program. Sadly, most of us can't manage it without liberal doses of sweetener. However, try it with a spoonful of honey and a dollop of yogurt—it makes a refreshing pudding.

A FEW THINGS TO WATCH

• Alcohol can put on weight very easily and very unattractively—where do you think beer bellies come from? If you cut down your alcohol consumption you will certainly see a weight loss. You don't have to give it up altogether, but while you're trying to lose weight I would suggest you have no more than two or three glasses of wine (or the equivalent in spirits or beer) a week.

• There is bound to be something that isn't covered in this food program that you positively crave. It could be chocolate; it could be ice cream; it might be crisps, sausages, pastry, or thick rich creamy sauces. If you're addicted to a particular food, there is probably either an allergy problem involved (check with a nutritionist) or an emotional issue. If it's the latter, you'll never be satisfied with the low-calorie options, and if you try to ignore it altogether, you are probably consigning yourself to failure. What I do is accept that once in a while I can have whatever I like—be it a bar of chocolate or a thick crusty pastry pie (horribly unhealthy I know). I don't do it that often, but when I do, I simply eat it, savor it, and enjoy it. No guilt, no draconian purgings the day after. Afterward, just get back into your healthy eating program as per normal.

• Specially prepared diet meals may look appealing, but I wouldn't honestly recommend them. They are expensive, overly processed and, to my mind, meager. The portions are small because they usually involve some sort of sauce which invariably kicks in the calories. Personally, I'd rather have a large bowl of something without the creamy sauce than a tiny taste. I also think it's really important when you're trying to lose weight that you don't become frightened of food. One of the most liberating things about following the kind of program I've outlined is that you can eat a lot of food—a veritable plateful each mealtime if you choose—and still lose weight. So you don't feel deprived. And gradually, your body will start to relax. You will be sending it a message that it's OK to eat; that it's even OK to eat quite large amounts of food and that these large amounts of food are going to keep on coming. At first your body will still be suspicious—after all, you've starved it or yo-yoed with it for so many years—and will hold on to weight in case you suddenly decide to plunge it back into self-preservation mode. But gradually, as the food keeps coming, it will learn that it can let go of the extra stores and keep just what it needs.

• If you feel you need more support then I would certainly suggest you join a club like Weight Watchers. People tend to ridicule such clubs, but I think they can be a very positive experience. Firstly, they focus on good, sensible eating habits rather than crash diets—they will only want you to lose the recommended one to two pounds a week. And, secondly, it can be very reassuring and motivating to meet up every week with people who are trying to do exactly the same as you.

My only reservations are that, although their guidelines are sensible (and in many cases very similar to the ones given here), they often stress the use of "diet" foods such as artificial sweeteners and convenience foods. Their emphasis is purely on weight loss, whereas I would like you to be more aware of the vital nourishment in the foods you eat. Some other slimming clubs also talk about "sin" foods, which I don't think is very helpful. The last thing you need when you're trying to get back into sensible eating is to think of food, any food, as *sinful*—rather you need to become aware of which foods will help your health (and your weight) and which are less useful. Again, Weight Watchers is quite good here—they say you can eat any food but that some must only be eaten in strict moderation. If you are addicted to cakes and sweets, you will be allowed to eat them on a Weight Watchers program. Frankly, I don't see that as a problem at all. Obviously, in an ideal world, you wouldn't eat too much sweet, sugary stuff but if you're craving it then eat it— under control in this way. As you lose weight and become happier with your body and with your self-esteem, you may find you don't need the sweets any more.

Kati Cottrell-Blanc has an interesting observation on sweet foods: she says that virtually every client who has had a fixation on sweet things has an unresolved issue with their mother. She advises such people to look at their relationship with their mother (whether she is still living or deceased) and ponder this.

If weight isn't an issue for you, I suggest you keep an eye on your food intake nonetheless—some of the slimmest people I know eat the worst junk food imaginable. They may be genetically able to handle it but, equally, it may catch up with them in later years. Whether we have to watch our weight or not, we all still need to make sure we are eating a sensible, natural, healthy, balanced diet.

June

There's something lovely about June. It's the prelude to summer—a young, clear, fresh and joyous promise of the fullness to come. June can be unpredictable; it can be warm and clear but equally chill and fractious. It's the month when spring pivots into summer at the time of the solstice on June 21. Since I started living in the country I have adored June. It's the month of village fêtes, of prizes for the best jam and the dog with the waggiest tail. There is a steady stream of children wanting to be sponsored for charity walks, and proud gardeners with green fingers open their plots to the world to show off their heroic battles against slugs and weeds. In my garden in June the weeds multiply with merry abandon, shooting up behind my back, and the sorrel defies gravity as it virtually grows before my very eyes.

June is sociable with all its community activities. We may think it's merely quaint but in fact they all serve an important need. The summer solstice is the time for looking at our place in society; how we fit into the community and how we handle our relationships. It's a great time for families; for getting out into the country or the park and having picnics; for heading off to open-air concerts; for having parties in the garden. Not surprisingly, when you think of these connotations, June is the big wedding month when couples pledge their vows and seal their most personal relationship in full view of their family, friends and the local community.

Nowadays we seem to have lost our sense of community. When I lived in London there were long periods in which I didn't even know the names of my next-door neighbors. I'm not saying you have to live in your neighbors' pockets—far from it. But if you can join in with community activities in some small way, you will probably find you get a lot out of it.

Now is the time to start looking at the emotional side of your life, at how you relate to other people, how you fit into the larger wheel of society.

Looking at Your Emotions

Where do you begin? It's a bit of a chicken and egg situation since every individual will be utterly different and probably need a different solution. However, I have found, on the whole, that perhaps the best place to begin is with the body. This works quite nicely at this point in the year as we are only just coming out of spring and so the physical is still very much uppermost. It is quite likely that if you have tried any of the forms of massage or flexibility work suggested in the earlier chapters, you might already have found old emotions surfacing or issues coming up to be dealt with. At first this can seem very puzzling. How can physical forms of exercise or massage affect our emotions? How can moving in a certain way or having your muscles probed in a particular spot bring back old thoughts and feelings?

I admit it sounds bizarre—to put it mildly. However, in the future, I am quite convinced that science will prove what virtually everyone who works with bodies already knows—we hold our memories, our emotions, our hurts and anguishes, our fears and traumas all over our bodies. Not just tucked away in our minds, but also in the muscles, the tendons, the connective tissue (the fascia), the organs, the very bones of our bodies. Our subconscious, if you like, is spread throughout our physical beings quite as much as it is held in our heads.

Almost all bodyworkers—whether osteopaths and chiropractors, masseurs and aromatherapists, or shiatsu and acupressure practitioners—have found that in the course of their physical work, emotions will often arise. However, certain forms of bodywork will bring emotions to the surface more readily than others. Which you choose is totally up to you. Some can be quite painful; others use only the barest touch.

Godlieve Denys-Struyf, a physiotherapist and osteopath who has tutored at the British School of Osteopathy, now teaches at her own school in Brussels. She insists that every person will need something different but, first and foremost, she believes we need to become more in touch with our own bodies. The treatment needs to suit not only the physical problem but the individual's personality.

"Some people like to be touched and other people dislike it," explains Virginie Holst, a physiotherapist who trained with Denys-Struyf. "Some people like to move while others don't; some are very rational, they like explanations and you have to explain what you are doing; other people aren't interested." She goes on to explain the link between body and mind, stressing that a large proportion of our physical problems start when the mind begins to use the body as a dustbin for its emotions.

"You have stress and you don't know how to cope with it," she says, "so you offload the stress you can't deal with on to your body. The body will begin to build up tensions in the same place and will eventually create a permanent tension. You will find you can hardly move your neck, or your digestion becomes bad, or you can't breathe properly." This, she says, is the psychosomatic stage, when we begin to become slaves of our bodies.

However, the next stage, which Virginie calls the somatopsychic, is even worse. "All this stress in the body starts to affect your mind. People start to become angry because they cannot move their bodies freely, or they become depressed or anxious. It is a bad state—the body is like a prison and people become unhappy living in it."

So the importance of this kind of work is not just in the mind. By freeing the emotions stuck in the body you will be easing your physical body as well. The result should be better health and happiness in all areas. This mind-body approach is becoming very popular in France, and Virginie hopes that British physiotherapists will follow suit. She suggests the following two exercises to help you begin to become more aware, more conscious of your body.

1. BODY AWARENESS: Wearing loose clothes and no shoes, lie on the floor on your back. Become aware of your body lying on the floor—feel the floor under you and where it supports your body. Now put your attention into your feet—imagine the bones of your feet, the muscles, the tendons, the skin. Are they hot or cold? Do you feel any difference between each foot? Are they light or heavy? Now gradually work up the body, repeating the questions, becoming aware of how different parts of your body feel. Move up your legs into the hips, up the body and down the arms, finishing with your head and face.

2. BONE-VIBRATING: We often forget about our bones. Virginie points out that if we aren't aware of our bones, we can hardly expect to move properly. She tells her clients to work on putting gentle vibration through the body. Use either your lightly clenched fists or the fingers of your hand and swiftly tap over your hip bones and pelvis. Listen to the sound it makes, and feel the vibration in your body. Move down your legs, listening and feeling for changes in sound and feeling. Try the soles of your feet. Work over all the bones in your body, noting any differences.

The Most Effective Bodywork Systems for Freeing Emotions

If you specifically want to get in touch with hidden emotions, these are the therapies I would recommend. They will also have a quite distinct effect on your physical body.

ROLFING AND HELLERWORK

Rolfing and Hellerwork are both very powerful systems of body-work which can alter the entire shape of your body and your posture. They can correct long-standing physical problems and create a sense of ease in the body. They are also superlative for releasing repressed emotions.

Both techniques are given in courses (Rolfing has ten sessions per course; Hellerwork eleven), and all graduates say that afterward they look different, more upright, more centered, more relaxed. They also report physical benefits such as release from long-term aches and pains; chronic headaches often vanish and there's a general consensus that energy levels soar. Minds follow close behind: on the emotional plane people swear it has given them increased confidence, a greater feeling of poise and balance, the ability to deal with people and to confront issues. It seems to make people more whole.

At first sight, Rolfing and Hellerwork appear little more than a deep form of massage. So how do their practitioners achieve such deep effects? The answer, says Rolfer Jenny Crewdson, lies in the fascia. Deep-tissue bodyworkers bypass muscles, and head instead for the connective tissue which contains and links the muscles. Not only does fascia house every muscle and muscle fiber but it also thickens to form the tendons and ligaments. It keeps our whole structure, muscle and bone, in place.

Yet the fascial system had been generally ignored until around fifty years ago when American biochemist Dr. Ida Rolf discovered that the fascia will adapt to support whatever patterns of movement and posture the body adopts. If you put more weight on one leg than the other, the fascia will bunch and shorten to compensate; if you hunch your shoulders, the fascia will knot to accommodate and hold your posture. If we put our bodies into imbalance the fascia will obediently change to hold us in that position. But, as Dr. Rolf soon discovered, if the fascia can change once, they can change again. And by manipulating and stretching the fascia back into their original position, she could reprogram neurological pathways and return her patient to alignment. The technique became known as Rolfing.

But it didn't stop on the physical level. Rolf also found that when she changed the body on a physiological level, her patients changed on a mental and emotional level as well. "When you change patterns on one level you change patterns on all levels," explains Jenny Crewdson. "There's a lot of evidence to show that memory isn't just held in the brain but in the muscles and tissue as well. Sometimes when you're Rolfing you'll touch an area and the person will scream and say something like: 'That reminds me of when my brother hit me when I was seven.' It's quite amazing. The tissue actually seems to retain memory, so that by releasing structural holding you release emotional holding."

Rolfing was the first technique I'd heard about which could apparently release emotions in this way, and I confess that at first I found the claim a little far-fetched. When I went along to Jenny Crewdson's practice I was also slightly nervous because Rolfing has a reputation of being remarkably painful. Somewhat self-conscious in bra and pants, I stood as Jenny scrutinized my body and posture. "You hold yourself up with your shoulders," she noted. "You have a rotation of the left hip and your left leg is shorter than your right." She then asked me to lie on the couch and started to work on my body.

Sometimes the Rolfing touch feels like a strong pressing movement; at others the hands seem to push inexorably into the body. It's insistent and occasionally very tender, but it's certainly not unbearable. In fact, if anything, I found it curiously releasing as old strains and stresses were stretched and straightened. But as Jenny worked around my shoulder blade she suddenly hit a sore point I hadn't even realized was there. And, clear as a movie, I suddenly "saw" the bright green grass of my childhood back garden. I was learning to ride a bike and kept falling off. It was a scene I had completely forgotten.

After my session I felt deeply relaxed but otherwise not that much different. However, when I looked in the mirror at home my shoulders had noticeably moved several inches away from my ears to a more civilized position. And over the next few days I noticed emotional changes too: memories of old hurts and disappointments would suddenly pop into my head as if to let me take a last look before they disappeared again. And, as I ran up the third escalator on the tube I suddenly realized my energy levels were higher than they had been for years.

To try out the other side of the deep-tissue coin, I paid a visit to Hellerworker Terry Petersen. Hellerwork was founded by

Joseph Heller who had trained with Ida Rolf before leaving to found his own form of bodywork. He wanted to concentrate more on movement and on the emotional side of treatment. But, as Terry Petersen explains, nowadays the differences between Hellerwork and Rolfing are very few.

At the start of my Hellerwork session I spent about twenty minutes learning how to sit, stand and walk in a more balanced way. Wearing just my pants I felt rather exposed and was very relieved to hear that Terry had not yet started to video her clients. However, both Rolfers and Hellerworkers take "before" and "after" pictures to show how rounded shoulders can straighten and protruding bottoms can tuck in following a course of treatment.

The Hellerwork touch is almost indistinguishable from Rolfing, although I found it slightly more painful in places. The main difference is in emphasis. Rolfing seemed more of an internal experience, with Jenny only making the occasional supportive comment or asking the odd question. Hellerwork demands far more participation. Each session has a "theme," and the practitioner will engage the client in a dialogue while working on the body. The first session is called Inspiration, and while she was probing into my back Terry asked me questions like, "What inspires you?" and "What would you like to be doing that you don't have time for in your life?"

Both practitioners insist they are not psychologists and that if any really deep emotional issues come up in the course of the work, they will refer the client to a trained counselor. "Sometimes it can be a little painful," says Terry Petersen. "One man had been in a car crash as a child. He had lost a couple of ribs and both his parents had been killed. When we worked on his chest he started hyperventilating and went into a memory of the accident. He needed to talk about it and have a cry but it was a release and he felt much better after it."

Jenny Crewdson says that in America bodyworkers work very effectively with shock and trauma victims—both from accidents and from rape and severe abuse. But, for the time being, no one in the UK really works at that level. In fact, there are very few Rolfers and Hellerworkers practicing at all—no more than a dozen in the whole country, mostly based in the London area.

It's a great pity because, although the treatments involve a fair commitment of time and money (regular weekly appointments are the ideal and sessions are quite expensive), the benefits really do seem worth the outlay and the slight discomfort. As Terry Petersen says, "The changes are quite noticeable. Physically you see it in the posture, the fascia, the skin tone. More subtly, you notice changes in presentation, vitality, confidence and energy. When people start, they look as if they are just hanging in there; by the end there is a sense of vitality and energy. It's very exciting."

LOOYENWORK

A more recent development is Looyenwork, which gains its name from its founder, Ted Looyen, a Dutch-born psychotherapist who turned to bodywork after a severe back problem. He tried massage and manipulation and found they didn't quite hit the spot, so he moved to California to sample a broader spectrum of bodywork but still none of them quite clicked. He felt that much bodywork didn't take into account the degree to which our posture and pain is often dictated by our personalities, our past emotions, our traumas.

Just as the physical pain of an accident can be stored in the tissues of the body, so can the psychological trauma of death, divorce, rejection, fear, shame, internalized anger. As a result, Looyen worked very slowly, very carefully and counseled his clients about the changes that could occur to their emotions when he untied the knots in their bodies. While Rolfing and Hellerwork are focused primarily toward easing physical problems, Looyen's emphasis is first and foremost on the emotional aspect (although undoubtedly physical changes occur as well).

A skilled Looyenworker can almost "read" your personality by the way you stand and sit; by the way your muscles tighten and loosen. Like Rolfing and Hellerwork, Looyenwork is a precise system of deep-tissue body therapy which is designed to realign the body, to release chronic tension and to restore natural balance and grace. Again, devotees claim the system gives them fresh boosts of confidence and self-esteem; they become less shy, more forceful and much more able to concentrate. They learn to stand fair and square against the rigors of the world.

One person who discovered how effective Looyen's work could be is Ingrid Martin, as yet the only practitioner of Looyen-work in Europe. She was traveling through the desert from New Mexico to California when her car suddenly shot off the road and cartwheeled four times. She suffered severe whiplash and was bruised from head to toe; when she met Ted Looyen she was in agony. However, by the end of a week her whiplash had vanished and, although she was still black and blue, she had no pain and actually felt more balanced than before the accident. She also noticed profound emotional changes. "I used to be very round-shouldered," says Ingrid, "but Ted sent me out into the street to walk around with my shoulders back and my whole chest area open. It was one of the scariest things I have ever done—I felt so open and unprotected."

However, she says, she did manage to change her posture and it has made her far more confident, far more outgoing. She stresses that any marked changes in posture need careful handling. "It can be very scary when your whole posture changes," she says, "because immediately you are interacting differently with the world. You are giving out different messages, and so people treat you differently." It can be one of the major reasons why people often don't continue with bodywork or why old problems frequently resurface. "You can work on someone and affect a big change in their posture, but they will change straight back because they found it too frightening, too unfamiliar."

Ingrid always talks to her clients about deep changes and sometimes refers them to a counselor if they need to come to terms with new emotions, new ways of looking at the world. Equally she might encourage them to express their emotions in quite physical ways. "I often tell people to scream, or to bash a pillow. I told one client to go home and wrestle with her boyfriend."

But Looyenwork does not just affect change in the emotions; it has precise, tangible effects in the body too. Neck, shoulder and lower back pain can vanish; it works well on frozen shoulders and repetitive strain injuries and can even relieve digestive problems and relax the breathing in asthmatics (although Ingrid stresses that it doesn't *cure* asthma). She often finds people appear to lose weight when their bodies become realigned, and many clients do actually lose weight as their body image and self-confidence improve (remember what we said earlier about weight loss and self-esteem?).

Although on paper Looyenwork sounds a dead ringer for its older cousins Rolfing and Hellerwork, in practice, it is really quite different. So I decided to put it to the test. A session starts with questions about past injuries and present pains. Then Ingrid asked me to stand up so she could assess my body. Unusually, she didn't ask me to strip to underwear or beyond (because many people find it uncomfortable, she explained). "You've got a slight case of what we call 'Superwoman about to take off,' " she smiled. "Your body slants forward, held by the shoulders. It's as if you're permanently geared for action, to take on the world."

She asked me to strip down as far as I felt comfortable and to lie on the couch with a large towel over me. Looyenworkers will work with whatever level of undress makes you feel comfortable, but you can quite happily strip if you choose, as Looyenwork is conducted more like a massage than a deep-tissue session: only the bit of body that is being worked on is left uncovered. Ingrid mixed a light oil with drops of essential oils to relax the muscles and then she began. Mostly she used a steady, static, downward pressure, working deeply into the body. When she did use movements, they were very slow and deliberate. But although Looyenwork is supposed to be much less painful than other deep-tissue work, I'm afraid to say it wasn't: some points were so very tender that Ingrid's touch, however careful, really made me wince. "You're very tense," she soothed but kept on pushing inexorably. Gradually, however, my recalcitrant body gave in and gave up the tension. Toward the end of my session I was quite comfortable and even relaxed enough to doze off. I wouldn't say it was a delicious experience but it was highly satisfying because, afterward, I could certainly tell something had happened—my shoulders stayed down of their own accord and my whole body felt easier.

Unlike Rolfing and Hellerwork, there are no set amount of sessions—Ingrid sees people for an average of seven to twelve sessions, although some people leave contented after one, while others continue having occasional treatments for years. The only people for whom Looyenwork is not suitable are pregnant women, those with cancer or osteoporosis, and anyone with inflammation. Apart from those, anyone can benefit and Ingrid's one regret is that people only tend to come when they have a problem. "I would love to see clients who haven't anything wrong with them," she says, "people who simply want to be more flexible, more in touch with their bodies." And, presumably, in touch with their emotions as well.

What is your body saying about your emotions?
Ingrid Martin says that we tend to store specific emotions in specific parts of the body. Although everyone varies, she has found the following to be common:

• If your calves are very tight and tense, you may well be storing anger.
• Tension in the lower back and hips can often indicate insecurity.
• A lot of tension in the pelvic region and lower abdomen can sometimes signify sexual abuse as a child. If the area has been touched without permission, it will inevitably tighten up in defense.
• Tension in shoulders is obviously a clear signal of stress.
• If you suffer pain in your neck, it could be that you tend to cut yourself off from your body, working through illness and stress and often eating the wrong foods and not exercising. Neck pain also often occurs in people who are stubborn.
• Tight hamstrings can indicate an unwillingness to really trust other people.
• Clenching the jaw is often a result of not being able to say what you mean or what you want to say.

Zero balancing
Most bodyworkers talk about emotions being held in the muscles of the fascia. Zero balancers, on the other hand, would say it is also held in the bone. If you would like a quite physical therapy but one which isn't as potentially painful as the previous three, then look at zero balancing. This might also appeal if you like the idea of energy-working—using the subtle energy of the body (chi) to clear away blockages.

It's common knowledge that too much rigidity in the body leads to stiffness, tension and often considerable discomfort or pain; we know we should keep our bodies flexible and relaxed.

But few of us ever think about the flexibility of our *energetic* body. For practitioners of zero balancing, however, your energetic body is just as important as the dense physical one, and when you lay on a zero balancer's couch you will be having not just your physical body adjusted but also its energetic counterpart.

The idea of an internal energy body lying alongside our physical frame is not new. The concept of the aura, a cocooning energy surrounding the body, goes back beyond biblical times. And the ancient Chinese and Indian systems of medicine have for thousands of years taught of the unseen lines of energy that underlie our veins and organs. Now even modern science is beginning to accept that there is more involved in organizing a body than mere sinew and bone.

Zero balancing was developed by Dr. Fritz Smith, an American physician, acupuncturist and osteopath who investigated a wide range of bodywork therapies and ancient energy systems before concluding that in order to effect real change he needed to combine the two approaches. The result is zero balancing, a system which works like esoteric engine oil, lubricating your body on every level, allowing your energy to flow steadily and easily. And it's not just your body which will appreciate a smoothly running energy system: tone up your vital energies, say the zero balancers, and your mind and emotions will undoubtedly follow suit.

It appears that our energetic system is just as complicated as our physical anatomy. Zero balancing teaches that there are three distinct kinds of energy vibrating through us: a background energy field (akin to the aura); a vertical energy flow which allows us to relate to the world around us; and an internal energy flow which circulates around the body. Within the internal flow there are three further, quite distinct levels: the deepest flows through the bone and bone marrow and brings together the skeleton as a complete functioning unit. The middle level runs through the muscles, nerves, blood and organs and corresponds directly with the Chinese concept of meridians, energy pathways connecting the soft tissue of the body. The superficial level controls the sweat glands and the energy in the tissues beneath the skin and acts as an insulation against the outside environment. If you regularly brush your skin (as described in MAY) you are doing your superficial energy level a great service: not only does skin brushing remove dead cells and tone your lymphatic system, it also clears and energizes this energetic system of your body.

With so much energy flying around the body it's no surprise to hear that problems can arise as easily in the energetic body as they can in the structural. Jeff Lennard, a zero balancer who works in London, explains that almost anything—from physical accidents to emotional traumas—can affect energy. A blow to the knee can cause physical damage but, long after the bruising has gone, the energy could remain twisted or stuck. And an emotional shock, such as bereavement, can equally remain caught in the energetic web, causing not just psychological stress but possibly physical stress and strain.

Lennard finds that zero balancing has a remarkable capacity to help people through times of change or difficulty. "It takes people very deeply into themselves," he says. "The minor chit-chat of the mind drops away and the clarity of an issue will often resolve itself. You come off the table knowing what you want." Its effects have been described as akin to deep meditation. But it's by no means purely mental. One of Lennard's clients, an Iyengar Yoga teacher, says one session on his couch is tantamount to two hours of vigorous yoga. And many people visit a zero balancer for quite mundane physical problems. Lennard has seen a singer who was told she was only using the muscles in one side of her neck—he found trapped energy caused her to hold her head undetectably to one side. Another client was a dancer suffering with a bad knee. To her surprise, as Lennard worked on her neck, she suddenly felt a release in the injured knee. Lennard was quite unfazed: "You don't ever know which part of the body will hold pain or trauma," he comments.

Zero balancing is a gentle, respectful therapy. All zero balancers must already hold recognized qualifications in other forms of health care, and many are registered osteopaths, acupuncturists, or masseurs. Treatment is given with the client fully clothed and there are no questionnaires to fill in, no need for painful soul-baring. Before my session, Lennard quietly asked me if there was anything I was concerned about or any part of my body causing me problems. Then he requested I take off my shoes and jewelry and sit on the couch while he felt my spine and gauged my energy.

After a few minutes I was invited to lie down on my back and relax. The zero balance touch is fundamental to the therapy: the practitioners seek to get into a dialogue with the client's energy system and together to balance the problem. The person undergoing treatment has as much to contribute to the process as the therapist. Lennard describes the touch as the "donkey-donkey touch." "It's like two donkeys walking up a hill," he says. "If they're on a steep slope, they will lean into each other to help get up the hill. Within this work we are doing it together."

Starting at the lower back, Lennard worked down my legs and into my feet and then up to the upper back and neck and then finished off back at the feet. Sometimes it felt like acupressure, shiatsu or osteopathy, at others akin to Rolfing or Hellerwork, but the touch *is* quite distinct. It goes deep, down to the bone, but is not at all painful. Lennard says one of its prime aims is to get people back in touch with their bodies and I could see what he meant. After a few minutes of his working on my lower back, I realized just how much stress and strain I hold there. And when he worked on my right knee I felt almost a buzzing in my head and recalled an old horse-riding accident which had left my right knee weak and liable to twist. More than anything, I felt very deeply relaxed. The zero balance touch is firm but comforting— it was as if my body took a deep breath and simply decided to flop into Lennard's hands, confident that it was safe and being nurtured.

Zero balancers are cautious people, loath to claim too much for their fledgling therapy. Lennard says it is not suitable for people with hip and knee replacements, those with epilepsy, ME or a history of cancer. "It doesn't make claims to heal serious illnesses," he insists, "and it is too much in its infancy to know if it could do that." However, if this is zero balancing in its childhood, it will be fascinating to see what this therapy will achieve once it grows up.

SHEN® THERAPY

Another new therapy which follows the energetic path is SHEN therapy. This involves even less bodily contact than zero balancing, so if you are not a very "physical" person or feel uneasy about even being touched, this could be for you. It's very, *very*

gentle—almost intangible. But the effects seem to be pretty powerful, nonetheless.

A scientifically researched form of energy healing, SHEN aims
to release emotions trapped in the body, allowing freedom from
pain and tension and a greater sense of confidence and ease into
the bargain. It has consistently good results with the kinds of
conditions that frequently won't respond to either medical or
psychiatric care; that is, any physical condition that has an emotional basis, be it chronic pain; irritable bowel syndrome; bulimia,
anorexia and other eating disorders; PMS; anxiety attacks and
phobias; post-traumatic stress syndrome and many cases of migraine. One of its most startling claims is that SHEN can halt
around sixty percent of migraines in the middle of an attack. Not
even powerful drugs can promise that.

So what is the secret of SHEN? At first sight, it appears no
different from numerous other complementary therapies. You lie
on a couch, fully clothed, while the practitioner merely lays his
or her hands on you in various positions. It seems just like spiritual healing or techniques such as reiki or jin shin jyutsu. The
difference, says Angela Renton who practices in Yeovil, Somerset,
is that SHEN is not mystical or God-given; it is precise and scientific, a happy marriage between the often inscrutable world of
ancient natural healing and highly sceptical modern science.

SHEN was developed by Richard Pavek, an American scientist
whose original disciplines were aeronautics, electronics and chemistry. His analytical mind found solutions for everything from
NASA's satellite launch vehicles, down to the humble television
set. However, living in America in the Sixties, Pavek was surrounded not only by science but also by a mind-boggling array of
alternative therapies and healing techniques. Intrigued but highly
sceptical, he decided to investigate. Healing, he realized, really
did seem to work in many cases but he was astonished to find
that the healers could not explain how or why their techniques
worked. The problem with healing, says Pavek, is that it shows
a "deplorable lack of science." He also pinpointed the one factor
that makes most doctors and scientists dismiss most alternative
and complementary medicine with its talk of "subtle energy,"
"life force energy" or "chi energy." "This energy has never been
directly measured with a measuring device," he states. "Technically, this is because no one has discovered a transducer [an

instrument which can convert energy into a measurable form] that will respond to this form of energy."

Fired by the challenge, he set out to discover the scientific rules behind healing. So far he has still not been able to precisely measure this elusive form of energy, but he has pinned it down further than most. Working on the laws of physics that state that magnetic and electrostatic fields move in a circulatory motion, Pavek reasoned that human energy patterns had to obey similar laws. He observed that all living things have an energy field which he calls the biofield. This biofield flows in certain set patterns. Observing thousands of healers he says, "We learned by trial and error that energy flows out of the right hand and into the left (in ninety-nine percent of people) and that the energy flows up the right-hand side of the body and down the left."

Having ascertained the nature of this energy, he became fascinated by the field of psychosomatic illness: disorders which have quite physiological symptoms but which cannot be traced to any mechanical, neurological or biochemical dysfunction in the body. It seemed clear that these conditions generally had an emotional component, but Pavek was unhappy with the idea, often held, that the patient was somehow mentally responsible for their condition. He noticed that while orthodox medicine and psychological approaches could do little for such patients, bodyworkers (whether masseurs or deep-tissue or bone manipulators) seemed to have the most success. This happened through the interesting by-product of their work that we have already discussed: while working on the body, they often found that they were releasing suppressed emotions alongside tense muscles or trapped nerves.

Pavek realized that when confronted by any shock or distress, whether physical or emotional, the body will often go into a kind of spasm, contracting around the pain or perceived hurt. Often the contraction will be automatically released but in many cases it becomes entrenched in the body. When this happens, over a period of time, quite physical changes occur: blood flow is impaired, toxins are unable to be released, tension and stress develop. However, because the brain has not been involved in the process, we are unable to release such contractions by conscious effort. Only by releasing the blockage with a clear flow of bioforce energy can the old hurt be released and the physical and emotional effects relieved. So while Rolfing *et al* shift the blockage by literally pressing and pushing it away, SHEN uses a more subtle energy.

The procedure is remarkably simple and actually very delightful. When I visited Angela Renton she explained how SHEN works and then asked me to fill in a surprisingly detailed questionnaire, quizzing me not only on my medical history but also on whether I had experienced any prolonged or unexpressed grief, any depression or insomnia, or any compulsive behavior, excessive worries or anxiety attacks. SHEN can treat almost anyone unless they are psychotic or suicidal. But practitioners won't treat you unless they are happy that you have a good support network at home or are working with a trained counselor or psychotherapist. The reason being that often old emotions can surface for days after the treatment and they need to be sure you will be supported if anything distressing comes up.

Next Angela invited me to take off my shoes and jewelry and lie on the couch, gently closing my eyes. I had driven for several hours before our meeting and was consequently feeling quite tense—I didn't think I'd be able to relax quickly, if at all. But within minutes I was totally de-stressed and floating in a kind of limbo, a curious half-dream, half-memory state. Scenes from my childhood unfolded alongside totally bizarre dream-like images. The SHEN touch is very light; there is no pressing or prodding, just a supportive feeling of holding as Angela moved from my head down my body. After a while I wasn't even aware of her hands, just of feeling totally relaxed and safe. I slid off the couch feeling deeply calm yet also alert and full of a quiet nourishing energy.

Angela stressed that it is hard to evaluate SHEN from one treatment and that practitioners like to give at least six closely spaced sessions before assessing how the treatment is progressing. However, I noticed quite perceptible—and surprising—results just a few days later. As a child I had a ferocious temper but over the years have gradually suppressed it until now I find it very difficult to express mild annoyance, let alone fully fledged anger. Yet, a few days after SHEN I found myself in the middle of Milan screaming my head off with righteous fury. It felt wonderful, as if I had rediscovered an essential part of my being. I shall certainly return to SHEN—who knows what I might rediscover next?

Where your emotions hit hardest

SHEN teaches that most emotions are held in the torso of the body. These are the main sites:

The heart The heart concerns our relationships with others; it is where we feel love but also pain, grief and the suppression of these emotions. When grief is not expressed fully, it has the potential to precipitate angina or more serious heart problems. Studies have shown that as many as sixty percent of patients in cardiac units suffered major grief within six months to a year prior to a heart attack. Suppressed grief can also lower T-cell activity—contractions around the heart suppress the activity of the thymus which activates the T-cells.

The solar plexus This relates to our relationship with the environment. This is the region where anger and fear are experienced. Repressed anger has long been suspected as a causal factor in stomach ulcers in which anger is turned inward and eats the self rather than the external antagonist. Anxiety attacks and phobias can often be healed after a few SHEN sessions focusing on deep-seated fears held in the solar plexus.

The kath (just below the navel) The kath deals with issues of your relationship with yourself and is the crucial center for self-confidence. It can also hold the bodily experiences of shame, lack of confidence, embarrassment, self-hatred and lack of self-worth. Often these feelings can be the root cause of PMS or colonic problems.

The root (the perineum) This concerns our existence on earth. It is affected by major life changes, moving house or relocating jobs. It also is activated by mortal, life-threatening terror. The root governs our most basic self-preservation urges. Post-traumatic stress syndrome is connected with this center, as is any kind of severe emotional shock. SHEN has even brought people out of comas, which have a strong emotional basis.

July

The fullness of the year, July, is the spirit of summer. Everything seems to be at its peak and passions are running high. Children have broken up from school; there are traffic jams on the motorways and queues to the seaside as a brief collective madness seems to sweep over the country. In the garden, summer assaults the senses—the sweet heavy scent of honeysuckle; the pure perfume of roses; the exotic miracle of passionflowers and the nose-twitching aroma of freshly cut lawns. For the Native Americans this is quite simply the Long Days Time.

If you can keep your cool and the temperatures don't rise too high, July can be a wonderful month, full of sheer *joie de vivre*. This is a good month to start thinking about your relationship with yourself, your levels of self-liking and self-esteem, and to start thinking about your relationships with others.

Boosting Self-esteem

If you have high self-esteem you can conquer the world. When you feel good about yourself, life becomes a challenge rather than a series of struggles; the world becomes a pleasant, exciting place rather than an alien, harsh, and dangerous environment. Our quota of self-esteem often dates back to our early years and the impressions we picked up as children. How our parents talked to us can affect everything from body image to social adeptness, while a schoolteacher's thoughtless behavior can totally scupper our future self-confidence in the workplace. By the time we reach adulthood we are frequently not even aware of how much or how little self-esteem we actually possess. Before you go any further, take a few minutes to answer the following questions honestly to discover your esteem quotient.

1. Is there a voice inside your head which exaggerates your weaknesses saying things like "you *always* say stupid things" or "you *never* make friends"?
2. Do you tend to devalue your work?
3. Do you find yourself "mind-reading" other people, imagining that they find you boring or are looking for excuses to leave?
4. Are you surrounded by people who treat you unfairly or take advantage of you?
5. Do you get angry or depressed if you are criticized?
6. Do you find it difficult to initiate sex or ask for what you want in bed?
7. Do you avoid challenges because you think you might fail?
8. Do you dwell on mistakes or missed opportunities?
9. Do you find yourself thinking everything would be better if you could only lose weight/get a new job/move house/ have children/get a better relationship?
10. Do you often give up your own interests in order to please other people?

If a large number of your responses are a resounding yes then you probably do have a problem with self-esteem. All the work you have already done should be helping (exercising, bodywork-ing, pampering, releasing emotions), but take some time also to think about the following.

AUDITING YOUR LIFE

Sit down with a large pad and mark each page with a different category: your appearance and body image; your personality; your work; your home life; your relationships; how you react socially and intellectually; and your sexuality. Then on one side of the page make a list of all your positive points, your virtues and strengths. On the other side list your negative points, your bad habits, vices and weaknesses.

Now examine your list.

• Which list is longest and in which areas are the negatives clustered? You may have good self-esteem in many areas but have one or two areas which need attention.
• Are your criticisms realistic or precise? Work through the list replacing negative words like "stupid" or "pathetic" with, for example, "I sometimes lack information" or "I get flustered in social situations."
• Take particular notice of your good points, amplify them and feel good about these aspects of your life.

THE INNER CRITIC

Our inner critic is the interior voice that monitors our every move and either approves or disapproves. A part of our brain that has usually been programmed in the past, the critic often links us to early authority figures such as parents.

Start to listen for the voice that tells you how stupid you are or what a failure you are or how ugly you are.

• Does it sound like anyone you know? Try to recognize the voice.
• Count the number of critical thoughts you have about yourself in a day and keep a thought diary for a while. At the end of the day, look at your list and work out the purpose behind

each thought. Was it goading you to do better, or was it giving you an excuse for not doing as well as you might? Was it protecting you from something?

• Start getting angry with your inner critic and silently shout at it every time it starts to attack. "Shut up!" often works, or simply recognize where the thought comes from—"this is just a lie my father/teacher/childhood friend told me."

REMODEL SUCCESS

Next make a list of your achievements in life, from learning to ride a bike or swimming a width, to having a baby or getting a new job. Write down half a dozen achievements and think back to how they made you feel. How exactly did you feel the day you passed your driving test? When you got the letter saying you'd got the job? When they put your baby in your arms? Remember precisely—how things looked, sounded, smelt, felt. Learn to recreate the feeling on demand and whenever you start to feel hopeless or useless bring back that feeling of achievement.

I always remember the surge of energy that ran through me when I heard my first feature was going to be published in a national newspaper. I put the phone down, punched the air and shouted "yes!" just like some salesman who's made a "killing." Shivers ran straight down my spine. Even all these years later, reconnecting with that precise feeling can totally alter my mood.

Your body image
Very few people feel totally happy with their bodies, and even top catwalk models can hate their shape. Mostly we have unrealistic expectations based on the images we see in magazines and on television.

• Look at the comments you made about your body in your audit. How realistic and specific are they? If you put down something like "I'm fat" ask what that really means. Change it to something like "I would ideally like to weigh ten stones" or "I have a thirty-four-inch waist."
• What is good about your body? Look in the mirror and, in-

stead of homing in on the "bad" bits, focus on the good parts.
Tell yourself you have great hair or lovely eyes, even superb feet.
• Pamper yourself. If we don't like something we tend to shut it
out, and many people treat their bodies like disliked machines. Think
about what your body really wants and needs, and then provide it:
nutritious, healthy food; ample, fun exercise; luxurious baths and
massages. You should be doing this by now anyhow. If you're not,
why not? What's stopping you? Ignore the voice (the inner critic again)
that says it's too expensive, too time-wasting, too self-indulgent.
Look on it as homework to begin with—something you *have* to do.

Your work

If your self-esteem plummets as soon as you walk through the
office door you need to pinpoint exactly why. Maybe you are
working with people who are critical or uncaring in their attitude
toward you. Ask why this has happened and whether you have,
in some way, invited the situation.

• Does the situation or the people involved remind you of
anything in your past? Many people find a strong link between
work and school.
• Ursula Markham, author of *How to Deal with Difficult People*,
advises that you analyze any criticisms and put-downs and work
out how much is justified. "If it's justified then accept the criticism
and put it right," she says, "but if it's judgmental, then ignore it.
No one has the right to personally attack you."
• At the end of each day write a list of your achievements.
Include everything, however small, and allow yourself to be impressed and approving of yourself.

Your social life

If you feel you go to pieces as soon as you enter a crowded
room, or that the moment you open your mouth you say something stupid, you're not alone. Most people feel, on some occasions, that they're simply not intelligent or interesting enough. I
won't lie and say that these tips will instantly turn you into a
social adept but they should help.

• Make sure you wear clothes which make you feel comfortable
and attractive. Don't use these occasions to try out your most

outrageous creation or to wear brand-new shoes which pinch. If in doubt, remember less is more and be discreet and polished rather than brash and over-the-top. Your clothes should serve you rather than take you over.

• "Recognize that being so self-conscious is actually selfish, because you are thinking of you and not of other people," says Ursula Markham. She advises that you visualize yourself feeling confident and talking happily with people.

• Pick out a person who is obviously ill at ease (there is always someone else) and make a beeline for them. Ask them questions and really listen to their answers. Do your best to make them feel comfortable, and you'll feel better in return.

• Check out your body language before you walk in a room. Imagine how you would look and feel if you really *were* confident. How would you walk? How would you hold yourself? Ten to one as you think about this you are automatically straightening your back and holding up your head. Paul Z. Jackson, who teaches people how to become more confident and self-assured, promises that it is very easy to give people the impression that you are much more confident that you really are. He advises you loosen up your whole body (pay particular attention to your jaw, hands, neck and shoulders) before you walk in anywhere— shake, stretch, yawn widely. Then walk in with a smile, attempting to make easy eye contact with people.

Your sexuality

Sadly our lack of self-esteem in this area is generally based on someone else's view, not our own. "Usually you can put it down to a former partner," says Ursula Markham. "It's not necessarily what that person actually said, it's what you told yourself when they went away."

• Reprogram your subconscious. Pick a phrase that strikes a chord, such as "I love myself and my sexuality." Repeat it silently to yourself over and over again. You may feel stupid but persist. Your subconscious will eventually pick up the message and start to act on it.

VISUALIZATION AND AFFIRMATION

These two techniques, says Ursula Markham, are very effective in building self-esteem. Both work directly on the subconscious mind, retraining it into a more positive outlook.

• Visualization simply involves imagining yourself in the situation in which you lack self-esteem. Take a few deep breaths and see yourself in your mind's eye making a brilliant speech at a meeting or chatting easily with people at a party. Really throw yourself into the scene, imagining the sounds, scents and feelings associated with it. See yourself succeeding—completely, utterly. Go back to this scene regularly.

• Affirmations are simply positive statements about yourself which you either repeat to yourself or write down regularly. They *sound* rather woolly but they do work. The most effective for self-esteem is the simple mantra "I love myself; I approve of myself." Repeat it silently to yourself as often as you like—some people do it around 200 times a day. Or stick up notes around the house or office to remind yourself how good you are: "People like me"; "I always succeed in my work"; "I have a beautiful, sexy body" all sound daft but can seriously change your subconscious beliefs about yourself. There will be more about affirmations later on.

Singing Yourself Happy

Back in May I talked about how to get in touch with your body and your emotions through dance. Now it's time to look at another art form: music, voice and song. Once again, you might be itching to skip on to the next section—the idea of singing is anathema to some people. I think that's really rather tragic. When we were children we sang for joy. We yelled if we were angry and we wailed if we got hurt. And yet, as adults, we rarely use a fraction of our voice. We learn not to cry or groan; we hate having to speak in public and if, for any reason, we have to sing, most of us squeak like mice or simply mouth the words.

And yet a growing band of researchers believe that by refusing to vocalize we are missing out on a simple, free and easy way to release stress, improve our moods and even heal ourselves. Learning how to express ourselves fully is an essential part of healing our emotions. Learning how to use our voices fully is the first step.

"Our voice is unique," says Susan Lever, who teaches people how to rediscover their natural voice. "It says so much about who we are; it's so personal that often people try to distort it. So many people try to copy other people's voices, have 'telephone' voices or try to get rid of dialects. They do it because often they have been given a lot of early messages that it's not OK to be who they are." A false voice is a stressed voice and, if we are straining our speaking voice, we are often massacring our singing voice. Lever points out that in earlier times, singing was a natural part of daily life: our predecessors sang as they worked, sang as they worshipped and sang for pleasure. There were songs for sowing, songs for harvesting; songs for work and songs for pleasure; songs of joy and songs of sorrow. Nowadays, with personal stereos, television and dwindling congregations in church, most people only sing if they go to harvest festival or midnight mass—or if they have one sherry too many.

"It's a great shame," says Lever, "because making sound can really change your mood. If you feel low and you make happy sounds, it will lift you without a doubt. Your breathing will automatically change and so will your physiological state. You will find you have a lot more energy, a lot more confidence and that you have a lot less stress."

Workshops are one way to get back into tune but Susan Lever points out that anyone can get off to a rousing start at home. The prime factor is to find your natural voice and relearn how to speak and sing without strain or effort. Often that involves relaxing and teaching yourself to let the voice come naturally from the whole body, rather than holding it tight in the throat. Learn to resonate. Once this happens, she warns, you might find some surprising side effects. "Often it starts to release long-standing blocks and tensions," she says. "If you have always spoken or sung from your throat, it is probably a protection mechanism. Start singing from your heart or your abdomen and you might find something else coming up—old grief, hurt, anger . . ." It sounds a little far-fetched, but in comparison to the latest theories in sound healing, it becomes quite banal. Researchers now believe that sound could be, quite literally, the medicine of the future.

"Disease is simply part of our body vibrating out of tune," says Jonathan Goldman, author of *Healing Sounds*. "Every organ, bone, tissue and other part of the body has a healthy resonant frequency. When that frequency alters, that part of the body vibrates out of harmony and that is what is termed disease. If it were possible to determine the correct resonant frequency for a healthy organ and then project it into that part which is diseased, the organ should return to its normal frequency and a healing should occur." He believes that by creating sounds which are harmonious with the "correct" frequency of the healthy organ, we could all learn how to heal ourselves, bringing our bodies back into balance. He and other sound researchers have been focusing most of their attentions on the sacred chants of varying traditions, believing that the high-frequency harmonics which most of them share could be having profound effects on both the mind and body.

Dr. Alfred Tomatis, a French physician and sound researcher, believes that Gregorian chants could actually have a neurophysiological effect which charges the brain. On researching sacred chanting around the world, he discovered that many of the chants were employing very high frequencies (around 8,000 Hz) which were capable of stimulating the central nervous system and the cortex of the brain. Dr. Tomatis himself says that he manages with less than four hours of sleep a night purely as a consequence of listening to four hours a day of harmonic sounds.

Dr. Mark Ryder of the Southern Methodist University in the USA discovered more benefits. By merely *listening* to music that was high in harmonic content his subjects reduced respiration and heart rate, calming and relaxing the entire brain and body. If you actually *make* the sounds yourself, the effects are even greater.

I tested out the theory with Jonathan Goldman's tape *Harmonic Journeys*. Sitting at my desk, wide awake and insomniac late at night, in a highly analytical (and somewhat sceptical) mode, I followed his instructions and joined him in toning different vowel sounds, imagining the sound coming from varying parts of the body. It started with a deep "uuh" sound resonating at the base of the spine and moved right through the body ending with a high "iiiii" from the top of the head. Within minutes I was deeply relaxed and it soon began to feel as though the sound was resonating *me* rather than I resonating the sound. I'm not sure how long the tape lasted because I totally lost track of time but, having finished it, I went straight to bed and had the best night's sleep I've had in months.

"Sound is vibration," says Goldman, "and everything in the universe is in a state of vibration." You can break a glass by matching its vibration and bring down a bridge by stamping out a rhythm over it, so he reasons that if you can destroy with sound, then there is no reason why you can't heal as well. Start with the odd hum, a few rounds of Bruce Springsteen in the bath and see where it ends. You could find yourself tuning up your whole life.

HUM YOURSELF HAPPY; SING YOURSELF SANE— DIY SOUND TECHNIQUES

- Humming is a good way of calming yourself. If you're feeling stressed, anxious or nervous just sit quietly and hum very gently. Feel the hum resonating through your body. Where can you feel it? Does it change if you alter the note of the hum?
- Exaggerated yawning is ideal if you're feeling tired. We hold a lot of tension in our jaws and mouths, and stretching the mouth releases tension. Give a good stretch as well to really wake up the whole body.
- If you're feeling irritable and tense, try an elongated, noisy sigh. Chris James, the Australian workshop leader, recommends deep groaning as well to release any negative emotions. The key is to forget about being polite and really let go.
- Take every opportunity to sing. Sing with the radio, while you're doing the housework, while you're in the bath or, even better, while you're driving in your car. Don't worry about what your voice sounds like, simply enjoy really belting it out.
- Try singing the different vowel sounds—uuuh, ooo, oooh, aaah, eeeeh, iiii. Where do you feel them in your body? How do they make you feel?
- Play with mantras—you don't need to do "Omm" or anything spiritual—simply try singing positive statements, repeating them

with different tunes. If you're feeling tense, try singing "I'm calm,
I'm calm"; if you need to feel more assertive, try "I've got a right
to be heard."

• Experiment with listening to different music and work out
what effect it has on your moods. Try listening to some of the
sacred chants available on tape for deep relaxation and a profound sense of peace.

The Power of Play

As this time of the year is the natural time for holidays and fun,
the "work" for this month and August are really intended to be
carried out in a very light-hearted fashion. However, just because
they may seem frivolous doesn't mean that they won't have deep
effects on your life. A case in point is play. Quite seriously, I
would love you to try to introduce more play into your life, more
silliness, more frivolity. If it sounds like another dose of born-
again childhood following swiftly after the singing and groaning
exercises, that's exactly the idea.

When we were very young we imagined there were fairies at
the bottom of the garden. We read books by torchlight under
the covers and raided the fridge for midnight feasts. Every new
day was an adventure; the world seemed packed with wonder
and life was full of play. Then we grew up. The fairies moved
out and noisy neighbors moved in. We took business reports to
bed and gave up disgusting habits like scoffing jam sandwiches
at midnight. In the adult world playtime seems as extinct as the
dinosaurs. We're all working too hard and too long; we're too
busy hanging on to our jobs to think about hanging upside down
on a climbing frame. And when we *do* take time off work we
call it leisure or sport and work damn hard at that too: stoically
pounding the stairmaster at the gym to lose weight; hurling ourselves around the squash court; drinking ourselves silly as we
desperately try to relax. And do we feel better? Unlikely.

Many therapists and psychologists say that the best thing we
could do is to relearn how to play. It's not a case of being childish
but rather of seeing the world from a childlike perspective—as

a place of endless wonder and joy. Far from opting out, it's about choosing to live life at full tilt, giving it your all and getting the lion's share back.

Play is taken very seriously and studiously in the academic world. Scientists have found that if you possess the ability to look life in the eye and giggle you will probably be far more confident and creative; you are also more likely to possess a comforting sense of spiritual peace. What's more, researchers at the universities of Texas and Southern Illinois found that a healthy sense of play could promote "cohesiveness within a couple's relationship" and that "the loss of playfulness in a marriage was strongly correlated with the onset of marital dysfunction." Take away the psychobabble and what they are saying is that those who play together, stay together.

Play works in the office as well. Tests have shown that working with a relaxed, playful attitude can help people solve problems, master new skills and cope more effectively with difficult new situations. And when creative people such as engineers and designers are put in a more playful, more relaxed work environment, tests prove they produce higher quality work and far more original ideas.

Robert Holden, who pioneered the Stressbuster Clinics and is the author of *Laughter, The Best Medicine,* is not surprised. "Life is often described as a classroom," he says, "but it is also a playground. The spirit of fun can be our greatest resource for inspiration, energy, creativity, self-realization, development and growth." He is so convinced by the power of play that he frequently prescribes it as essential medicine for chronically stressed and sick patients. "Play can be a therapy, a medicine and a natural healer that promotes humor, happiness and wholeness," he insists. "An absence of fun, little or no playtime and a lack of laughter are common symptoms of stress, sickness and disease."

But why do we stop playing? Isn't it just a natural part of growing up? "We stop playing because society tells us we can't do these things any more," says David Sumeray who runs "Play World" workshops designed to get people back in touch with the spirit of play. "It's a legacy that has been handed down for generations—work is the important thing and play is something you do in your spare time." Psychologist Ann-Marie Woodall says the conditioning starts very young: "We're taught as kids to be careful, to watch out, so the world out there becomes frightening and serious. As we grow up that idea becomes lodged and makes us scared of letting go and playing."

The result, says Woodall, is that we become blocked from enjoying life to the full and from realizing our true potential. She firmly believes that rediscovering spontaneity and playfulness can make even the modern world a place where dreams come true. However, she points out, it's not just a case of putting on a silly hat and going through the motions. You really need to access that deep, hidden part of yourself that knows how to laugh with innocence and play with total abandon.

TAPPING INTO THE MIRACLE MIND

To rediscover our sense of play, says Woodall, we need to distinguish between what she calls the "ego mind" and the "miracle mind." According to Woodall, the miracle mind is the "real" us, the part of us that knows, deep down, that we are good enough, that we can succeed. As children it was the part of our minds that allowed us to reach out, to explore and play; it gave us our sense of self. Truly creative and successful people hang on to the miracle mind and tap into it through adult life as well. It's the miracle mind that let's them take chances with life and win; that prompts them to say "Let's go for it," rather than "Well, I'm not sure . . ."

On the other hand, the majority of us spend our lives being controlled by the "ego mind." The ego mind has a valid role—to save us from dangerous situations—but often it becomes over-developed in childhood and takes over our lives, making us scared of new challenges, wary of new people and terrified of making idiots of ourselves. Woodall laments that we all carry subconscious messages of childhood locked in our heads—"Act your age"; "Don't be stupid"; "Sit down and be quiet." But, she says, if we learn to listen to the miracle mind and trust its urges and desires then the whole world becomes one vast playground.

Both Woodall and Sumeray warn, however, that even grownup play might just end in tears before bedtime. "Starting to play again is not all just good simple fun," says Sumeray. "It's about listening to our hearts and finding out what we really want from life. And when we do that the changes can be radical." He has often seen people change career paths after learning how to play. Some also alter, or even end, their relationships. "When people get in touch with parts of themselves they have denied for years, sometimes they can't continue with their normal lifestyle," he says. "Yes, relationships can end, jobs can end. It can change your life."

LEARNING TO PLAY AGAIN

Don't expect to change your life overnight or to become abundantly playful by making purely cosmetic changes.

• Check out your play quotient. How much do you play in your life right now? When did you last do something just for fun, just for the hell of it? Do you play in certain areas of your life but not in others? Do you have fun and games with friends while your relationship is strictly serious? Can you behave like an idiot at home but turn strait-laced and tight-lipped when you walk into the office?

• Get in touch with your miracle mind. In her workshops, Ann-Marie Woodall gives everyone a sock which is turned into an "ego snake" by adding large eyes and a forked tongue. "Use it as a reminder of what's really holding you back," she says. "Whenever you feel you can't do something or can't let go and enjoy something, look at your ego sock-snake and ask yourself what's stopping you—is it really you or is it just the part of your mind that censors you?" Keep the sock on your desk or on top of the fridge or somewhere close as a reminder of what stops you enjoying life.

• Robert Holden recommends you start every day with what he calls the "Newness of Life" game. He suggests we try to see each day as a newborn child would see the day—as a new day that has never happened before. He recommends that we ask ourselves "What can I look for, listen for, think about and do that is new today?"

• Cultivate spontaneity. Every day, allow yourself to do at least one thing that you want to do "just for the hell of it." "Be yourself," urges Ann-Marie Woodall, "even if it's only for five minutes a day."

• What did you enjoy most when you were a child? Did you paint or act or sing or dance? Why not take them up again? Often we feel we can't be creative as adults because we're "not good enough." Drop the idea of perfection or competition and just enjoy yourself. Or did you enjoy sports—netball, hockey, cross-country running, football? Play them again—you don't have to win, simply enjoy the game.

• Turn your work into a fun factory. Fun may still be a dirty word to many companies and if your boss or colleagues look like they permanently suck lemons, simply play solo. Imagine the people you work with as just a bunch of kids in the playground—they will seem more human, and dealing with them will become far easier. If you hate your boss, imagine her or him when they were young, as a schoolkid—it will put them in perspective and might give you an insight into their behavior.

• Use creative stupidity in your work. When you have to come up with plans or ideas, don't limit yourself to thinking in the normal, logical, sensible way. Instead, make yourself invent the most ridiculous things as well. "Being silly helps to keep the mind young, fresh, alive and relatively unconditioned," says Robert Holden. "It often inspires creativity, original thought, invention and innovation." And, if you're the boss, never ever shout someone down for "being silly"—encourage even sillier ideas. One might just be the next Coca-Cola or Wonderbra.

• Above all, don't work too hard at learning to play—that defeats the whole object. Simply open up a small corner for play in your life and see what happens. It won't ever be quite the same as it was when you were six but you could just capture a fragment of the joy and wonder and enchantment. And, as you play more and more, the fragments could join up until, once again, the world becomes a joyful place in which to live.

RETURNING TO THE PLAYGROUND

Start small. Try the following suggestions as tiny steps to reintroduce play into your life.

For yourself
• Reread a favorite childhood book, or all of your old favorites.
• Get out videos of your favorite childhood movies and watch them in the afternoon with a choc ice, a bottle of pop and a bag of popcorn (OK, it's not very healthy but once in a blue moon it won't hurt).
• Sing while you drive the car—at the top of your voice.
• Dance to records on the radio; grab a hairbrush and pretend you're the lead singer.
• Wear a wig or hat—it changes the way you feel and act.
• Plant mustard and cress in the shape of your name and watch it grow.
• Play mermaids in the bath.

At work
• Smile and greet everyone as you come in the office.
• Find something to compliment in all of your workmates.
• Bring in a huge tray of cakes or cookies and have a tea party with your morning or afternoon break. You could ice people's names on their "own" cakes. Yes, it's sugary things again, I know, but the trouble is that these were our "treats" as kids. Once again, the odd occasion won't hurt. You could always try to find a healthier alternative—I can't quite think of one myself!
• At meetings suggest that you have five minutes for "utterly ridiculous" ideas. Often the most creative ideas come when people stop trying to be sensible.
• Pin your favorite cartoon to your computer or noticeboard.
• Surround yourself with things that make you smile or giggle.
• Do little things that help your workmates but keep them secret.

With friends
• Spend a day at the seaside—with buckets and spades. (If it's cold, don't let that put you off—just wrap up.)
• Go to a funfair and try all the rides and all the sideshows. Eat toffee apples (yes, once again!) and get sticky.
• Buy a kite and go flying.
• Play ping-pong instead of squash. Play charades instead of chess.
• Find a pool with slides and wave machines, and frolic.

• Sing opera—even if you can't sing. Turn normal conversations into operatic nonsense.

With your partner
• Find a wild moor or a local park and play Cathy and Heathcliff.
• When you meet in a cafe or bar, pretend you're meeting for the first time and that it's passion/lust/love at first sight.
• Draw pictures with your fingers on each other's back and get the other person to guess what you're drawing.
• Indulge in more and more ridiculous pet names and keep changing them.
• Tell each other about your childhood. Get out the old photos and really reminisce.
• Hide under the bedcovers and tell each other ghost stories.
• Find out what your partner's favorite toy was as a child and buy him/her one for his/her birthday or Christmas.

Holidays, Health and Happiness

Of course holidays are (or should be) the ultimate form of play. Ten to one at this stage of the year your mind may be skipping off the idea of shifting emotions and purifying diets and veering off to warm seas and blue skies. All quite natural as this is the start of the great holiday season. Hopefully, you'll be so into eating well and exercising by now that you'll want to continue on holiday. Most people imagine that for some reason holidays are, by necessity, times when you eat appallingly and pile on weight and toxins. Not necessarily. Most of our favorite holiday destinations are renowned for their wonderful healthy cuisine. Generally speaking, eat where the locals eat; go easy on the ice cream and the local liqueurs and you shouldn't go too far wrong. Take the opportunity to have fun with exercise. Whether you go for long walks, swim in the pool or take up a new and exciting sport, there are plenty of opportunities to enjoy yourself while keeping fit. Inevitably you will probably eat and drink more than you would at home—that's part of the fun of being away, so don't beat yourself up about it. And if all you feel like doing is collapsing on a beach mat, then go ahead and do it.

Interestingly, you may find that although you are not consciously trying to think about your emotions or your life, thoughts may well come up. Holidays can often be a time when we take stock of our lives. The normal everyday clamor and clutter is removed and we are left with ourselves. Often it is the only time we have the luxury to sit and do absolutely nothing. And when we do nothing is often the time that thoughts and feelings emerge.

Generally, this is a good and positive occurrence. You might find it useful to keep a notebook with you and jot down any thoughts that crop up and to take notice of any strange or vivid dreams you have. Sometimes, however, holidays can cause less positive reactions and, without wanting to sound like a killjoy, its worth at this point, briefly outlining the potential problems that can occur. Forewarned is forearmed.

How many times have you set off on holiday perfectly healthy and then fallen down with flu on the second day? Mainstream doctors would say it's just coincidence or a bug you pick up at the airport, but alternative practitioners accept that the body's energy levels and immune system can be affected by a sudden change of environment. They are far more cautious about advising overstressed clients to fly off and collapse in the sun for a mini-break. Acupuncturist Felicity Moir explains the syndrome: "When you are working you keep pushing yourself. Despite the fact that you are under stress and overtired your energy keeps flowing. However, when you stop suddenly you lose that energy flow and you get to your base energy level which may be very weak. That is when it is easy for illness to get in." In Western medical terms we would say our immune system is weakened; in the Chinese system it is considered that the body is out of balance, when the "evils" of damp, cold, heat and wind have a chance to manifest.

The most frequent holiday sicknesses are simple but debilitating colds and flu, although Felicity Moir also points to other common ailments. "It is well known amongst Chinese practitioners that fluids can accumulate in the body and these manifest on holiday as sinus problems, coughs and chest infections."

Felicity also agrees that life issues and emotional problems can also be highlighted on holiday: "When you are working you don't have time to stop and think about your life. When you go away you suddenly have time to think about what's going on in your life and frequently people don't like what they find out."

The problem, it seems, is that the odd week or two a year of holiday is simply not enough. Nowadays we are working so hard (not necessarily physically harder than in the past but certainly mentally and stressfully) that we do not allow ourselves enough rest and recuperation time throughout the year. "People don't rest properly after a cold or flu," points out Felicity. "They race back to work because we have this ridiculous work ethic. It's not a good idea in the long term because the immune system cannot recover and even if the acute symptoms have gone, illnesses will lock into the system and manifest at a later date.

"People push themselves beyond reasonable limits: they work nights and weekends or take work home; they work through lunch; they eat late or on the run. Then, if they just stop, the body is thrown into imbalance."

Stressed-out workaholics should learn how to relax in easy stages. Psychotherapist Kati Cottrell-Blanc recommends you ease yourself into rest. "Do it gradually," she says. "Start by taking an afternoon off for a swim, then ease yourself into exercise. Progress to taking weekends off and finally a whole week. You have to ease the body into rest rather than shock it."

Felicity Moir suggests that if you can only take a week's break you should opt for an active holiday. "Go skiing or, better still, take a walking holiday. You get the benefit of the holiday because you are changing your environment and you're not doing mental work. You rest the mind but keep the energy moving."

In a perfect world, she says, we would have at least five weeks' holiday a year: "Two one-week holidays which are active. If you can afford it a week, say, skiing at Christmas and a week swimming and walking at Easter would be ideal. Then you need a good three-week holiday. You need one week to be ill, one to recover and one more to build up your energy."

It sounds mad doesn't it? Only now in the paranoid run-up to the millennium could we have holiday trauma! Yet think about it. In the old days the problem didn't arise because, firstly, we didn't lead such highly stressed lives. People worked hard, but it was mainly physical work rather than continued, concentrated mental effort. It's much easier to relax your body than your brain. Secondly, if people went away on holiday at all it was to resorts in this country and they traveled by car or train. Now we jet off without a thought: our bodies are used to British summertime and we throw them suddenly into Caribbean heatwave or Nordic chill. No wonder they get thrown off balance. Obviously I'm not going to suggest you swap your hard-earned break in the Bahamas for a couple of weeks in Bournemouth (although there are plenty of beautiful places to discover in the British Isles). But just be aware of the potential problems and try to forestall them before they arise.

HOW TO AVOID THE SUN, SEA AND STRESS SYNDROME

Stress-management consultant Ursula Markham suggests the following ten-point plan for holiday relaxation.

1. Give yourself plenty of time to put things in order before you leave. Arrange for your work to be covered, someone to feed the cat and water the plants. Don't leave it to the last minute and panic.
2. When you arrive, don't race straight out and drink to relax. Lie down and slow yourself down, do a relaxation exercise and then, and only then, have that drink—and really enjoy it.
3. Don't take work on holiday with you. Read something you really enjoy and make sure it's escapist—nothing to do with reality.
4. Wear clothes that are completely different from your usual attire. If you normally wear sober suits, take something bright and cheerful.
5. For the first few days it's quite usual for worries to come into your mind, but develop a system of mentally putting things on one side. As each worry surfaces, actually write it down so you can see it in black and white. Then either deal with it or decide it's out of your control. Once you've made your decision throw the paper away.
6. If you just can't switch off, practice simple relaxation techniques. Make yourself comfortable and shut your eyes.

Start by breathing deeply and easily; go systematically through the body, relaxing all your muscles, and then imagine yourself in a beautiful, calm, safe place (for once with these kinds of exercises you are quite likely to be physically in a beautiful place as well). Stay there for ten minutes or so and then slowly bring yourself back. If you find this hard there are plenty of relaxation and visualization tapes which can help.

7. Remind yourself that life will go on without you. People like to think they're indispensable, but reassure yourself that there is very little which can go wrong that cannot be corrected.

8. Exercise can be a good source of relaxation but only do what you find fun and what makes you feel good.

9. Don't forget that essential play factor—splash in the water, build sandcastles, lose your inhibitions. If you've got children, you have the ideal opportunity to join in with them and go back to being a child.

10. As long as you aren't hurting anyone else, a certain amount of self-indulgence on holiday is a good thing. Whether it's getting up at silly times or eating the odd rich meal when you're on a diet it won't hurt.

WATCH OUT: HOW HOLIDAYS CAN BE BAD FOR YOUR HEALTH

1. Exposure to the sun accounts for eighty percent of skin aging, and melanoma is becoming one of the most common cancers amongst Caucasians. Follow the guidelines given earlier on keeping safe in the sun.

2. Unprotected exposure to UVB light can trigger cataracts and other ocular problems. Eye strain and headaches can also appear on holiday. "There is more glare abroad," says Bob Hutchinson of the Federation of Ophthalmic and Dispensing Opticians. "We are not used to reflections off buildings and the sea and they make us peer and squint. Also, if someone has bad eyesight and is faced with a new environment they could strain their eyes." Make sure your sunglasses are good quality and that they filter both UVA

and UVB light. Again, wear a hat or baseball cap to minimize the glare.

3. Jet lag dries the skin, dehydrates your body and can cause
   irregular sleeping patterns. It can make your feet swell and
   cause your joints to ache and become stiff. Try to avoid
   drinking alcohol or caffeine on the flight. Stick to pure
   mineral water and lots of it. Wear loose comfortable
   clothes and slip off your shoes while you fly (pack a warm
   pair of socks in your hand luggage in case your feet get
   cold). Aromatherapy can help. Aromatherapist Valerie Ann
   Worwood suggests that before you leave for your flight
   you should have a bath with a couple of drops of peppermint or eucalyptus. When you arrive at your destination
   she advises you stay awake until local bedtime and have
   a bath with a drop each of lavender and geranium before
   you go to bed. Continue with this routine (peppermint or
   eucalyptus in the morning and lavender and geranium at
   night) until your body adapts to local time. If you prefer
   to shower, then put the oils in your hand (added to a few
   milliliters of base oil such as almond) and rub them all
   over your body after you have showered but before you
   dry off.

August

The year has ripened, come to its zenith and now arrives the harvesting season. The Native Americans called the first part of August the Ripening Time and then, as it slides into September, the Harvesting Time. In the countryside these names come to life: the fields bustle with activity; combine harvesters lumber like dinosaurs through the golden acres; big bales of corn balance on tractors which rumble slowly along the high-hedged lanes. There are rabbits darting everywhere and larks flying up from the stubble as you walk. In the garden, the pure blues and pinks of early summer are shifting into warmer tones—deep reds and yellows, the purple of Michaelmas daisies and the overindulgent overblown deep blue of morning glory clambering through the trees. The nights are long and balmy, hazy with warmth and only marred by the clouds of midges and buzzing and biting of persistent mosquitoes.

Despite the activity in the fields, August is somehow a lazy month. It's almost a point of stasis—nothing can get any bigger, any fuller, so for a brief moment you just luxuriate and enjoy. It's a time of sensuality—a sense of ease pervades the body and the emotions. Properly speaking, with the festival of Lammas launching this month, it's also a time of thanksgiving, a time to think about your life with a sense of deep gratitude. A time to ponder on what you take from life and what you can possibly give back in return. August is a gathering month in all senses of the word. While the corn is being gathered from the fields it's also a time for you to gather your thoughts in readiness for the next big shift of the year. This is a time to start thinking about what you demand from life, from your body, from the people around you, from yourself—and what you give back. Maybe it's also a time to start to consider what you need to do to change.

The festival of Lammas which falls on August 1 is the festival of Harvest. It is also known in the Celtic tradition as Lughnasadh. Lammas is a Saxon name which comes from Loafmas, the first loaf of the harvest, made from the new corn. The old traditions suggest that we think deeply about what we take from life. Every day, life forms have to die to keep us alive, even if we are vegetarians. There's nothing wrong in this and no guilt implied; it's simply that this is a good time to give thanks for our life and the lives that are given to nourish us. It's a little like a major version of a blessing before eating. Incidentally, blessing your food before mealtimes is a lovely little ritual that keeps this festival alive throughout the year. Offering thanks for our "daily bread" is a ceremony that is carried out throughout the world, in almost all religions. It doesn't have to be a standard blessing— in fact it's probably better to avoid simply galloping through "For what we are about to receive may the Lord make us truly thankful" which has become almost meaningless to most of us. Take it in turns to say thank you in whatever way you like. Children might like to find a short poem; adults might simply like a few seconds silence or a quiet thank you. Extend your thanks to the cook as well! But keep it short and sweet—no one wants a cold dinner.

Pagan priestess and therapist Shan suggests that this is also a good time to think about the people who give to you (whether physically or emotionally) throughout the year. Is there any way you can give anything back to them? Or maybe you could just show your appreciation with a special thank you or a little card or note. Equally, she says, we can give back to nature, to the special places we love. If you have a favorite spot you like to visit, can you do anything to help it? Perhaps you could clear some rubbish? One lovely little ritual is to make a little posy of flowers or choose a particularly beautiful pebble or make a ring of twigs and leave it as a present for any place you find particularly sacred or special. There are certain places I visit which are very magical for me—small spots which always seem to recharge my batteries and give me a shot of love and courage. It may sound silly or fanciful but they really do make a difference to the way I feel. And I always take something with me: a daisy chain to lay on the water of a natural spring; a beautiful leaf or a speckled stone to set in the middle of a copse.

The Joy of Juice

Make sure you enjoy the abundance of August in all its ways. Soft fruits are plentiful now, and there can be nothing more delicious than a bowl of freshly picked strawberries or raspberries. As it's August, go on and have a dollop of cream or, if one dollop is never enough, choose healthier options (but still delicious) such as crème fraîche or creamy Greek yogurt.

We've talked about juices already in this book but it's worth recapping and introducing some more information here. August is a good month to discover (if you haven't already) the wonder of fresh juicing. Not just the traditional fruit juices but vegetables as well. Not only are they delicious but they are a great way to get lots of vitamins (particularly those essential antioxidants) without having to chomp your way through pounds of steamed vegetables. They also have individual health-giving properties of their own.

Many naturopaths say that a day a week on a diet of vegetable juices will be beneficial to anyone. They usually recommend you have about 500–700 ml up to a liter a day. Take the juice in sips throughout the day, don't just gulp it down. In addition make sure you drink plenty of water. You could also supplement the juice with weak rose hip tea to help elimination through the kidneys. But why is vegetable juice so wonderful? In general, vegetables are highly alkaline in their nature and have the ability to bind acids and eliminate them through the kidneys and urine.

So it's not surprising that alkaline vegetable juice can be so useful for people who suffer from rheumatism and arthritis.

THE SUPER-JUICES

Carrot juice Carrot juice really is a bright orange miracle. The essential oils in carrots have an effect on the mucous membranes of the body and stimulate the circulation of blood in the stomach and intestinal tissues. Because of this balancing action, carrot juice is also good for constipation and diarrhea and all sorts of digestive problems. Often when the digestion is sorted out, other problems disappear. Many people find their headaches, eczema and bad skin all vanish when the digestion is functioning properly. If you suffer from frequent coughs and colds, remember carrot juice—it is refreshing and soothing and helps battle against infectious diseases. Packed full of antioxidant vitamins, it is a feisty fighter against the free radicals that cause disease and aging. And its rich supplies of carotene (provitamin A) improve the eyesight and stimulate the production of rhodopsin (visual purple), the lack of which causes night-blindness. As if all that were not enough, carrot juice is said to help balance your weight and to give a beautiful complexion—certainly worth trying.

Beetroot juice The dark purple juice may look unappetizing, but don't let its appearance put you off. Beetroot contains betaine which stimulates the function of the liver cells, protecting the liver and bile ducts. One-hundred millligrams of beetroot juice contains 5 mg of iron in addition to trace elements which encourage the absorption of iron in the blood. Everyone can benefit from beetroot juice but it is particularly recommended in the first two years of life, during puberty, during pregnancy, when breast-feeding and during the menopause. Children from six months to two years need only a teaspoon of juice before meals.

Celery juice Celery is alkaline and encourages elimination and so it is recommended for any diseases or problems connected with an accumulation of wastes and toxins, for instance rheumatic and arthritic ailments. It also regulates the water balance in our bodies and is superb for elderly people.

Tomato juice Tomato juice is acidic, so it is not recommended for arthritic or rheumatic conditions. In addition, quite a large number of people find they are intolerant of tomato. However, it has interesting properties. The old herbalist say it can help with overtiredness and combat unpleasant body odor. They also suggest it is a protection against premature aging. It is a lovely refreshing juice which cleanses the body

Of course you can experiment with a wide variety of juices. Naturopaths will often recommend particular combinations, and polarity therapy, a therapy that combines elements of naturopathy, Ayurveda and other Eastern influences strongly advocates the use of fresh natural fruit and vegetable juices to aid healing and general health. The following are recommended by the founder of polarity therapy, Randolph Stone:

For constipation: cabbage, spinach, celery and lemon juice.
For skin conditions: carrot, beetroot and celery juice.
For arthritis: carrot, celery and cabbage juice.
For high blood pressure: celery, beetroot and carrot juice.
For low blood pressure: carrot, beetroot and dandelion juice.
For asthma and catarrhal conditions: carrot and radish juice.
To open up sinuses and air passages: horseradish and lemon juice (100 g of horseradish and 50 ml of lemon juice, combined with one teaspoon of garlic juice and a tablespoon of honey; take a teaspoonful four times daily).
To help you sleep: celery juice.
To soothe the nerves: lemon and lime juice.
For sore throats and colds: lemon, lime and pineapple juice.

Living Your Life with Passion

The whole natural world is full to bursting in August: nothing is held back, nothing is begrudged or stinted. And we can learn a lot by watching this wholesale giving. There are times when we need to conserve our physical energy but this isn't one of them. And it is certainly not a time to hold back emotionally. In fact, if we learn to live life with pure passion and joy, we could find life a much more delightful place. Reclaim the passionate part of your inner self, and life will become more vivid, more exciting, more lucrative and definitely more sensual.

We have all been amazed and impressed by passionate people—the kind who are so full of life and the joys of living that they virtually leave us breathless. Well, why shouldn't we all have that sense of wonder and delight? It doesn't mean that we have to become different people, we just need to introduce a little verve and enthusiasm into our daily lives. If you followed the guidelines for reintroducing play into your life which I outlined in July, this should be pretty easy. If not, you might like to go back and look at the two in tandem because really they are two sides of the same coin. It may sound strange but passion and play go hand in glove. People think of passion as something that has inevitably to do with sex, with wild romance, plunging necklines and scorching kisses. Well yes, it is, but passion itself is much deeper than just sex. It should touch every corner of our lives.

I learned a great deal about the power of passion from the American lecturer and workshop leader Denise Linn, who is the living embodiment of passion. A five-minute conversation with her is enough to kick-start your whole week. Denise travels the world teaching everyday timid souls how to let rip and let passion rule. "A lot of people associate passion with sex," she agrees, "and that *is* part of it but it's far more. Passion is about living life to the full; it's about excitement; about making life really worth living."

But surely passion is something you simply either have or you don't have? How can you *learn* to be passionate? Linn explains that the problem is that although as children we are naturally passionate creatures, as we go through our teens and into adult life we gradually learn *not* to be passionate. We are taught that to be an adult is to be calm, in control, rational, considered—even cynical. The passion is inexorably drawn out of us until we have forgotten what it means to cry at a sunset, to become lost in a painting, to giggle like a child.

"We get caught with cultural conditioning," says Linn. "We're told we should be responsible, we shouldn't have too much fun. We learn that life is supposed to be serious and, if you're having fun, then you're not taking care of your responsibilities." Society regards passion as emotion out of control, as an irrational force

that, left to run wild, would grind industry to a halt within the
day. In fact, says Linn, quite the opposite is true. Live your life
with passion and you will become more effective in your work,
more pleasant to live with and, most importantly, you will enjoy
life to the full.

Her workshops have evolved over almost twenty years, ex-
panding from short seminars into full two-day weekend workshops. The one I attended started off inauspiciously: around fifty
people of all ages sitting quietly and politely in a large hall.
Hardly anyone was talking and, apart from one woman in a
bright red flamenco skirt, no one looked even remotely passionate. But Linn swiftly had us divide into small groups and asked
us to find out what made each other passionate. Looks are decep-
tive, and once our group warmed up, they transformed. One
woman talked about her children, about how she had put her
whole life into them but how, in quiet moments, she wished she
could still paint and draw. A man in a somber business suit talked
quietly but emotionally about his father, a strong quiet man who
had been a farmer all his life and had died a few years ago. Ten
minutes into the workshop and people were laughing, even crying and the whole room was full of noise and emotion.

Linn teaches at a fast pace and always through direct involve-
ment. If you don't like talking to strangers or cringe at the idea of
doing stupid things in public, then this isn't for you—or maybe,
perversely, it is *exactly* what you really need. Certainly, at times,
I would have wished myself a million miles away. Part of reclaiming passion involves learning how to take risks, how to dare
to make a fool of yourself and just let go. So we found ourselves
making stupid faces in one process, feeding each other food in
another. One strategy had us simply standing in front of the
group, saying nothing. It sounds easy, but for some people having fifty pairs of eyes boring into them was just too much. One
woman almost fainted; a man had to rush out the room to be
sick.

Quite what this has to do with passion may seem unclear, but
Linn insists that by learning to confront our fears of looking stupid, of making fools of ourselves, we can begin to take risks in
life. Once we believe we can stretch ourselves and do more, we
can start to find out what we really want to do with our lives;

instead of living life safely, we will begin living passionately, to the full.

Linn uses every technique she can summon up to put people in touch with their feelings: from creative visualization to past life regression (see JANUARY). After the event, people report many changes. Some simply allow themselves to take up hobbies they had dropped through lack of time or because they thought they were frivolous. One woman took up opera singing and now spends all her spare time with her local amateur opera group; another always fancied belly-dancing and now regularly transforms her living-room into a scene from the Arabian nights. Some simply give themselves time and permission to enjoy life a little more—taking in a movie, enjoying a massage, sitting doing nothing for an hour or so. But others find their lives totally transformed. One businessman gave up his high-powered city job and went traveling for a year. When he returned he retrained and became a teacher. He earns a sixth of the salary but loves every moment of his days. Other people re-evaluate their relationships and make profound changes; most say simply that their relationships improve, but occasionally someone finds that after the workshop, they need to leave the relationship altogether.

THE TEN-POINT PLAN FOR RECLAIMING PASSION

1. Look back and remember what made you passionate as a child. Tune in to that sense of childhood joy and maybe try reclaiming some of those activities.
2. Think about what you are passionate about now. What activities make you really "lose" yourself? What causes are you passionate about? Get involved.
3. What stops you from being passionate? Work out what beliefs or anxieties prevent you from living with passion.
4. Take risks. Even small risks help you to push through your fear boundaries and gain confidence. Be willing to make mistakes.
5. Be kind. Random acts of kindness (leaving a flower on a desk at work, feeding a stranger's parking meter if it's run out) have a chain reaction, making everyone feel good.

6. Make a commitment to incorporate activities you really enjoy into your life.
7. If you hate your job, find something—however small—that you can enjoy in it.
8. Imagine you were at the end of your life, looking back. What would have given you fulfilment that you didn't do? What would you regret not having done? Why not do it now?
9. Maintain passionate relationships by keeping your imagination alive. Be spontaneous every so often—whisk your partner off for a picnic, buy a surprise present.
10. Get in touch with your body. Experiment with movement and music. Jitterbug around your kitchen, pretend you're Torville and Dean. Dance is a wonderful means of freeing our straitjacket self.

Biodynamic Therapy and Watsu: Two Unusual Ways of Touching Your Emotions

Throughout the summer you should have come to a better understanding of your emotions. Don't expect to do it all at once. There is no way you will change years of conditioned behavior and hidden subconscious messages overnight or even within the year timespan of this book. But you should, hopefully, have made a start. And the departure of summer certainly does not herald the end of work on the emotional side of life. What you have set in motion will continue and grow throughout the months—and years—that follow. Throughout autumn and winter there will be many more suggestions on how to access the emotional side of your life. However, there are two therapies I would like to introduce at this stage. They fall in between camps really: biodynamic therapy is a mixture of bodywork and psychotherapy, while watsu is quite unique. They are not for everyone by any means, but both are quite intriguing and can have very deep effects.

BIODYNAMIC THERAPY

It could well be that this month's emphasis on play and passion has irritated you beyond belief. You might look at your life and think the only way to get through is not with all this fun and games but simply by muddling through. The only true solution is to grit your teeth and put a brave face on it. But while gritting your teeth gets you through the days, it is, according to biodynamic therapists, slowly destroying your true self. The "brave face" is a mask that we initially put on as protection but which, over the years, becomes a form of armor, cutting us off from our true emotions and banishing any real sense of joy. Take away the mask and see through the eyes of your true self, and the world will become a far brighter place: more vibrant, more intense, more alive.

Biodynamic therapists are in fundamental agreement with the play experts, believing that as children we live only in our true self (which they call the primary personality)—spontaneous, exuberant, intuitive, really "alive." But as we get older we gradually learn to hide our feelings from the world for fear of ridicule or disapproval—we literally build a secondary personality to shield us from the "dangers" of society. The aim of biodynamic therapy is to put you back in touch with the primary personality. It doesn't mean regressing to a childlike state of unfocused tantrums and unbridled fantasy but rather learning when it's appropriate to let down the barriers and allow your real self to come out to play. As a result, many people find they have the courage to take up new challenges, to take calculated risks, to dare to change their lives. If you don't feel you have the nerve to reintroduce passion and play into your life on your own, this might well be the helping hand you need.

It's a totally unique therapy which uses a variety of techniques. One week you could find yourself sitting in a chair talking about your life, just like regular psychotherapy. The next session you might end up pummeling your fists into a mattress on the floor. And then again, you are equally likely to spend an hour on a massage couch with your therapist giving you a deep bodywork session. The massage is perhaps the most famous (or infamous) part of biodynamic: it's singular in that the therapist gauges the effect of the bodywork by listening intently to your stomach through an anaesthescope. The rumblings of the digestive system, they believe, give a clear indication of whether or not you are releasing emotional blocks. It sounds so bizarre that it puts many people off, fearing it's nothing less than sheer idiocy concocted out of thin air by a complete lunatic.

But Norwegian-born Gerda Boyesen, who developed biodynamic therapy over thirty years ago, is certainly no lunatic. A psychologist and physiotherapist, she realized that she could get even better results in her psychotherapy by working on the body as well as the mind. While most therapists either opt for a totally cerebral approach (by talking as we'll discuss next month) or a purely physical approach (in bodywork techniques such as Rolfing, Hellerwork and Looyenwork), Boyesen combined the two. She found, like many other bodyworkers, that emotions were held in the body and that through certain kinds of deep massage they could be released. But she also noticed that the greatest release came when the gut started rumbling. She listened, experimented and finally developed what she called psychoperistalsis, a finely tuned technique which encourages the body to literally "digest" emotional stress through deep powerful massage. "It sounds crazy," admits biodynamic therapist Gillie Gilbert, "but we're not the only people who listen to the sounds of the alimentary canal. Anaesthetists listen to the gut when they are anaesthetizing someone."

There is no such thing as a typical biodynamic session. On my first visit to Gillie, we simply sat and talked to begin with. She explained the biodynamic theory: how over the years we suppress our true selves and, in so doing, prevent vital healing energy from being allowed to flow freely through the body. As the energy becomes "stuck" so we build up what she calls "armor," a straitjacket of rigid muscles and tense internal tissue. "We believe your body is the library of your life," she says. "It stores your whole history. So we start by working with the body to bring back energy into it. With massage we can dissolve the stuck chemistry, take the muscle tissue and manipulate it to increase the blood circulation. Then the extra oxygen and water will diffuse into the tissue and disperse the block."

I was very keen to experience the massage and Gillie agreed that it would be helpful. Generally the therapist will suggest what form each session takes, but the client is always given the chance to ask for an alternative. "You have the inner knowing," says Gillie. "At a deep level you know what you need to do."

So I lay on the couch, fully clothed, and waited. Gillie started work on the neck and shoulders, my head and upper spine. It's a very deep touch, quite painful in places—in fact, if I'm honest, it really hurt at first. But you soon acclimatize and, within minutes, I was barely aware of anything except deep, deep relaxation. Normally I flit in and out of consciousness during a massage, often lightly dreaming, but this time I was knocked out completely: there were no dreams, no thoughts. After forty minutes I emerged and Gillie told me my digestive system had been making quite satisfactory noises, so clearly something had been shifted. I smiled and left, far from convinced: it had been a great massage but I didn't see it changing my life. But the next day I found myself a different person: lighter, brighter, as if a huge load had been taken off of my shoulders. It lasted several days.

The second session was to be what biodynamic therapists term vegetotherapy. Gillie asked me to lie down on my back on a large mattress and to relax, slowing down my breathing and becoming aware of my body. At first I felt uncomfortable and slightly embarrassed: it all seemed a bit pointless. Then I felt my fingers start to twitch, almost as if they wanted to claw at something. The feelings of irritation grew and I found myself thinking about how often I suppress my true feelings in order to keep other people happy. My session was very quiet but Gillie was pleased. If I were to continue with the therapy, she explained, she would ask me to explore the feelings in my hands and see what happened if I exaggerated the movement. Quite likely, she said, I would have clawed the mattress or turned my hands into fists and pounded it. People often find they can use the vegetotherapy couch to excise deep emotional blocks, acting out their feelings as old hurts and anguishes surface.

"Your ability to control and suppress your feelings reduces when you're on the mattress," explains Gillie. "It can be fascinating for people to see what emerges when they take away the superego, the controlling part of the mind."

She has treated people for a large variety of problems. Some people come for a few sessions of massage to clear headaches and migraine. Others look on the therapy as a long-term commitment to deep-seated change. Gillie has several clients who see her for terminal shyness. Two are high-powered business people who found that their careers were being blocked by their inability to communicate in front of crowds. Biodynamic therapy is steadily ironing out the problem. Others come to rid themselves of long-term depression or anxiety. But equally, she says, many come because they simply feel there has to be more to life. "They have reached their late twenties or thirties, are climbing the ladder at work and have relationships and families," says Gillie. "But they had come to the fundamental realization that the potential they had as a child and the reality as an adult simply don't match."

Biodynamic therapy slowly allows the secondary personality to relinquish power a little and allow the true self to emerge, like a butterfly finally emerging from its thick, hard, rigid chrysalis. And when the true self frees itself of its old restrictions and beliefs, it can stretch its wings and simply fly.

WATSU: FREEING THE EMOTIONS IN WATER

The second therapy is new and quite controversial but can, I feel, be very useful for certain people, providing it is given by the right therapist. It is called watsu and is quite unique. Watsu is the latest buzzword in smart American spas, but it is certainly not simply a panacea for the rich and fashionable. A long, intense session of massage and manipulation techniques, carried out while you float in a warm pool, watsu promises to heal you in mind, body *and* spirit. Fans claim it has remarkable regenerative qualities; that it can release stress, muscle tension and pain like no other treatment. They also say that, equally, it can release emotional anguish, giving you back that elusive sense of childhood innocence and joy. Its practitioners say it can even help heal the deep wounds of childhood abuse, incest and other early traumas. However, not everyone is convinced about watsu: a few detractors claim watsu is too invasive, too intimate a therapy. So what is watsu all about?

Watsu is the brainchild of Harold Dull, an American poet who became fascinated with the Japanese acupressure massage and stretching therapy, shiatsu. Having studied in San Francisco and Japan in the Seventies, he wanted to combine the therapeutic effects of shiatsu with the healing properties of water. At first he tried giving massage on a padded board set up in a hot tub, but when he moved to Harbin Hot Springs, California, he soon realized that he could achieve far better, far deeper effects by floating his client in water, working on their body while cradling the head above water. His watsu techniques had such good results that they were taken up by the Timpany Center in San Jose where the therapy is still used to help people who are severely mentally, emotionally and physically disabled.

Intense research over the last ten years has shown watsu to have a host of benefits. Water takes the weight off the vertebrae and relaxes the muscles so that the practitioner can move the spine in ways that would be impossible on land. The effect is far greater freedom and mobility in the body. Harold Dull puts it this way: "In the Orient, stretching is an even older therapy than acupuncture. It strengthens muscles and increases flexibility and range of motion. I found that these effects can be amplified and made more profound by stretching someone while floating them in warm water. Without pain the body can move beyond the limitations that fear would otherwise impose. New life is stretched into long neglected connective tissue, and the restricted body is shown new possibilities of freedom."

Tests have also shown watsu influences the body in other ways too: it decreases muscular tension, increases superficial circulation and lymphatic function; strengthens the immune system and can aid digestion and respiratory difficulties. Many people find it helps insomnia and anxiety, that it can release deeply held stress and improve posture. In California it has been used successfully to help people with addictions and, paradoxically, it can even help people get over a fear of water.

One of the patients at the Timpany Center had suffered injuries in the last San Francisco earthquake. Mary, sixty-two, had muscle spasms in her right shoulder and was in constant pain. Physiotherapy and ultrasound had not worked, but exercise in water seemed to help so it was decided to try watsu. After five treatments, her right shoulder showed a dramatic increase in flexibility, and her posture and breathing were much improved. But, more importantly, to her great delight, the pain had vanished by session three. "I came to the third session in a great deal of pain," she recalls. "The pain had kept me awake all night. But approximately two-thirds through the session I realized that the pain was gone. I felt like laughing out loud."

However, Mary admits that the therapy does take some getting used to. "The intimacy seems greater than that of being massaged," she says, "perhaps because you are both in swimsuits, both in the water." And many people have shied away from watsu because of this "intimacy." However, Harold Dull insists that the close contact between practitioner and client is an essential aspect of the therapy; that it allows for the deep emotional healing that can take place. Clients have to lie back and trust themselves to the practitioner. "A person's very life, their connection to the life-sustaining breath, is entrusted to the arms of the watsuer," explains Dull. "Many people get in touch with a sadness at not having been held so before." Many also find the close, nurturing touch, brings up old memories—sometimes good, sometimes bad, sometimes almost unbearable.

But is watsu simply too intimate, too close for comfort? To find out I took the plunge and visited Pim de Gryff who, alongside his wife, Sally Bryant-de Gryff, studied with Dull. They have now set up the first watsu practice in the UK in Totnes, Devon. The pool they use at present is a small hydrotherapy pool in a residential nursing home. The first thing that hit me was the heat— the room was warm, very warm. Before we entered the pool, Pym asked me a series of questions. Watsu can be used safely on most people (whatever their age or size) but practitioners need to know whether clients are pregnant (certain moves aren't used) or have spinal problems, implants or any serious health or psychological problems. Some people who suffer from motion sickness find watsu uncomfortable and it cannot be used when there are open wounds, skin conditions or infectious diseases.

Having completed the health check, we descended into the pool. Pym took my head in his hands and asked me to lie back, relax and float. Throughout a watsu session you are encouraged to breathe deeply and evenly, using your mouth alone, and to keep your eyes gently closed. The water felt lovely but it took some time before I realized that my head wasn't going to go under, however Pym twisted and moved my body. The breathing also felt unnatural to begin with and my mouth frequently became dry. And, yes, it *did* feel very strange and even a little embarrassing being cradled in water by a virtual stranger. But after maybe fifteen to twenty minutes, it was as if my body and mind decided to give in, relax and trust. Then time simply vanished and with it all sense of where I was, even who I was. Some people say watsu feels like returning to the womb and I can understand what they mean. All my everyday cares and concerns simply fell away and, in a paradoxical fashion, although my body was being intensely worked upon, at times it felt as if I had no body at all.

Most of the time, watsu is delicious; a wonderful sense of release came as Pym stretched, rocked and manipulated my body. My spine arched and undulated like an otter's as he freed its knots. But at other times, I must confess, I was in agony: I groaned and wailed while he undid painful tension in my hands and feet. "Keep breathing," encouraged Pym. "Let the tension go." After nearly two hours I emerged from the pool quite frankly speechless. I estimated I could bend almost two inches further than normal and my whole body felt liberated. But what surprised me even more was that I felt emotionally moved and even quite tearful. Being held so closely, particularly by a stranger, is simply not part of our culture. It had felt like being a tiny child again, soothed and rocked by a loving parent. Personally I found it a very gentle, comforting, and healing experience; however, I could easily see why some people find watsu so confrontational, even frightening. And, without doubt, the power of watsu to affect not just the body but the emotions as well means that it will need to be very carefully controlled and monitored for the simple reason that when you step into a watsu pool, you are putting your very life and soul into someone else's hands.

AUTUMN

The Season of the Mind

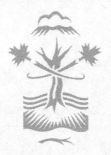

KEY FOCUS
Finding your path in life; tackling the outside world.

SECONDARY FOCUS
Strengthening your body.

TASKS
Assessing your career; soothing your mind; fine-tuning your environment; becoming organized; managing stress.

QUESTIONS
What do I want from life? Am I willing to change my life for the better? Do I handle stress? Am I hiding from anything in life?

CHALLENGES
Dare to make changes in your life; start to trust your intuition; dare to say no—become assertive.

FESTIVALS AND CELEBRATIONS
Autumn equinox, Samhain/Halloween.

You know the instant autumn has arrived. It's almost impercep-
tible, but one morning you wake up and walk outside and it's
there—not quite a scent, more of a feeling. A slight chill, a defi-
nite shift: the "roundedness" of summer has been sharpened. We
may regret the passing of summer, the warmth and laziness of
the days, but still there is something exhilarating about autumn.
The nip in the air, the frost on the lawn, the cool wind on
your face may all be harbingers of the cold winter to come but,
nonetheless, they are welcome. For a few months nature puts on
another of her extravaganzas: an artist's palette of color falls over
the trees; ruby-red berries sparkle in the hedgerows and on urban
hedges. Mists hang low over the fields and there is a freshness
about the world again.

Autumn shouts "wake-up" to the psyche—it's time to dust
yourself off after the languor of summer and take life head on
once again. After spring this is the most dynamic season of the
year, another case of blowing away the cobwebs and kicking
yourself into action. In spring you started to ask yourself lots of
questions about your life, your path and your desires. Now is
the time to get them going, to take action, to shift your external

world. Autumn is the season of the mind, but it also concerns our relationship with the environment, with the world outside, the bigger picture.

Up to now in the year we have been dealing with our selves, our bodies and emotions and our close personal relationships. Obviously these continue throughout the year but now the picture starts to widen. Autumn is a perfect time to decide what you want to make of your life; what you want to achieve; where you want to be; how you want to work. It is the key time for deciding on your life path or making moves toward it. That may sound frightening, even offputting, but it needn't be. Often we automatically find ourselves making changes, shifts, in the autumn. We may not be totally instinctual beings any more but deep within we are still moved by the rhythms of the year. Our hearts and souls still beat to the ancient drum. It is no real surprise that schools and colleges use the beginning of autumn as their starting point for the academic year. What better time to make a fresh intellectual start than at the beginning of the season of the mind?

This is the perfect time to get your life in order and to start looking for answers to the questions you posed yourself back in spring. If you need to shake your life around a bit, this is the time to do it. Don't feel you have to change for the sake of it. It's more a case that if you have been looking for a change, this is a good time to think about putting things into motion. You should be in good shape to do so. You will, by now, hopefully be feeling connected in your body and clearer in your emotions. You should be feeling more able to make choices and changes from a position of clarity and strength, rather than being panicked into change. As always, if the time doesn't feel right, don't do anything. I'm certainly not suggesting that everyone should go out and get a new job or a new relationship or move house or emigrate on September 1! Simply that if you feel there are changes in your life (however small) you might want to make, the energy at this time of year will help you make those changes. It's like a car being given a dose of high-octane fuel or a horse being given a feed of oats—you should be feeling frisky and full of energy.

But let's look at the basics first. As with all the seasons, there are shifts and changes to make in your basic lifestyle. After all,

you need to be in good shape if you are going to keep all this
life-force energy moving healthily.

Indian Summer: The Harbinger of Autumn

Before we launch into autumn proper we need to look briefly
at the inbetween time that often occurs—the Indian summer that
can last into the first weeks of autumn. In the ancient systems
this is considered a separate season of its own: the Chinese say
this is the fulcrum of the year, a time of perfect balance when
the fire energy of summer burns down and begins to mellow
and transform into the balanced energy of earth. Neither *yin* nor
yang can hold power at this time of the year—the year is held
like scales in perfect balance. The color associated with this time
of year is yellow, the color of sun and earth combined. In the
human system it is connected with the stomach, the spleen and
the pancreas. If earth is unbalanced in your system you will
probably have problems with digestion.

This is a transitional time when you need to keep balanced
and centered, just like the year itself. But it is also a time when
the powers of creation are coming up again—from the clear energy of fire comes the manifestation implied by earth—not just
the harvesting of the fields but all kinds of creation, new beginnings, the start of something different. Earth energy allows us to
form views, thoughts and opinions. It can kick-start you into new
directions and differing ways of living life.

However, be careful that your thoughts don't become obsessive—imbalanced earth can lead to obsession, stubbornness, ob-
stinacy, a refusal to see any other view than your own. And while
imbalances in earth can cause havoc with your digestion, they
can also give difficulties with the menstrual cycle and the spleen.
The spleen is said to govern the memory, our ability to form
opinions and our willpower, so any trouble in the spleen may
cause anxiety, lack of decision-making powers and forgetfulness.

In the early part of autumn you should begin a building and
toning diet to prepare you for the cooler weather to come. This
involves adding a little more fat than in spring and summer and

more protein-rich foods. Generally you can add a little more dairy produce to your diet (unless your *prakuti* forbids it). You can increase your consumption of fish and poultry and add a little red meat. Plenty of grains will help to fortify the system without making you feel full and heavy.

The ayurvedic physicians say that this is a pivotal time when all the energies of the body can be disturbed. They advise eating a diet of cooked foods rather than raw and making sure your diet is well-balanced. They also recommend you shift to wearing light but warm clothes and take oil baths and massages to gently begin to warm the body.

The Season of Metal, Air, and the Dry Evil

The Chinese see autumn proper as a time when the energy of earth transforms into metal, a time when energy once again begins to withdraw and pull back. They describe it as condensing, as contracting inward so that it can begin to accumulate its powers and store them for the lean times to come. Metal energy governs the lungs, the organs that take vital energy from the air and get rid of the waste products from our blood. It also governs the large intestine which takes vital nutrients and water from our food while eliminating the toxins and unnecessary matter.

So, not surprisingly, to the Chinese view, autumn is a time for storing what is necessary and getting rid of what is no longer needed. It's a time of clarity; of dumping the dross, of getting rid of things both physical and emotional which no longer have a place in your life. It's time for a second big clear-out, an "autumn-clean" if you like (more details in the SEPTEMBER section). The color of metal and autumn is clear white, the color of clarity and purity. According to the Chinese philosophy, if you cling sentimentally to old attachments and desires you will end up feeling anxiety, grief and a profound feeling of melancholy. These feelings, in turn, will affect your body—predominantly your lungs and large intestine. The result will be flu, colds and a general case of low resistance, of feeling under par. If the problem goes deeper it might bring breathing difficulties, chest pains, skin conditions and other unpleasant results. Better to shed the old emotions and attachments!

The "evil" of autumn is dryness. Caused by insufficient moisture in the air, it can be particularly damaging to the lungs. When combined with cold, dryness can bring on headaches and a blocked-up nose. When combined with heat, dryness will cause excessive thirst and profuse sweat, a sort throat and dry nose. Both forms of dry evil will make your skin feel hard and dry, your lips become chapped and will generally cause constipation. Avoiding dry evil, however, is particularly tricky as it is caused generally by air conditioning and central heating. Smoking is also a major cause of dry evil. Counteract it by keeping some fresh air circulating even when it's really cold. An ionizer will help and so will bowls of water to increase humidity.

The Native Americans talk of air as being associated with self-sufficiency, with a gathering of strength from within and a chance to prepare for the future. They see autumn as the season of gathering in information and knowledge—a time to organize your life once again.

Metal is very similar to the element air in the Indian ayurvedic tradition. The association of air with autumn is quite obvious. Air produces the wind that blows the leaves from the trees—it is the governing element of the ayurvedic *dosha vata*. The ayurvedic tradition also associates autumn and air/metal with the color white and talks of it being expressed in the inner workings and activities of the mind. Ayurvedic sages say it directly governs all aspects of the mind, particularly those connected with developing ideas, writing and speaking. They also echo the Chinese by saying that air imbalances often give rise to coughing and problems with breathing and agree that autumn and air/metal governs the lungs, large intestine and also the skin and body hair. Breathing is considered very important to good health by the ayurvedic sages, hence the emphasis in yoga on *pranayama* or correct breathing. They see the breath not just on a physical level as a means of taking in new air and expelling waste products but also on an energetic and emotional level, of taking in new energy and breathing out the spent; of taking in hope and expansive spirit and breathing out everything that is stagnant and repugnant for the soul. On a symbolic level, this tradition sees coughing as the body trying to expel anything it doesn't want—not just mucus and phlegm but old emotions or an unwelcome change too. The lungs are the organs which most closely put us in touch with the world outside—they are the great mediator. No wonder this is the season when we examine our wider relationships.

The Autumn Diet

The autumn diet regime aims to reduce any accumulation of fire energy from the summer and to prepare the body gently for the colder harsher season of winter. In ayurvedic terms, the diet should consist of warm, moist, well-lubricated foods with a greater emphasis on foods which are sweet and sour in taste. Take advantage of the wonderful crop of autumn berries—the late raspberries and luscious blackberries. Fresh figs start to come into the shops and are utterly delicious and very healthy. If you have problems with constipation, try figs (sweetcorn is also very helpful). Soaked prunes are another bowel-mover. If, however, your bowels move in the opposite direction, obviously it's better to steer clear of figs and prunes. Also, if you are trying to lose weight, bear in mind that both are quite high in calories when compared to other fruits, so don't overdo them. Continuing the fruit theme, this is a good time of year to start introducing gently cooked fruits—stewed apples and rhubarb, peaches and plums are all perfect for autumn. Add a handful of blackberries for piquancy.

Vegetables at this time of year benefit from being gently cooked—steamed or stir-fried or added to soups and light autumn casseroles. The choice is large: plenty of lightly cooked spinach, peas, leeks, cauliflower, cabbage, beetroot (try cooking it as a vegetable rather than always consigning it to the salad bowl) and the perennial flavor-enhancers and immune-boosters onion and garlic. Seasonal crops include green beans, parsnips, carrots and tomatoes. Pumpkins are always associated with Halloween but don't throw away the innards—use them for smooth creamy soups or in the traditional pumpkin pie. Other squashes are also becoming popular now and are available from most supermarkets—experiment with these unusual fruits of autumn.

Foods can be slightly sweeter now, but always choose natural sweeteners and don't overdo them: fruit juices, honey, molasses and maple syrup can be taken in small amounts, but go easy if you are keeping an eye on your weight. In general, as at the beginning of autumn, you can continue to take a little more dairy produce and eat a little more meat, adding seasonal game (which is low in cholesterol), duck and darker meats. However, as always, don't allow meat to dominate your diet. Vegetarians can enjoy warming stews and bakes with lentils, any of the dhal family (mung dhal, tur dhal and urad dhal), and soya products. Tofu and Quorn work well for vegetarians and nonvegetarians alike.

Autumn is the season for nuts and these too will boost the vegetarian diet and give variation for meat-eaters. Fresh walnuts, filberts, hazelnuts and chestnuts appear in the shops, followed by the more exotic brazils, pistachios, macadamias and cashews. They are all delicious and nutritious, but be warned: firstly, some people are allergic to nuts and, secondly, all nuts, except chestnuts, are high in fat and calories. So eat them sparingly if you are trying to lose weight and always check with guests that they or their children do not have allergies to nuts.

SPICING UP AUTUMN

Autumn is also a great time to start to spice up your food in preparation for the cold winter ahead. Most of us use spices without thinking, obediently following recipes or enjoying the odd curry takeaway. Yet the huge range of spices all have remarkable health-giving benefits and you can help to warm and fortify your body by incorporating them into your everyday cooking. You don't have to make every meal into a vindaloo—most spices are very subtle and delicate and can be used just as effectively in sweet dishes as in savory. Here is a run-down of the most useful, effective and delicious. Use them particularly toward the end of autumn as the colder weather approaches.

Cardamom
Ayurveda prizes cardamom very highly and rates it as a superlative spice for autumn as it is sweet and warm in its nature and

tends to gently stimulate our energy. The volatile oils in cardamom can help stimulate the digestion and relieve wind (often
very useful in the windy *vata* season of autumn!). It can also be
used to ease indigestion. Cardamom is the delicious scent and
taste in many Indian sweets as well as a classic ingredient in
curry.

Cinnamon

Cinnamon is one of the most widely used spices—and with good
reason. It is pungent and warming and so excellent at this time
of year. It will ward off colds and flus, help stomach chills and
soothe arthritis and rheumatism. The Chinese consider cinnamon
a strong *yang* tonic which can help the *chi* to circulate freely. It
is famed as a strengthener and also a sexual tonic!

Cinnamon is also used specifically to calm the nerves, to warm
the internal organs and to treat headaches and fever. It is said to
relieve tension in the neck and shoulders by dispersing energy
blocks in that area. Practitioners of Chinese medicine claim that
cinnamon will clear the skin of blemishes and give you a more
youthful complexion. So add cinnamon into your cooking and
also pop it in warming drinks—it is lovely added to nighttime
milky drinks (so is cardamom) and is a staple ingredient (with
cloves) in mulled wine.

You don't have to limit cinnamon to your cooking either—use
the essential oil too. Put five drops of pure essential oil in a bowl
of just-boiled water and inhale the steam (put a towel over your
head and the bowl) to relieve coughs and respiratory problems.
Dilute 10 ml of cinnamon in 25 ml of almond oil and use as a
massage oil for stomach chills, diarrhea and colicky pains. A
couple of drops in the bath will warm the whole body if you
feel chilled.

Warning: cinnamon can act as a uterine stimulant so do not
take large amounts during pregnancy. Do not use it if you are
overheated or feverish.

Cayenne

Cayenne, the red-hot chili, is another supreme warmer, a stimulant and tonic which is wonderful in the run-up to winter. It is
very hot, very pungent and it affects the whole body—increasing
blood flow, tonifying the nervous system, increasing the appetite

and easing indigestion. Once again, it is a *yang* tonic. Cayenne (its botanical name is *Capsicum frutescens*) has been used to treat headaches, to soothe the pain of rheumatism and arthritis and to reduce fat in the blood. Some people believe that cayenne can also trigger the release of endorphins, the brain chemicals that relieve pain and produce a feeling of mild euphoria and well being. So add a pinch (no more) of fiery cayenne to dishes when the weather starts getting cold—it can also keep colds and flus at bay and seems to have a beneficial effect on sore throats as well. However, although cayenne can be used medically for a host of problems—for migraine, shingles, tonsillitis, ulcers, rheumatic pains and even depression—it is best to consult a qualified herbalist as cayenne is very powerful.

Warning: cayenne should not be used in therapeutic doses during pregnancy or breast-feeding, and excessive consumption could lead to gastroenteritis, kidney and liver damage. The seeds can be toxic so avoid them.

Fenugreek

We may not be as familiar with fenugreek as with cinnamon, cayenne or cardamom but it is one of the oldest therapeutic spices known. It was used in ancient Egypt to ease childbirth and increase milk flow and is still used today in Egypt as a remedy for period pains and for stomach cramps caused by the dreaded "traveler's tummy." The Chinese agree and have used it for centuries for all kinds of abdominal pain.

Again, it is a very warming spice which is pungent and bitter in its taste. It has a generally anti-inflammatory action; it acts as a digestive tonic, a uterine stimulant and is said to be an aphrodisiac. It also reduces blood sugar levels. In China, fenugreek is used to treat male impotence, period pains, menopausal problems and diabetes. It is also used externally for skin inflammations. You will find small amounts of fenugreek in many Chinese and Indian recipes but don't overdo the amounts as it is very bitter.

Warning: avoid fenugreek during pregnancy because of its uterine-stimulating effects. Consult a medical herbalist for serious conditions and for using fenugreek medicinally, particularly in cases of diabetes.

Garlic

If you use no other herb or spice, then at the very least try garlic. It is absolutely wonderful for your health and will add a great kick to your cooking. Garlic is hot and dry in its nature and pungent in taste. It is rich in B vitamins, minerals and flavonoids and has volatile oils with a variety of beneficial effects. Garlic is known to be an antibiotic, an expectorant, an anticoagulant, an antihistaminic and antiparasitic. It promotes sweating and reduces blood pressure, blood cholesterol levels and blood sugar levels. It tonifies and boosts the immune system. Medical herbalists use it widely for chest infections and problems, for digestive disorders and fungal problems like thrush. It is useful in cases of late-onset diabetes and can help skin infections and acne. Even orthodox doctors will admit that it can reduce the likelihood of heart attacks and other cardiovascular problems.

So, if it is so wonderful, why aren't we eating more? Mainly because of the smell, I suspect. There's no denying that garlic's pungency will creep out of even the pores of your skin and without doubt float on your breath. The best defense is to make sure the whole family eats it (you don't notice the smell on others when you've had it as well) and that you eat fresh parsley afterward (it tends to diminish or eliminate the smell).

Don't limit garlic to your cooking either. In fact, the fresher the garlic, the better the effects. Rub the fresh cloves on acne, mash the cloves and put on verrucas or warts or corns. A couple of crushed cloves added to a morning drink of fresh juice will ward off colds and coughs and all kinds of infections. See a medical herbalist if you feel you need garlic for serious heart problems, diabetes and severe digestive problems.

Warning: although using garlic in food should be quite safe, be careful of overdosing on garlic if you are pregnant or breastfeeding. Like many adults, some babies dislike the taste of garlic and it will undoubtedly be tasted in breast milk!

Ginger

Ginger is another spice we are so familiar with that we overlook its amazing healing properties. Ginger has been used therapeutically for thousands of years in China, India, and in the West as well. Another winter warmer, ginger is pungent, hot and dry in its nature and acts as a stimulant to the circulation, an expectorant, antiseptic and antispasmodic. It promotes sweating and prevents vomiting. Ginger increases blood flow and so has been used as a superb circulatory stimulant. The fresh root can now be bought in most supermarkets and is delicious in stir-fries, stews and all kinds of curries. It will help ward off colds and chills and is superlative for indigestion, nausea and flatulence. Ginger will also ease travel sickness (buy the capsules and take one or two before you travel).

The Chinese see ginger as another *yang* tonic and use it to warm and stimulate the stomach and lungs (useful at this time of year when these organs are at their most sensitive). Recent trials have also found it very useful for morning sickness (take no more than 1 g a day).

The essential oil is a useful friend as well. Add up to ten drops of pure ginger essential oil to around 25 ml of almond oil and use as a massage oil for rheumatic conditions. It can also help with stomach upsets and menstrual cramps—simply massage into the stomach. And again, if you feel very cold or chilled, add a few drops of ginger oil to your bath to help get your circulation moving again and to prevent chills and colds setting in.

Warning: it is not advisable to use ginger if you suffer from conditions such as peptic ulcers or other hot conditions in the stomach. Do not use excessive amounts of ginger in early pregnancy (the amount given above for morning sickness is safe).

Nutmeg

A sprinkle of nutmeg on rice pudding is how most of us use nutmeg, but it's a powerful and useful spice, although one that needs to be treated with great respect. Nutmeg can stimulate the appetite and the digestion in general; it is also very useful for diarrhea. The essential oil is used for rheumatic pain and even to help toothache. The outer part of the fruit, known as mace, has been used as an ointment for rheumatism. Another pungent, warming spice, nutmeg can be used in many recipes to add a subtle kick.

Warning: large doses of nutmeg are very dangerous. It can be a hallucinogen, and produce palpitations and convulsions.

Turmeric

Bright yellow turmeric brightens up curries but did you realize that it is a potent antibacterial spice? Ayurvedic physicians have used turmeric for thousands of years as a treatment for obesity, and it now appears that the spice can have a strengthening and tonifying effect on the liver, stimulating the flow of bile and breaking down fats. It was also used for menstrual problems and stomach disorders. Modern research seems to agree on turmeric's powers—it appears it can help to strengthen and tonify the gall bladder and prevent disease. It helps to prevent blood clots and because of its anti-inflammatory properties, it also helps in cases of arthritis. So keep adding it to the pot!

KICHADI: DELICIOUS MEDICINE IN A POT

In Ayurveda there is one dish that surpasses all others. A simple *kichadi* (or *kitcheri* or any number of variations of spelling but basically a stew) or rice and mung dhal with spices and vegetables is used to balance all the *doshas* and to ease almost every problem. *Kichadi* is used extensively in ayurvedic cooking and can be particularly useful at this time of year to soothe all the *doshas* and to prepare your body for the cooler weather. The best news is that this meal in a pot is also delicious.

The prime ingredients are simple: basmati rice and split mung dhal which you will usually find in Indian supermarkets and health food shops. Spices such as the ones we have already discussed are used freely and often vegetables are added. The other staple ingredient is ghee, the clarified butter used in Indian cooking. Many supermarkets now sell it but it's easy to prepare yourself. Simply heat unsalted butter in a heavy saucepan over a medium heat. It will begin to bubble, and allow it to bubble over a medium heat for around fifteen to twenty minutes. Just before it is ready, milk solids will start to collect at the bottom of the pan. Wait and watch carefully until the liquid suddenly becomes clear and stops bubbling, then quickly take it off the heat. Allow it to cool slightly and pour through a metal strainer into a glass or plastic container. Keep at room temperature rather than in the fridge—if it has been prepared properly it will keep well.

A Basic Receipt for Kichadi
Use around 30 g of rice and 15 g of mung beans per person. Mix the rice and beans together and wash in cold water. Melt a

tablespoon of ghee in a pan and add half a teaspoon each of fennel, cumin and coriander seeds. Cook for a minute or two. Then add half a teaspoon each of powdered ginger and turmeric plus the drained rice and beans. Allow them to become well coated with the ghee and then add enough water to cover the ingredients well with a few inches to spare and bring to the boil. Then cover and simmer gently, stirring occasionally, making sure the mixture does not dry out or stick. It should take about one hour to cook. If you like, you can add vegetables. Root vegetables should be cooked from the beginning, leafy vegetables should be added toward the end of the cooking time.

Variations: you can adapt *kichadi* to suit almost any condition and taste. A warming variation which is good for this time of year uses the following combination of spices: one teaspoon each of cardamom seeds, cumin seeds and coriander seeds; one teaspoon of black peppercorns; three-quarters of a teaspoon of cinnamon, half a teaspoon of ground cumin, one teaspoon turmeric, quarter of a teaspoon of ground cloves, one tablespoon of fresh grated ginger, two cloves of garlic, one bay leaf.

As before, wash the rice and mung beans and heat a tablespoon of ghee. Add the cumin seeds and lightly brown. Then add the rice, mung beans and water and bring to the boil. Simmer for around forty-five minutes. Meanwhile, warm two tablespoons of ghee in another saucepan and add the coriander, cardamom, peppercorns and bay leaf, sauté for a few minutes and then stir in the rest of the spices and the garlic, plus a chopped onion. Transfer these all to a blender with a little water and grind well. Then pour the mixture into the pot with the rice and mung bean mixture. Add vegetables (carrots, beans, courgettes, cabbage or whatever is fresh and available) and allow to cook for a further twenty minutes. This is wonderful for the digestion and circulation.

Exercise for Autumn

Autumn brings a fresh influx of energy and it can be a wonderful time to try a new sport or move your workouts up a notch.

However, equally, you might find that, as the weather starts to get colder and the nights draw in that you have less natural inclination to get out and do something. Autumn is a good time therefore to investigate team sports or to persuade a friend to join you in your training or exercise program. It's much easier to stay curled up by the fire or in front of the television when it's only yourself you're letting down—if you know there is a partner waiting for a workout or a team waiting for you to play, there's far less chance for excuses. Also team sports can be brilliant fun and a great way to get to know people. The list is endless and you will find most represented at your local sports center. It's well worth trying sports you played at school: netball can be a revelation; five-a-side football is wildly energetic and other sports like hockey, lacrosse and volleyball can be exhilarating too. You'll be surprised how your view of such sports changes when you are doing them out of choice rather than being bullied by a draconian sports teacher. However, try to balance these energetic forms with quieter kinds of exercise too. Yoga, t'ai-chi, chi kung are all excellent.

Whatever kind of exercise you do, make sure you warm up properly before launching yourself into hearty exercise and that you stretch fully both before and after exertion. Many of the injuries people get from exercise are caused because they hurl cold muscles into intense exercise. If you have been to a good aerobics class you will know the score: you start off with movements designed to warm up the muscles without straining them and then have a period of stretching before the pace hots up. At the end you gently slow down again and stretch fully before stopping. Whatever your sport, you should follow a similar routine. If you aren't sure about stretching, refer back to the APRIL section. It's also worth going to a class to learn how to do it properly and thoroughly—it will save you a lot of grief.

Looking at Your Life Path

Now the hard work begins. At the beginning of the book you will have answered questions about your life path and how you feel about your position in the world. Take a few minutes now to look back at what you wrote. Has anything changed? Is there anything you feel you should add? If you didn't fill it out then, take some time out to do so now.

How many of us, hands on heart, are in jobs we really love? I'm willing to bet the answer is very few. And yet our work is how we spend the vast majority of our lives. Doesn't it therefore seem a little strange that we are quite resigned to the fact that work is usually a drag? So many of us buy into the "Protestant work ethic" idea that work *should* be hard, difficult and relatively unpleasant. Earning money must, by its very definition, be something serious. Why? Why shouldn't we enjoy our work? Why shouldn't we look forward to each working day? Why should we dread Monday morning and mutter "Thank God it's Friday" at the end of the working week? Some people say they even start feeling depressed on Sunday morning because they know they have to go back to work the next day. It's insane.

And yet how can you change the situation? Surely it's just too dangerous out there to think about changing career midstream, of launching into the unknown. Well, yes and no. No one in their right mind would simply hand in their notice and stomp out without a contingency plan. But work takes up such a hefty chunk of our lives that it seems criminal to continue with a job that makes us actively unhappy.

Few of us take the time to analyze precisely why we do the work we do and where exactly the problems lie. We often make career decisions in haste, in panic, at the drop of a hat. And, although you may insist "I hate my job," it is worth sitting down and asking *exactly* what it is you hate about it. It might well be only one element of your work you dislike. Armed with that knowledge, you are in a much better position to decide whether to alter the kind of work you do in the same organization or whether to change both your job *and* your company.

You *do* have a choice. The trouble is that we have often ended up in a job through force of circumstances and then believe that we can't change. Old-style career counseling hardly helped: it merely focused on what jobs you should be doing. If I had followed the advice of my careers counselor I would now be either snowed under in industrial relations or managing a hotel. I'm not sure either would really suit me. However, why not fit what you *enjoy* being good at with the ideal career? By analyzing precisely what constitutes your "job personality" you can make your working life more profitable, more involving and much more fun.

It's worth setting aside a day, or a couple of evenings, to solely work on you and your career. Put the answerphone on, tell family or friends you need some undisturbed time. Arrange for children or dependents to be looked after. It is important to give yourself your undivided attention. Before you start, try to get into a relaxed state. Take some deep breaths, stretch, roll your neck slowly around. Detach yourself from your normal work and commitments. Don't look on these exercises as a chore. Pretend it's a game, have fun, feel free to use colored crayons, paints, huge pieces of paper—whatever suits you. If you want to draw pictures, that's great. Above all, be honest. Remember no one needs to see this except you. Put down everything you can think of, however silly or unrelated it may appear. Some people have made incredible careers by unearthing skills and pleasures from things they did at school or at the youth club.

OUR FAMILY SCRIPT

"But work isn't *supposed* to be fun" is our knee-jerk reaction. Says who? Generally our parents, our schoolteachers, our religious instructors, everyone we come into contact with at an early age. We learn many of our deep-seated beliefs about work at a very young age from previous generations for whom the concept of work was often intrinsically bound up with notions of duty, of discipline, of hard slog.

Women have another prejudice to battle—most of us have the early imprinted idea that we either don't deserve to be in the workplace (we should be full-time mothers and housewives) or that we have to work twice as hard as men to achieve success. On the other hand, men don't have it easy either: their subscript runs that they should get a "proper" job, a "manly" job which will bring in enough money to support the family. Men are under pressure to perform better than women, to earn more than women, to reach higher positions than women. Yes, even now.

Consequently, we are almost all following other people's work scripts, obeying decisions we made *almost subconsciously* about work before we even entered the workplace. By becoming aware of your scripts you can let go of a large number of preconceptions about the nature of work, about the kind of job you are in and your expectations from work.

• Ask yourself your thoughts about work. For example, do you think "I never get what I really want"; "I always get to be the deputy, never the boss"; "I have to fight and be tough to make myself heard"? "I have to have a 'proper' professional career, like a doctor or lawyer"?
• Write down whatever comes to mind, however silly it may seem and spend some time pondering where those thoughts originally came from. Did you feel unsatisfied at school, perhaps? Or was your father never promoted beyond a certain level? Did your parents tell you how much your education was costing and that you owed it to them to get a sensible job?
• Look at your thoughts logically and decide whether they are appropriate thoughts for you now. If not, be willing to let them go. Merely by being aware of your internal script you can reassess your work pattern.

FINDING YOUR JOB PERSONALITY

Having realized that most of your hard-wired conclusions about the kind of work you *should* be doing are based on other people's decisions, not your own, you can now look at what you really want from a career, what will support *you*.

It may sound egocentric, you may well think "Oh but the workplace doesn't work like that," but the most successful organizations now encourage the "entrepreneur" attitude amongst staff, finding that employees who are the most fulfilled and happy contribute the most to the organization.

• Make an audit of all your skills, your knowledge, your attributes and qualities, your hobbies. Start from as early as you like and put down everything you can think of. Include the subjects you learned at school and college; the jobs and careers you have followed and the skills and qualities they called for; the extra-

curricular activities and hobbies you enjoyed; any workshops
or trainings.

• Don't judge what you are writing, don't think that acting in
school plays is irrelevant if you're an accountant. Everything is
important, from playing in the netball team to enjoying caring
for your younger siblings.

• Look at your list and see if there are any patterns, any subjects
you have always enjoyed; any skills that you have used throughout your life and which you enjoy. Decide which are your favorite three skills and your favorite three areas of knowledge.

• Flesh out each skill and subject with stories from your past:
how you used this skill; what the situation was; who was there;
how did it feel? Can you think of any skills you enjoyed using
on lots of occasions? Say you like organizing: be very precise
about how *exactly* you enjoy organizing. Is it organizing people,
or data or things? Organizing in a methodical, logical way or
using your intuition and gut reactions? Were you part of a team,
alone, managing the team?

• Look at your stories and decide which are your favorites.

You will now have a good idea of where your skills and areas
of expertise lie. You may well feel you would like to develop a
skill or start using an old skill again. You might consider that
your present job really doesn't represent your true skills and
breadth of knowledge. Jot down any thoughts that come into
your head and then move on.

THE IDEAL WORKPLACE

You might well have found that your present job does use all
your skills and knowledge but that you are still unhappy. It could
well be *where* you are working. Once you know what your skills
are you must question the context in which you want to use
them.

• Look back at your audit and make a list of the environments
in which you have either worked or learned. For each stage of
your life ask yourself about the kind of organization you worked
for: was it large or small, public or private sector? What did it

produce (did it make things, disseminate information, help people, etc.)? Was the workforce primarily male, female or mixed? Did you work alone, in a small team, as part of a large structure?

• Note any patterns. Were you always happiest working primarily on your own but reporting to a small group of co-workers? Do you like to feel part of a large but organized team involved in caring?

• Ask yourself what you really want from a workplace. Do you like working for established businesses, for new growing concerns, for non-profit-making organizations? Do you like working for an organization that manufactures things (and, if so, what kind of things?); or that processes information (how do you like to deal with information?); or that works with people (exactly what kind of people? What age range, what background? Individuals or groups? Easy-going or difficult people?).

• Would you be happy if you changed your work environment? If, instead of teaching large groups of adults, you could give one-to-one help to children with special needs? If you were working for a small, personal company with huge challenges rather than an established large safe firm? Or maybe you simply need to change the way you work. If you are lonely working on your own, perhaps you could suggest that you become part of a team or under the auspices of a larger department which would give support and feedback.

YOUR WORK LANGUAGE

What kind of language do you listen to all day long in your workplace? Do you spend your days talking in accountant-speak, or library-lingo, or teacher-talk? More to the point, do you enjoy the language of your workplace? Lots of people have discovered that they enjoy the skills they use but hate the language they have to speak. But a solicitor does not have to just speak "solicitese": he or she could also speak the language of film or theater; of medicine; of psychology; of shipping, depending on the environment in which he or she chooses to pursue her skills. An administrator might love the job, might feel very happy with the size and structure of the organization for which he or she works but simply hate the fact that it deals in military uniforms because, over the last few years, their views on defense have fundamentally changed. You can never be happy in a job if you wince every time you hear certain words or phrases.

Look at your subject list, your list of areas of knowledge, and note down any that you couldn't stand working with all day long. Which are your favorites? Which would you be happy talking in and listening to all day long?

CREATING YOUR IDEAL JOB

Now you should have most of the information you require to discover your ideal work situation. Pull it all together and find the anatomy of your ideal job.

• Make a list of your three favorite skills, your three favorite subjects, the kind of place you would like to work (its three primary qualities), the kind of co-workers you like, the kind of people you would like to deal with, the goals you want to bring to your career.

• Think about anything you might have missed in all the previous exercises. Ask yourself what your dreams are: if this were the last day of your life what would you regret not ever having done? Incorporate any answers into your job anatomy.

• Indulge in some playful thinking around matching your favorite things to possible jobs. Be inventive, be silly, don't analyze. Try to think of ways to link even the most incongruous qualities; use it as a test of your lateral thinking.

MAKING LINKS

Now is the time to start thinking about the external factors: what is out there and how to match what employers want with what you have to offer.

Don't immediately fly to the nearest employment agency or job pages. Richard Nelson Bolles, author of *What Color Is Your Parachute? A Practical Manual for Job Hunters & Career-Changers,* points out that people who think in unorthodox patterns stand far more chance of success. If you reply to an advertisement in a paper, your odds are pretty slim; you could be competing against hundreds of applicants. If you go for a job from an employment agency you will still be up against a fair few. But, as Bolles points out, if you target yourself at a specific organization and convince them that you are tailor-made for them, you are competing against nobody.

OK, you might argue, but there is no job vacancy. Perhaps not, but people who know precisely what they want and have matched their skills to a specific organization are quite often irresistible. I personally know several people who have had jobs literally created for them after offering their services to the ideal employer.

• Spend some time asking yourself the following questions. Which of my skills are transferable and could be used in a variety of occupations? Which jobs would allow me to use my favorite skills in a field based on my favorite subjects or areas of knowledge? Which organizations or companies employ people in these careers? Which of these organizations do I like? Which of these organizations need my skills and knowledge?

• Ask friends or family to give some input. Show them your list of criteria and see if they have any thoughts or hunches.

MAKING CHANGE

By following this process you should have emerged with some clear indications of where your working life is going wrong and what needs to be adjusted or changed to make it better. You may feel the need to visit your personnel department and see if there is any position which would utilize more of your skills or clarify whether you should move direction or take on more responsibility. You might be ready to take the leap and work for yourself or to work from home.

The cardinal rule at this stage is to look before you leap. Think about the implications of any change. If you would need to re-train, or take more training, would you be willing to lose your spare time, or your weekends? Would you be willing to pay for courses? Would you be willing to take a cut in salary to achieve your new job? How would your partner or family feel?

Changing career is always risky, and there is no way to completely avoid the risk. Simply make sure your risks are manageable. Talk to people who already pursue the career you want to try. Think about the positive *and* the negative aspects of it.

One small but important footnote: don't write job applications when you are feeling down or angry or miserable. Your mood will automatically communicate itself to the employer. If you always seem to be depressed, try getting a friend around to boost you up before you get to work, or go for a run, have a swim or do a workout. And do write plenty of job applications at the same time. Never just send off one and then wait for the result before trying another. Keep the energy and the momentum going.

September

Back to school, back to work, back to reality. September sweeps in with a sharp breath of clean crisp fresh air, businesslike after the lazy languor of summer. The first leaves are falling and the air is freshening. Out in the garden the borders are glowing with rich reds, burnt oranges and deep yellows—the tones of autumn reflected first in the flowers, soon to transfer to the leaves of the trees. There is ploughing in the fields, the busy sowing of winter crops.

For the Native Americans September witnesses the end of the Harvesting Time and the ushering in of the Falling Leaves Time. It is seen as a time of organization, of preparing for the future, of gathering in—not only the fruits of the harvest against the winter ahead but also of our inner resources. They believe it should be a time of information and of knowledge, a more intellectual focus than the warmth of summer.

September is equally a month of letting go. The autumn equinox which falls on September 21 is seen in the pagan tradition as a festival of purification. In South America the women and children wear white and float white flowers on the sea under the soft glow of the moon. They are offering them to the great goddess, the mother of nature, who at this time begins her descent from the earth into the quiet depths of the underworld. There is a sense of sorrow at this time of year: we are having to say goodbye to the summer and also bid farewell to parts of ourselves that no longer serve us. It is a purging, cleansing time when it is good to decide what we want from life and what we don't. That can be hard and painful but, in the end, it will serve us well.

Back in March we talked about space clearing and the importance of having a clear, pure space around you in which to live your life. Now, at this important transition of the year, it is time to go back and fine-tune your living and working space (we will also do some more of this in winter). Throughout the summer you will have been spending more time outdoors. The windows will have been open, allowing air to flood through your home. But now, as you start to batten down the hatches for the approach of winter, it is time to focus once more on how your inside surroundings can best serve you. This time I would like to introduce the Eastern art and science of feng shui, which I mentioned briefly at the beginning of this book. There has been a lot of interest in this over the last few years and you may well be familiar with it. If not, it will probably sound very strange. Bear with me, it is well worth trying out.

Feng Shui: Esoteric Interior Design

You may well think that what happens to you in life is purely luck or chance. Health, wealth and happiness? Fame and good fortune? Simply the luck of the draw. Others might consider that we make our own luck just as easily as we can make our own money—by hard work or simply by adopting a positive attitude. However, how many of us would consider that our surroundings have a large part to play in whether we swan through life with ease and pleasure or fight tooth and nail every step of the way? According to the ancient Oriental science of feng shui, we can bring about sweeping changes in our lives simply by making small changes in our homes and offices—from where we place our bed to how we arrange our desks.

The easiest way to describe feng shui is as a sort of subtle interior design which works rather like acupuncture for houses. An essential part of Far Eastern life, it is now becoming wildly popular in the West as people realize there's more to interior design than having the right curtains and the right furniture: you need the right energy as well.

As we've already discussed, the ancient Chinese discovered that there were invisible but powerful lines of energy (known as *chi*) running through the human body: if the energy ran smoothly and freely, the person enjoyed good health but if the energy became stuck or imbalanced, disease and illness followed. Similarly, they came to realize that the same energy ran through the environment and that it could become stuck or imbalanced in houses and offices just as easily as in the body. Stagnant or unchannelled energy could result in all manner of problems from lack of money and lack of promotion to family arguments and family ill health.

"It was discovered by minute observation, over three thousand years ago in China," explains Sarah Shurety, one of the small but growing band of UK feng shui consultants. "First of all they realized that certain places were auspicious, the energy flowed well, whereas in other places it was sluggish or too undisciplined. The same applied to buildings, but here they could be even more specific: they found that certain areas of the house were related to different areas of life." Gradually they developed a map, known as the *ba-gua*, which plots eight different areas in a house relating to career, inner knowledge, family, wealth, fame, marriage, children and helpful people. If an area is missing or the layout of a room is badly planned, then the corresponding area of your life could suffer.

It sounds fanciful but feng shui consultants can read your house as a palmist reads your palm, pointing out your strengths and weaknesses, warning of potential pitfalls. They can be uncannily accurate. I first came across feng shui several years ago when I was living in a Victorian terraced house in London which, like many such buildings, had a rough L-shape. Money was always tight, but I never dreamt of blaming my house—until I talked to international feng shui consultant William Spear who informed me that my wealth area was totally missing, lost out in the back garden. The "cure," he soothed me over the telephone from New

York, was to position a large green shrub in a huge terracotta pot in the garden where the missing corner should have been. I felt a bit foolish but followed the advice and within a month my income had quadrupled without any extra effort on my part.

Total coincidence? Possibly. But when I moved to a new house in the country and life didn't seem to be going well I decided to take no chances and asked Sarah Shurety to take a look. She had never met me before and knew nothing of my life but as soon as she walked through the door she looked alarmed. "Have you noticed changes in your life since you moved here?" she asked. "Accidents, bad luck, lots of drama?" Well, only two car accidents, a fire, a leaking roof, several deaths in the family—all in the last nine months. "I'm not surprised," she said with sympathy. Apparently my main problem lies in the straight line of four doors leading from the front door right through to the other side of the house. This, says Shurety, allows energy to rush unimpeded through the house, creating havoc and chaos.

As she walked through the house I was given a shopping list of alterations: painting my study blue and placing a large plant by my computer; adding wind chimes to the dining room; placing a heavy curtain across one of the offending doors in the hallway and even popping a mirror in the yew tree in the garden to put a brake on the energy which apparently races down the lane opposite. The main bedroom was a disaster, she said, and if I wanted my marriage to last, it would need to be almost totally redesigned. But at least, she soothed, I didn't have a beam over the bed. Beams, she warns, are bad news in feng shui.

One woman she consulted was on the verge of divorcing her husband; they were barely talking. Shurety soon found the reason: a large beam ran down the middle of the ceiling over their bed. "They were literally sleeping on either side of it—it was causing a terrible division." She advised that they move the bed, and now the couple are "madly in love again." Another client had suffered from mysterious stomach problems for three years. She too had a beam over her bed—this time over her stomach area. As on this occasion there was nowhere else to move the bed, Shurety advised her to cover the beam with dried flowers. She obeyed and within three weeks all her symptoms had gone.

But how, I asked, can something as trivial as covering a beam have such a profound effect? "Energy is very subtle," says Shur-

ety. "Think of how just putting a small twig in a stream can affect
the whole water: it sends ripples out and alters the entire flow.
So simple changes in your home can bring profound changes in
your life." Cynics might say that simply by focusing on the problem, you start to subconsciously work out your own solutions.
Shurety shrugs in agreement: who cares how it precisely works
when it patently does work?

People often consult Shurety when they want to move home
or when they have problems selling houses. She has helped people to get publicity for pet projects and parents to sort out problems with their children. Curiously enough, however, most of her
work lies in advising businesses. Feng shui is so effective that
many firms are now consulting experts like Shurety to ensure
that profits stay high, that employees will work well together and
that the company will achieve a high profile. "Lots of bankers
and stockbrokers use it," she says, "although they don't often
advertise the fact. I'm never quite sure whether it's because they
don't want the competition to cotton on or simply that they think
it sounds too weird."

Before you race off to hire your own feng shui consultant, I
have to warn you that they don't come cheap by any means.
However, they would argue that the visit will usually pay for
itself within a short space of time (by ushering in extra income)
or be beyond price (if it helps to salvage a relationship or help
your health). Nevertheless, there are plenty of things you can try
for yourself before calling in the experts.

DIY FENG SHUI FOR HEALTH, WEALTH AND HAPPINESS

William Spear advises that before you launch into DIY feng shui
and hang the mirrors and crystal balls which are traditionally
used to "cure" problems all around your house, you need to
spend some time thinking about what you want to change in
your life. In other words, it is pretty much the same process you
carried out when you filled in the questionnaire at the beginning
of this book. However, at this juncture think about what precisely
you want to change or shift. It might be an improvement in your
income or your relationships, or you might need a complete
makeover following a separation or loss, years of difficulty, and

a long stream of "bad luck." Setting goals will help you gain a perspective.

In feng shui life is divided into nine sections. Spend a little time recapping these areas of your life.

1. Your career (Spear calls this The Journey). How do you feel about the work you do? Are you fulfilled by your career? Or are you not working or in a job you hate or which does not satisfy you?
2. Marriage and other close relationships. How are the partnerships in your life? Your spouse or partner, your friends, your colleagues? Are you surrounded by solid, healthy relationships or is your personal and social life a desert?
3. Family (particularly your relationship with older people). What kind of relationship do you have with your parents? Your grandparents? Do you have respect and love for them or do you avoid them at all costs? If they are dead what kind of memories do you have—good or bad?
4. Wealth. Is money a real problem for you or do you always have enough cash to go around? Do you feel you are lucky or do you seem to attract a string of bad luck?
5. Unity. This is the central core of the universe and life. There is no direct way to evaluate this section.
6. Helpful people. Are there lots of people you can rely on or do you often feel quite alone? Do you, in turn, help other people or volunteer your time?
7. Children (although this can refer to creativity in general). Does your life bubble with creativity, or do you feel less creative than a block of wood? If you have children, are they a source of joy or a permanent headache? Do you want to conceive but find you can't?
8. Knowledge. What is your relationship with the spiritual world? Is your life full of spiritual meaning or are you too busy or too skeptical to look at life beyond the material?
9. Fame. Are you recognized in your work and fulfilled in your life? Or do you worry that people see you in a bad light; do you feel people don't respect you and your work enough?

Completing this exercise should show you which areas need attention. Each of these sections relates to a different area in our homes. By shifting the energy in the appropriate area of your home you can alter that part of your life. To discover which part of your house corresponds to which of the nine sections, feng shui uses a kind of map called the *ba-gua*. Imagine an octagon (eight-sided) shape divided into nine segments: the center is known as unity and fanning out from it are eight equal segments. It's a little like the points of a compass. At the top (the north position) is the area governing fame; northeast is marriage; east is children; southeast is helpful people; south is career; southwest is knowledge; west is family and northwest is wealth. To work out which part of your home corresponds to which area simply imagine the ba-gua superimposed on your house (your front door will lie along the south line—either directly south, or southeast or southwest). Then you will see that the room in the far left-hand corner will correspond to wealth; that in the far right-hand corner will relate to marriage and so on. Sometimes you can instantly see what is wrong. If you have a lavatory in the area of wealth you could, quite literally, be flushing money down the toilet. If your house is built so that the marriage corner of the ba-gua is missing, you may well have problems with your relationship. If your hall (which often corresponds to career) is cluttered and full of rubbish you may never truly succeed in your work.

Individual houses need individual solutions. Often when you start to think about feng shui the answers will come quite sponta-

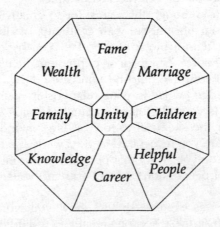

neously and intuitively. However, there are certain things everyone can consider in their home.

First impressions are important. Walk into your home as if you were a stranger.

- What is the first thing you see when you arrive?
- What is the first aroma you notice in the house?
- What did you hear when you arrived?
- What did you notice that needed fixing?
- Overall, what was your impression of the place?

If your first impression is of clutter and chaos, then that is what you will have in your life. If your hall feels cramped and dark, that will govern the whole of your life. Equally, a clear light yet comfortable first impression will most probably reflect a clear comfortable life. Pay attention to your front door, above all—it is the entrance to your interior world. It should be well-kept and in good working order. Houses where doors stick have occupants with loads of frustrations.

THE CURES

Feng shui uses a battery of "cures" to help move energy around the home, to clear "stuck" energy and to calm too much energy.

Mirrors Mirrors can be very helpful but need to be placed with care. Do not use small mirrored tiles that fragment your image. Equally, steer clear of mirrors that divide your image (for example on wardrobe doors). Mirrors should reflect something pleasant—a pond or garden, treetops or the sky. Do not place a mirror where it reflects dustbins or the bathroom. Mirrors are used in feng shui to replace negative space so if you are missing an area in a room or house, mirrors can be placed on the walls that border the negative space. They also help to increase space and energy. If you have a cramped narrow passageway use a mirror on the walls. If a corridor ends with a blank wall put a mirror on the wall—perhaps even a convex one to spread light and energy.

Silver Balls These are small round balls which are often sold as jewelry. They are used to deflect harmful energy. If a road leads directly toward your house, or a large building looms over it or faces it (for instance, a church, a tower block, a larger house), you may suffer from "cutting *chi*" which can affect the health and happiness of the inhabitants. Place a ball or a small octagonal mirror (from Chinese stores) to hang in a window that faces the road or building. Hanging a silver ball from the mirror inside your car is said to help keep you safe from accidents— providing you still drive carefully.

Crystals Crystals activate energy: choose clear man-made glass or lead crystals in symmetrical shapes (orbs, diamonds or teardrops). Buy them from gift shops or charity catalogues. Put them in any corner of the room to stimulate the energy in that area. However, do not use them in combination with other cures.

Wind Chimes Wind chimes moderate or change *chi* flow. Use them if you have a series of doors in a line to break up the energy or between two distinct spaces (for example, the living room and dining area). If a neighbor sometimes plays loud music try putting wind chimes in a window that faces them. If they *constantly* play loud music you will need the silver orb instead!

Plants Healthy green living plants can help to harmonize the energy in a house or office. If you want to stimulate a particular area, put a large green plant in that particular corner. However, only use plants with sharply pointed leaves where there is plenty of room—if the space is small use plants with soft rounded leaves. Equally, avoid cacti in cramped areas.

Water Water symbolizes good fortune to the Chinese. A bubbling aquarium with healthy goldfish will bring good fortune. Placing a birdbath outside the home, particularly if there is negative space, will activate the missing energy. However, keep it clean and well-maintained. Stagnant water creates confusion.

A Few General Tips

• Make sure you are still clutter-free. Ten to one the piles of papers, old clothes, broken toys, general rubbish have grown again since March. For *chi* energy to circulate freely, rooms should be clean, bright and clear.

• Always keep the lavatory seat down; otherwise you could be flushing away money and good energy. Put a notice above it to request that your visitors do the same (it's bound to provide a talking point as well!).

• Make sure the basics are working well in your house: gas leaks, clogged plumbing and blown fuses can all affect your health. So can broken window panes and creaky, stuck doors and windows.

• Mirrors are good for feng shui but they should not be tarnished. Also ensure they are hung at the right height. If they are too high, people feel uncomfortable; too low, and they could create headaches.

• Spiral staircases can cause health problems. Grow a vine or other climbing plant around the banisters and install a light on the ceiling above the stairway to shine from the top floor to the bottom.

• If you have a beam over the head of your bed you might suffer from migraine or headaches; a beam over the stomach can cause ulcers, and if the beam crosses your feet you might find your mobility limited. Again break up the energy of the beam by decking it with something soft like a swag of fabric or a garland of dried hops.

• A blocked door or window symbolizes something blocked in your life or health. It can be as literal as bad constipation! The energy should be able to flow freely throughout the house. If a door has to be blocked, cover it with an ornamental curtain or hanging.

• If the windows outnumber the doors in your house by a three to one ratio, you can expect cheeky children who always talk back. Hang a bell or wind chime near your front door.

• Young children should always sleep in the "children" position (see the ba-gua) in their bedrooms. Alternatively, place something white (e.g., a soft toy or flowers) in that position.

• Teenagers need to have their beds in the "knowledge" position, or place something black or green there instead.

• When children go job hunting, enhance the "career" and "helpful people" positions with wind chimes or things which are black and green.

• Doors which are overly large for a house or room can cause money to disperse. Place a heavy object at the entrance, near the door.

• Bathrooms should not face the kitchen or money will be flushed away. Hang a mirror on the outside of the bathroom door.

• Beams over your stove or dining area indicate financial loss, in particular lent money will not be returned. Attach a red fringe along the beam.

• Couples should sleep with their bed in the "marriage" position of their bedroom, or place something red in that spot.

• If the relationship is rocky, check the "marriage" positions both in your house in general and also in the bedroom. Try putting a green plant there.

• Stones or statues can help stabilize a volatile relationship. Place in the "marriage" position of the house or bedroom.

• At work, your desk should always be positioned diagonally opposite the door, with you facing the door.

• If the boss sits too close to the door, she or he will be treated as an underling and lose respect. Workers in more advantageous positions will become insubordinate.

• If you sit directly in front of, or behind, your boss, place either a crystal paperweight or a bowl of water on your desk.

• Workers who sit close to the door will leave early and avoid overtime.

• Computer workers who have their backs to the door will become stressed. Sitting with your back to the door can even cause you to be demoted or made redundant. If you really can't move, position a small mirror on your desk so that you can see the door.

• To attract more money into the office, put a plant or fish tank in the "money" position.

• Fish in offices can bring good luck and help to prevent accidents. A tank with a bubbling aerator is most effective.

A Final Word on Feng Shui

Feng shui may still sound absolutely daft but please give it a go. Just try a few of the DIY suggestions and see what happens. If you find it fascinating then it is well worth investing in one or two books which go into this vast subject in greater depth. I've listed the most useful ones at the back of this book.

September, to my mind, is a very practical month. Esoteric though it may seem, feng shui always seems inordinately sensible and down-to-earth to me. You shift something in your house and something shifts accordingly in your life. Cause and effect— wonderful. The other most helpful suggestion I feel I can give you this month is also wildly practical. It is a simple series of techniques which will give you more time to get things done in your life. It's called, quite obviously, time management.

From Managing Space to Managing Time

Time management sounds hideously boring and very corporate. Surely, you might think, it's the kind of thing only men in pin-striped suits do. Well, yes—and no. Everyone can, to my mind, do with a few extra hours in the day, and who needs time management more than a busy mother or a frenetic schoolchild? Really it's very simple but exceedingly effective. Personally, I have found it a life-saver. I have always had piles of paper reproducing in my bag, in the car, on the kitchen table, in numerous drawers, by the side of the sofa. My Post-it notes tend to breed faster than rabbits and I have been known to manage my life from two diaries, four calendars, six notebooks and a filing system from hell. The result? A life of barely suppressed panic.

I'm sure it's not just me. Time, it seems, is our greatest modern enemy. Admit it, how many times have you muttered, "If only I had more hours in the day"; "If only I had time to retrain, to learn that language, to write a book—*then* life would be great." But does it have to be that way? A few years back I interviewed businesswoman Peggy Czyzak-Dannenbaum. She had four sons, a great marriage, ran a six-million-pound company, was vice-chairman of a hospital trust, did "a bit of charity work" and played soccer in her spare time. Yet when I talked to her she seemed to have all the time in the world—how? "You have to learn how to think, to sort out the unimportant from the important," she told me. "You have to learn how to create priorities and you have to learn how to manage your time."

Time management is the key to ending panic, learning how to run our lives rather than letting our lives run us. The concept is not new, but what *is* new are the numbers of people flocking to take courses in this science of managing your life. I tried one out in London, run by one of the largest companies, Time Manager International.

"Time is a line running through your life and we don't know how long our line is," was the merry pronouncement that greeted fifty of us from our trainer Frits Dirks, an ebullient Dutchman. "If you knew how long your line was, would you live your life as you do now?" An uncomfortable silence filled the room as we contemplated mortality and long empty stretches of well-wasted time. Most of us, he pointed out, either lived in the past ("if only I had . . .") or in the future ("when I get . . ."). "It's no good talking about something," he lectured. "If you want to influence the future you have to take action NOW!"

The Time Manager course is predominantly aimed at people in management and uses a sophisticated form of Filofax system to make effective use of time. But the principles it teaches apply to anyone who needs to manage their life and time, and you don't need a fancy system to make time your ally rather than the enemy within. I found the following points really useful. Hopefully you will too.

IDENTIFY YOUR GOALS

Where were you five years ago? What were you doing, who were you with and what were your goals, your dreams? And where are you *now*? Are you in the same place with your goals transferred or have you achieved your dreams and are setting new ones? Are you still seeing people you don't really like that much or are you frustrated because you don't have the time to see the people who are important to you? These were the first questions Frits put to us. "Ask yourself what are you doing and why," he advised. "Without awareness you have no choice, so have regular goal-setting times, establish what you want on a regular basis."

Goals can be short term or long term, anything from writing a report or hitting deadlines, starting up your own business or learning a language, to losing weight, spring-cleaning the house or playing regular squash.

The key is to spend regular set time checking them: a few minutes each day and every week, a little longer each month, and maybe set aside a day a year for long-term goals.

Make your goals clearly defined, realistic but challenging, and set a manageable timescale for achieving them: deadlines are essential.

Break down large tasks into manageable chunks and set sub-deadlines. The Olympic gold medallist John Neighbours cut his time by a seemingly impossible four seconds in four years by planning to cut his speed by 1/1200 of a second every hour! A successful dieter scheduled a weight loss of just two pounds a week and focused every week on her mini-goal and what she needed to do to achieve it. Within four months she was at her target weight.

PLANNING

Once you know what you want to do, you can concentrate on how to do it. Frits advised us to regard planning as a long-distance journey: you need an atlas (for overview), a road map (for more detail), and then to keep looking around as you actually drive while frequently checking the road map and the atlas. What's going on ahead, are there brake lights? By looking ahead we can avoid crises in the future.

As with your goals, you should aim to set aside periods for planning. Again, do this regularly: every year (for an overview); monthly (for middle-distance); weekly (for closer focus) and daily (for an action plan). Ask yourself what you want to get out of the period ahead; what are your goals; your most important tasks; how much time you have already committed (for example, to holidays, courses, family, meetings) and what long-term large projects you have.

A PLANNING SESSION A DAY

Long-term planning is important but daily planning will make an instantly noticeable effect on your life. It only takes around five minutes at the end of each day to prepare for the next, but it could save you hours. Having a clear plan for the day ahead focuses the mind like nothing else; you instantly feel in control which boosts your energy and your performance. Frits believes it could do even more: "With a clear awareness of the tasks and problems of tomorrow, you can put your subconscious brain to work and it will start to produce ideas and solutions—even while you sleep." Whether or not the answer to your prayers arrives in the morning post, you will certainly find it easier to ward off interruptions and be far more efficient.

How do I know? Because I've tried it. Usually I have about four half-finished features on my desk, and every so often I wander off into a daydream. The phone rings and I natter for a while and lose my thread. Someone pops over for a chat and, before I know it, it's dark outside and I haven't achieved anything on my "to do" list. *This time* I threw out my endless "to do" list and worked out what I could reasonably achieve in a day. I set aside half an hour for calls, an hour for a sociable lunch, scheduled an appointment and set aside clear blocks of time for specific projects. I achieved more in a day than I normally do in a week! Try the following tips:

• Just before you finish work ask yourself what regular scheduled tasks you have for tomorrow—block them off in your diary.
• What is your major task, what *must* you do tomorrow? Set aside a realistic block of time.
• If you still have time left, ask what you would *like* to achieve and how much time each thing would take? Schedule them in. Remember to add in any traveling time.
• In addition, make a list of short one-off tasks (phone calls/letters/birthday cards) that could be slotted in. If you find you have overestimated your time and have a few spare minutes, use them for these tasks.
• Don't make long lists of everything you have to do. It is demoralizing and causes lack of concentration. Instead, analyze what has priority and plan accordingly.
• Finally, spend a few minutes getting everything ready: clothes, sports gear, papers, keys, travel pass.

EATING ELEPHANTS

Some people always just get by; they scrape deadlines, catch the odd aerobics class halfway through the stretch and bolt a sandwich on the run. Others always seem in control; they meet deadlines with ease, exercise every day, have a wonderful social life and cook gourmet three-course dinners and somehow contrive to learn Hindustani in their spare time. How? They have set their goals, planned their time and, finally, developed a technique for dealing with those seemingly impossible vast tasks, such as learning a language. Frits calls such monster tasks "elephants" and deals with them like this:

• First divide your "elephant" into "bite-size" pieces and schedule regular bites in your schedule.
• Secondly, make sure you "eat" a bite every day, in addition to your other tasks.
• And finally, make sure you finish your elephant and don't take on more than one or two elephants at a time.

So, if you wanted to learn Hindustani, you would not only schedule in your weekly classes but also commit yourself to learning ten new words a day. It doesn't sound like much but by the end of the year you would have learned 3,650 new words.

KEEP A BALANCE

"It's nice to do things efficiently and effectively and even better to do the right thing at the right time," says Frits. "But sometimes the last thing you want to be is efficient and effective." In other words don't become a monster, even if you are an efficient monster. Balance is the key, and effective time management is about giving yourself and the people you work with and live with better quality time: it is not about running your life like a spartan health camp. Used properly, it should mean that you find you have all the time you need to work effectively, to socialize and play, to work steadily toward fulfilling your goals and still have time to collapse on the sofa on a Sunday afternoon without feeling guilty. Relax, you've got all the time in the world.

THE BAD GUYS: TIME STEALERS

1. The telephone. Telephones have a horrible habit of ruling our lives. Try to keep calls during busy periods short and

to the point. Phone people just before lunch, before they leave work, before they take the kids to school—they won't keep you nattering so long! If you can, set aside phone-free periods for tasks that need concentration and bunch all your calls into set phone periods.

2. Drop-in visitors. People who always say "have you got a minute" and then chat for hours. Make it clear to people when you can be interrupted and when not. Use body language to dissuade persistent pests—stand up and look them straight in the eye rather than lolling at your desk. Keep them at the door rather than inviting them in to sit on the sofa.

3. Inefficient meetings. What is the meeting for? How long does it need to take? Is it really necessary? Be clear, concise and set a time limit.

4. Disorganization. Lack of planning, lack of priorities, papers all over the desk or all over the kitchen table. Keep clear, focused, direct and tidy.

5. Inability to say "no." Are you scared of offending people? Do you take on far more than you can logistically cope with? If you know how much available time you have, you can judge whether you can take on any more. If not, then say so clearly and politely.

6. Lack of self-discipline. You know you *should* be doing that report, attacking that pile of washing, writing that letter but you'll just have a small break, just make a quick call, just have lunch . . . Give yourself deadlines and stick to them, using your daily plan.

THE GOOD GUYS: TIME SAVERS

1. A clear desk or workspace. Keep only *one* thing, the thing you are actually working on, in front of you.

2. A large rubbish bin. Look at each piece of paper as it arrives and make a decision about it. Either deal with it, file it, or bin it—immediately.

3. Schedule "Me" time. If possible allow yourself certain periods each day when you won't be disturbed. Use them for

dealing with elephant tasks, for creative work or ideas, or simply for sitting quietly and refueling.

4. Become proactive rather than reactive. Decide what you will do and when. Plan what you will do and when; treat "appointments" with yourself just as appointments with someone else, only breaking them if absolutely unavoidable.

5. Take stretch breaks every hour. Just walk around for a few minutes and you will return refreshed and with your concentration replenished.

6. Look at your energy. Some of us are early birds, some night owls. When are you most creative, most organized? Schedule your day accordingly. When do you feel half asleep or on another planet? Don't attempt something major, use the time to make calls, catch up on small tasks.

With feng shui and time management working for you autumn should be getting off to a great start. However, there is one other subject I want to introduce now which is NLP or neuro-linguistic programming.

NLP is a series of techniques which can be highly useful for everyone because, at the simplest level, it helps you to communicate more clearly and effectively. It teaches how people perceive the world around them and how, by understanding the way they work, you can make more immediate and effective contact with them. It is used extensively now in business, in politics and in education. It can also help you on a far more basic level: understanding what makes your partner and children tick; how to deal most easily with difficult people at work; how to avoid unpleasant confrontations in daily life.

NLP: The Master Communicator

What makes one person succeed where another fails? How come some people can debate metaphysics in a foreign language while the rest of us are still stumbling over "Two beers, please?" Are we just genetically wired to be either super-achievers or also-rans, or can we change the program? Feng shui can help, so can organizing your time more effectively with time management, but advocates of NLP insist there's a scientific, precise technique that will stop you languishing in the mire of mediocrity. We can, they insist, all be super-people. If one person in the world can do it, instructs NLP, so can you. You just need to learn *precisely* how they do it and then copy them.

If it sounds far-fetched look at a practical example. Two women of similar height and build joined my gym at about the same time with the aim of getting fit and losing weight. After six months Jan is looking pretty good: she's lost about two stone and is getting trim and firm. Sally, on the other hand, has lost a few pounds but is beginning to think it's a waste of time. The difference could be their metabolism, it could be any number of excuses, but one obvious reason is noticeable on the aerobic studio floor. Jan stands at the front and copies the instructor move for move, putting in as much energy as she does, echoing precisely the way she moves her arms and legs. Sally meanwhile lurks at the back, half-heartedly following her own version of the class. Almost before the class has finished Sally races off to the showers while Jan stops to chat, asking how the instructor gets so much energy, what she eats, how she keeps fit herself.

What Jan is doing, more or less unconsciously, is following an NLP technique called "modeling" which can, if properly applied, give us a precise map to achieve the same excellence as the person we model.

NLP started in the 1970s in California when Richard Bandler (a mathematician and gestalt therapist) and John Grinder (a professor of linguistics) started to question what exactly made some people brilliant in their work while others remained mediocre. As an experiment, they picked three people who were acknowledged experts in their fields and "modeled" them, finding out exactly how they worked, how they thought, how they perceived, how they moved and spoke, what minute processes took place and exactly the sequence in which they happened.

Their findings were the start of NLP, not really a therapy but more a precise tool for understanding human communication and improving it; of working out what causes excellence and how we can each achieve it. Although their first models came from the field of therapy, Bandler and Grinder swiftly went on to model business people, athletes, dancers, teachers, even politicians. The results were so impressive that they put their findings together and called this new system for analyzing excellence as NLP.

Jo Hogg from the ANLP (Association for NLP) says: "The official definition of NLP is 'the study of the structure of subjective experience,' but it comes down to looking at what we do unconsciously and then being able to improve it. It's almost like taking an advanced driving test."

Anthony Robbins, an American-based workshop leader and author of several best-sellers, puts it like this: "The movers and shakers of the world are often professional modelers, people who have mastered the art of learning everything they can by following other people's experience rather than their own. They know how to save the one commodity none of us ever get enough of—time."

It sounds brilliant, but how exactly can we take the theory and put it into practice? Most good bookshops stock books on NLP but the procedures can be tricky to master from the printed page, so I went along to a weekend course to find out how to pursue excellence. Around fifty of us (a mixture of therapists, teachers, businesspeople and the simply curious) gathered at a hotel in Wembley, north London. The trainer, Emile Ratelband, is an ex-student of Anthony Robbins with an overload of energy who told us that since learning NLP he has swum with sharks, slept in cemeteries and sky-dived. "I can smash wood like a karate expert," he strutted. Well, bully for him but the rest of us wanted to learn something more directly applicable to everyday life. Ratelband obliged and we uncovered some of the skills of perfect communication.

The first lesson is that in order to effectively communicate with someone you have to know which "mode" they are in. Apparently we have three modes of functioning: visual, auditory and kinaesthetic (feeling). You can usually tell which mode a person is using at any time by their body posture, the speed of their speech, their breathing and even the words they use. NLP teaches that many of our misunderstandings occur when people communicate in different modes; say when a person in visual mode tries to communicate with someone in an auditory state. Good communicators "match" the person they are talking to. So if, for example, they are talking to a "visual" person they too will go into visual mode, speaking rapidly, breathing quite high in the chest and using "visual" words and phrases such as "I *look* at it this way," or "I *see* what you mean," "What's the overall *picture?*" Suddenly you are speaking the same language.

Following on from this is "rapport-building" in which by subtly mirroring the person you are talking to (adopting a similar posture/speaking at the same speed/breathing in synchronization) you can almost instantly put someone at ease. Basically it's all about learning how brains work and how different people's brains work in different ways. Simple techniques like the above can prove highly effective in any situation, from soothing the boss, getting through to the kids to communicating honestly with your partner.

Understanding how brains work is also fundamental to the ability to model. In order to copy someone exactly, it's not enough to merely mimic their physical moves, you have to get inside their head, to find out the processes behind an action. Anthony Robbins gives an example of the strategy athletes use to model the best in their field.

"If you wanted to model an expert skier, you might first watch carefully to see what his technique is," he advises. "As you watch, you might move your body in the same motions, until they feel like a part of you. Next, you would make an internal picture of an expert skiing. Then you would make a new visual internal image, this time a disassociated image of yourself skiing. It would be like watching a movie of yourself modeling the other person as precisely as possible. Next, you would step inside that picture and, in an associated way, experience how it would feel to perform the same action precisely the way the expert athlete did. You would repeat that as often as it would take for you to feel completely comfortable doing it. Thus you would have provided yourself with the specific neurological strategy that could help you move and perform at optimum levels. Then you would try it in the real world."

Back in Wembley, Emile Ratelband told us that by modeling fire-walkers we, too, could walk on burning coals. What's more, he says, we can actually test out our prowess—over five meters of red-hot embers. Trousers rolled up to knees, eyes held high, Ratelband clenched his fist and marched straight across the burn-

ing path, shouting, "Cool moss! cool moss! cool moss!" He arrived, totally unscathed, at the other side and then everyone in
turn followed him, fear turning into amazement turning into sheer
joy and high spirits. Mike, an actor, was ecstatic: "I feel I can do
anything now," he gushed. "If I can do the fire-walk then nothing
is impossible. I feel liberated, empowered, brilliant."

Scientists have, rather disappointingly, proved that the fire-
walk is perfectly possible without all the mantras and the
clenched fists, but Ratelband says that's not the point. "It's not
really about fire-walking," he insists. "It's about taking control.
When you walk across the fire you turn your fear into power."

Transformation is the key to NLP. Turn your fear into power;
your failure into success; your ailing backhand into a mesmeriz-
ing Arnie of a shot or your flabby body into a supermodel shape.

"If you want to achieve success, all you need to do is find a
way to model those who have already succeeded," concludes
Robbins. "That is, find out what actions they took, specifically
how they used their brain and body to produce the results you
desire to duplicate. If you want to be a better friend, a richer
person, a better parent, a better athlete, a more successful busi-
nessperson, all you need to do is find models of excellence."

ASSESSING CLUES

As we've learned, NLP teaches that we each favor a specific
"pathway" or mode of perceiving the world—visual, auditory or
kinaesthetic. But how can you tell? Here are some guidelines:

• Ask someone a question that requires them to recollect something in the past—for example, what did you do last weekend?
If, when the person answers, they look up to your right they are
predominantly visual. If their eyes slide from the left to the right
of your face, they are mainly auditory. If they look down and
to the left then right before answering, they are working in a
kinaesthetic pathway.
• How do you best learn a new subject? Do you need to memo-
rize a page of information (visual); repeat facts out loud (auditory) or write down what you are learning (kinaesthetic)?
• What kinds of words do you use to express yourself? Would

you talk in terms of seeing ("I see what you mean"; "The picture is quite clear"; "Look at me when I'm talking to you")—all primarily visual. Or in terms of hearing ("I hear what you're saying"; "I'd like to sound them out"; "Listen to me when I'm talking to you")—auditory. Or in terms of feeling ("I feel it in my bones"; "It really touched me"; "Can't you feel the difference?")—kinaesthetic.

• If you're assessing a child, there are other ways of gauging. When the child is angry do they look you in the eye with defiance (visual), scream and shout (auditory) or stamp their feet or throw themselves to the ground (kinaesthetic)? What would they notice first on a walk in the park? Other children, the birds and animals around (visual); the sound of music playing, dogs barking, people shouting (auditory) or the wind, the rain, the cold or the heat (kinaesthetic)?

This may all sound very interesting in theory, but what help is it practically? Well, if for example you were deciding to learn a new language it would be helpful to choose a method which allowed you to work in your most comfortable pathway. So a series of audio tapes would not be enough for a kinaesthetic person, while an auditory person would not do so well with a simple textbook. A visual person will always manage better with clear text and diagrams, an auditory person through spoken words and a kinaesthetic with practical examples. In an ideal learning situation all three pathways will be used.

NLP can also help you understand people. You will never sell a car to a kinaesthetic person by telling them to "Look at the fabulous styling" or to admire the color. They need to sit in it and *feel* the solidity, the comfort, the grip of the wheel. People find they get on much better with their boss or a difficult member of the family if they can talk the same language, picking up on which pathway the person works in and shifting your own language to match their own. It's subtle but highly effective and, if you are interested in good communication, well worth investigating in greater depth.

October

October is truly the heart of autumn, full of glorious color and a light bright sparky kind of energy. Mists shroud the hills and float low over the fields giving a ghostly feel to early morning walks. Spiders' webs are miracles touched by dew while the bright berries of the rowan and hawthorn and the gleaming hips of roses sparkle with frost that looks for all the world like caster sugar. Their glossy colors make up for the fact that everything else in the garden is dying back. One hard frost and it's farewell to brave lingering bedding plants while the bright and cheery nasturtiums wilt and shrink back away from its chill. Leaves continue to dance in the breezes and rustle in drifts along banks and pavements. Raking them up is great October exercise; rolling in them afterward is wonderful October fun.

This month in the Native American calendar sees the Falling Leaves Time give way to the Frost Time. We start to wrap up warm, to bring in logs to keep cozy around the fire. Trails of smoke snake from chimneys. Almost as evocative as the berries and turning leaves are the smells of autumn—the scent of woodsmoke, of burning leaves, of the cruel crisp frost.

In the country, October is a month of housekeeping, of husbandry, of stocking up and storekeeping. Vegetables are gathered

in to be stored, nuts are collected and mushrooms provide a free
harvest from the fields. The apple harvest waits to be transformed
into fragrant, heady cider. At this time of year the wisewomen
would brew their cordials and syrups for the winter months:
draughts of sloe berries against stomach cramps and diarrhea;
elderberry cordial for respiratory problems; rosehip syrup for
coughs and colds. The last of the lavender has been dried and
laid in the linen cupboards and amongst summer clothes to deter
moths and keep everything smelling sweet and fragrant. Corn
dollies are made and placed above the hearth to hold the spirit
of the corn alive and safe throughout the harsh winter and to
remind us that the cold will not last forever—spring and the new
year's sowing will come around once more. On the hills they are
starting to bring the animals down to pastures lower and safer.
Hedges are cut and ditches cleared. The bull appears in the fields
and sheep are mated for early lambs.

October may be beautiful but not everyone loves its charms.
Many people find autumn and the approach of winter a time of
anxiety and even fear. When you think about it, it's actually a
very natural feeling. Everything about us is in decay and decline.
The days are getting shorter and colder, there is less sunlight to
keep us cheerful and we tend to stay indoors more. The decay
of nature, the rotting of the leaves, can all put us in mind of our
own mortality, our own frailness. It's very reasonable and so
don't imagine these feelings should be suppressed as morbid or
unnatural. Who's to say we have to be perpetually cheerful and
bouncy? That would be as artificial as permanent summer.

Autumn is a natural time of reflection. It's the forerunner to
the contemplative season of winter in which we start to look at
our very souls. And bear in mind that while nature does rot and
decay, it never stays that way. The leaves of this year will provide
the rich leaf mold that will feed back into the earth to provide
nourishment for the next year's leaves. Truly nothing is lost in
life—we live in a perpetual round of recycling. Marian Green,
who has written wisely and beautifully about the seasons and
pagan life, reminds us that while we live in a society which sees
death as a cut-off point, a launch-pad to another existence, other
cultures see death as merely a pause in the chain of incarnation,
a time for rest and reflection.

So October is a strange, often unsettling month. On the one

hand it is still full of the light bright energy of early autumn, a time for bustling and sorting out, for rearranging your life and deciding to throw out the old in order to make space for welcoming in the new. And yet, as October moves toward November it becomes more reflective, more soulful. The shift from autumn to winter is more gradual than that from spring to summer and from summer to autumn. The two energies start to mingle. So this month's suggestions are a combination of these two forces.

Before we launch into winter soultime, we need to be able to calm ourselves enough to pause, to stop, to allow a little space in our worlds. We need to learn that there are times to throw ourselves into the world with energy and times to withdraw. We need to be able to relax and recharge. Hopefully the ideas on time management will allow you a few more hours in the day. It's not a bad idea to schedule in "quiet" time, especially around this time of year when the energies are shifting.

The Mid-Autumn Cleanse: Strengthening Your Body for Winter

We can recharge on a physical level too. This is another excellent time of the year to use a short spell of detoxing to cleanse and strengthen your body. By adapting your diet as suggested in the run-up to autumn you should have weathered the change of season quite well, but it is still a good idea to have a real clearout. It will help you on the mental level as well. By getting rid of accumulated waste and toxins you will be giving your body the message to "let go." This will, in turn, be passed on to the mind and emotions, helping you to push on with the great task for this part of the year—getting rid of all that no longer serves you to make room for the new and exciting.

I turned to Fiona Arrigo, psychotherapist and body worker who originated Stop the World, for advice on how best to ease yourself into a pre-winter clean-out. She suggests you follow this program for between five and seven days. However, if you're feeling really good on the regime, you can extend it to ten days.

As with the May detox, it's better if you can set aside time for yourself away from work and commitments. If that's impossible, just be as gentle on yourself as you can and say "no" to as much as you can. As Fiona says, "If you do this while you are working, make sure you have at least a reasonably stress-free week to do it in. It is hard work detoxing when you are stressed." I'd say it's hard work detoxing at any time—so make it as easy for yourself as you possibly can.

YOUR PRE-WINTER CLEAN-OUT PLAN

Days 1 and 2

On rising Take a mug of hot water and freshly squeezed lemon. If you have fresh mineral water so much the better; simply boil it and add the lemon. If you have to use tap water it's best to boil it for a good fifteen minutes. If you're hopeless first thing in the morning, you could make up a thermos flask the night before—providing it will keep the heat so it's still hot (rather than lukewarm) in the morning.

Half an hour before breakfast 120 ml fresh juice (start with apple and carrot). You really do need freshly made juice for this so buy or borrow a juicer if you don't already have one. Commercial juices often have added extras or, even if they don't, will never be packed full of all the vitamins of the fresh juice.

Breakfast Warm fruit (the warmth is important as the weather is getting colder). Choose from apples, kiwi fruit, oranges, etc. (but not bananas, and avoid dried fruits as they tend to have a high-sugar content). Don't overcook the fruit; you can gently warm it in a pan with a little juice so that it doesn't burn.

Half an hour before lunch 120 ml fresh juice as before (or you can alternate: try beetroot and apple; carrot, spinach and celery; carrot and beetroot).

Lunch Steamed vegetables (as many as you like). Try to avoid adding salt or commercial dressings. A little lemon juice, ginger and garlic will make a tasty dressing. They *are* boring, I know, but choose the vegetables you like best and think of all the good it's doing you.

Half an hour before dinner 120 ml fresh juice as before.

Dinner Any amount of vegetable soup that you like the sound

of. Again, stick to natural seasonings: celery will help you avoid
the need for salt. Add herbs or spices for flavoring.

Throughout the day You should drink a minimum of four liters
of water throughout the day. If you can take it hot (try making
up a thermos of boiled spring water), so much the better—it
seems to travel through the system and, according to Ayurveda,
will help to dislodge mucus and toxins. If you've tried it (and do
try it, honestly it's not as vile as it sounds) and still absolutely
hate it, stick to room temperature (not chilled) water.

You can also drink peppermint or fennel tea in abundance,
but steer clear of "normal" tea and coffee. In addition, Fiona says
to avoid salt, vinegar, dairy produce or dairy by-products, sugar,
canned or frozen foods, alcohol or meat.

Days 3 and 4
As before, but add in lots of whole grains at lunch: brown rice,
millet, couscous.

Day 4 Onward
As before, but a baked potato can be added to lunch if you wish.
If you continue beyond Day 7, you can now add porridge to
breakfast, made with water not milk.

This will all sound horribly bland and tasteless, particularly with
no salt to perk it up. However, you can add warming spices
such as cayenne, paprika, ginger and cardamom to give it zest.
Remember, as Fiona says, "The point is to keep the food as
warm, plain and digestible as possible to enable the system to
rest and recharge."

While you are detoxing, Fiona suggests you take a few supplements to help the process and support your immune system in
the run-up to the cold season. Take echinacea (either in tablet
or tincture form) which is readily available from health stores or
herbalists. Don't overdo echinacea, however. Use it just for the
duration of this detox. A strong vitamin C supplement will help
too (make sure you ask for a buffered version if you suffer from
gastric problems or ulcers). Fiona is also a fan of blue-green
algae (also available from health stores).

That is the food side of the equation but, to gain the optimum benefits, you need to add a little more. So, take on board the following.

• Take some slow, even exercise throughout the duration of the detox. It shouldn't be too taxing or exhausting, as you don't want to put extra strain on your body. Walking is excellent, particularly if you can get out into the fresh air of the countryside. Yoga is great; so is t'ai-chi. Psychocalisthenics (described in detail in *Supertherapies*) is a pretty wonderful swift form of exercise which gets to every muscle (both internal and external) in the body.

• Try some breathing exercises or meditation (or mindfulness— skip ahead to the WINTER section for details). Or all three. You are aiming to detox your mind as well as your body and nothing will help more than stilling it from the bustle of everyday life.

• Do anything, says Fiona, that has the quality of ease and relaxation. "I would suggest a lot of sleep," she says. Great idea. If you keep feeling drowsy and tired, go with it and let yourself sleep.

• In addition Fiona suggests listening to gentle music, investing in smells, oils, flowers, and burn scented candles to enhance your well-being. This is a time to feed all your senses and allow everything to rest and recover. So choose the kind of music that soothes you—probably not heavy rock or Wagner. It doesn't have to be "New Age" pipe music, didgeridoos or whale music (although if you like it, that's great); it could be gentle folk music, soft classical, mellow jazz. Choose aromatherapy oils which you love to scent the house. Treat yourself to flowers you adore— even better if they smell divine too. Splash out on scented candles (virtually every cosmetic house now produces them but make sure you like the scent). If in doubt, stick to aromatherapy favorites like lavender and geranium.

• Brush your skin regularly. Get into the habit of doing it before every bath or shower (incidentally baths are probably better during this process as they are more inclined to relax you). Use a body brush with natural bristles, or a damp flannel with a bicarbonate and salt mixture, and brush smoothly, always moving toward your heart. It is essential while you're detoxing because it allows the lymph to circulate and to remove toxins.

• On the first night, just before bedtime, give yourself an Epsom salts bath (providing you have no heart condition or high or low blood pressure). Use about 450 g of Epsom salts (available from chemists) and dissolve them in a warm bath. Relax for about twenty minutes (candlelight will help, as will some relaxing aromatherapy oils in a burner) and when you get out wrap up warmly, especially your feet. Get into bed and you'll find you'll sweat away even more toxins.

• Try to arrange at least two massages if you can afford them during your cleansing program. Aromatherapy is lovely, so is MLD (see MAY) which will help rid your body of the toxins it is shedding. If you can't afford a professional, try to persuade a friend or partner to give you a massage. Or, if all else fails, set aside time to massage yourself. It's not quite the same in the pampering stakes but it will still have a wonderfully beneficial effect on your body.

• A steam bath or sauna (if you have access to either) will be of great benefit around the midweek mark. And any beauty treatments you can afford won't go amiss either. This isn't just about cleansing, it's about giving yourself time out for you. So facials, body wraps, even manicures and pedicures will all be very worthwhile. Check if your local health farm or spa offers one-day packages. I occasionally dive into nearby Cedar Falls, where I live, for a "Top to Toe" day which gives me a facial, a massage, a steam and unlimited use of the facilities, including yoga classes and swimming pool: all ideal pursuits on a cleanse. Of course, you'd have to check that they could provide you with the raw provisions of your detox diet, but any health spa worth its name should be able to come up with fresh juices and steamed vegetables.

• Fiona's last prescription is to look into positive thoughts and affirmations, if you feel so inclined. You can skip ahead to December for more on these.

These guidelines are really just that, guidelines. As long as you're not pushing yourself, do whatever feels good. Learn to listen to what you really want and then give it a chance. You may well find, if you follow all these ideas, that you will experience side effects. On a physical level you might feel tired. You could find you get a terrible headache as you suffer withdrawal from stimulants like tea and coffee. It's possible you might find you get a little constipated. This is all quite natural but, if you feel uncomfortable or worried at any time, check with a naturopath or your doctor.

The side effects might not all be physical either. Often detoxing like this will bring up emotional issues, old problems, or even new ideas and plans. Sometimes this can feel a little unsettling and so make sure you have someone you can talk to, if necessary. Maybe a good counselor or simply a close friend who can be at the end of the phone.

Don't let this put you off: a good cleanse at this time of year is often harder than the spring version but the results can be very profound. So give it a try.

Halloween: Pulling Back the Veil Between the Worlds

Of course the whole of October is really limbering up to the great festival of Halloween, or Samhain as the Celts called it. For years Halloween has languished in the shadow of Guy Fawkes night in the UK, while in America it has become a formal institution with a huge marketing push behind it to sell all those masks and costumes, decorations and pumpkins. Now we seem to be following the same path. I would like to suggest we pause just a moment and see if we can get back to the original feel and meaning of Samhain. It doesn't mean the end of trick-or-treating or the banishing of ghost costumes—far from it. It's simply a case of remembering why we do these things in the first place.

In the olden days Halloween wasn't just confined to one night—on October 31; it was celebrated over the last couple of weeks in October. It was the time when families would come together for reunions, before the weather became so bad as to prevent travel. Those who lived the summer months up on the mountains or in faraway pastures looking after livestock would bring their animals down and themselves with them, returning home after long periods away. This was another great fire festival (like Beltane), and so it is quite easy to see how Bonfire Night or Guy Fawkes fits in. Originally the huge bonfire would have been simply a Samhain fire, a beacon to guide wanderers home and to welcome guests into the feast. It was also an homage to the sun, almost a reminder of what heat and warmth and light looks like, in the hope that the great sun would not be extinguished forever.

Nowadays many people see Halloween as a ghoulish, unpleasant, devilish festival with its demons and skeletons and eerily grinning lanterns. Some say it should be banned altogether because by dwelling on the dark, occult side of life we are inviting evil into our homes. Not so. Samhain *is* a dark festival, a festival of the dead, but that is no bad thing. Our ancient ancestors believed that this was the time of the year when the veil between this world and the shadowy world of spirits was at its thinnest. It was considered a time of remembrance, of the past, thinking about and honoring our ancestors who have passed away. But equally, it was a time for peering the other way through the shadowy curtain, into the future.

In the past, Samhain was a time to look forward as well, thinking about the children that will be born in the future. One old tradition is that not only can you see the spirits of the dead appearing in the bonfire smoke, but also the candles lit on Samhain call in the souls of the children who are waiting to be born in the coming year so they can inspect their future parents and look at their future home.

The traditions of Halloween/Samhain all have their roots in very ancient customs. The grinning lanterns are to scare away evil spirits while the dressing up in strange costumes was again a ploy to fool spirits or evil demons so that they wouldn't recognize you and follow you home. And while we may think "trick-or-treating" is a new-fangled American custom, its roots are very ancient. Samhain was a time for clearing debts and quarrels—a kind of rough-and-ready score-settling. Neighbors would offer a choice: you stopped doing whatever annoyed them or paid up your debt, or you took the consequences. Horses and cows might be hidden; gates removed, windows whitewashed. The "vengeance" was certainly not meager, but there were clear rules over which no one would step: you could not harm any person or distress any animals.

Many people find it odd that Halloween should be so

strongly associated with children. But, as pagan priestess and therapist Shan explains, Halloween is a wonderful opportunity for children to come to terms with scary ideas in a gentle and fun-filled way. It's a chance for them to explore and start to understand their fears of the dark, of death, of the unexplained, in a safe environment.

"One of the most important things Halloween does is to present children with their bogeys and help them get used to them," she says. Every year she organizes a festival for pagan Halloween and a central part is the children's fashion show. "Children come up with really grisly costumes," she smiles. "They don't know about cancer and leprosy and dying, but they are playing with the images. By playing with them they can get used to the fact that life has its ugly side and learn to live with that."

However, it's not just for children. Halloween is a chance for us all to allow our deep, dark repressed fears to come harmlessly to the surface. Its aim is to help all of us to understand death and its place in the cycle of life. It helps us face our fears. The pagan belief is that we focus too much on life and try to shut out, to exclude, death. That is neither healthy for our psyches nor is it practical. Halloween is all about accepting that there is a time for ending. Just as the year dies, so too, at some point, will we. But hopefully, like the ever-spinning year, we too will return—if not to this world then to somewhere or something else.

Having discussed the more serious side of Halloween, it's time to look at another fascinating custom of this time of the year. As I've already said, Halloween was a traditional time for looking to the future as much as revering the past. People looked into bonfires and candles to see spirits, and there are myriad customs for peering behind the veils of time to see a peek of the future—generally to see the face of a potential lover! This is the time for divination; for tarot cards, for runes, for all manner of oracles and auguries.

Divination: How the Future Can Help You with the Present

Many people are terrified of oracles, of divination and the whole process of looking into the future. They say it's unnatural, dangerous and terrifying. I wouldn't agree. However, I would say that you should approach this whole area with as much respect as you would approach a doctor or therapist—it's not a parlor game. People have consulted oracles since time immemorial. There is nothing new in it. Nor need it be frightening. Certainly divination can seem uncanny; sometimes the cards or runes or whatever can almost precisely mirror your situation. However, at other times, they can be quite wrong. The main point about any form of divination is to take it in the right way. Truly speaking, it is not about seeing the future. Rather it is about looking at a problem or situation in a nonlinear way—it's like a kind of lateral thinking.

A common response to any question of divination is the old one about the tarot: "What if I get the death card?" Well, there are two issues here. Firstly, the so-called "death card" in the tarot pack is not necessarily or even probably about death. Its meaning is transformation, a change, a shift in life. Obviously, you could argue that death is the ultimate transformation but, in truth, it very rarely presages death. And secondly, people presume that the reading they get is carved in stone; that it will happen, no matter what. Again totally untrue. It seems that systems like the tarot or the runes deal in possibilities, not certainties. When you lay out the cards you are really tapping into a complex web of possibilities. The cards are saying that given the present situation and your attitude, your state of mind, this is the *most likely* outcome. People who use divinatory tools properly see them as opportunities for growth, for development. They would look at a potentially unlucky spread and ask what they could do to improve the situation, how they could avoid anything unfortunate. Those who are truly enlightened will use it as a tool for personal development and not be at all interested in the predictive powers of the cards.

It is these last aspects that I am most interested in here. I have little time for "fortune-tellers" who tell you what will happen in the future. Firstly, I do not believe anything is written in stone—we always have choice and free will. Secondly, they are often wrong, very wrong. And what is most worrying is that if people believe their predictions they might even make them come true because of their own conviction. I'll give you an example. A few years ago, just before I was due to get married, a friend badgered me into seeing a tarot card reader. Being a natural skeptic, I took off my engagement ring before I went in. First the man told me I was a nurse (which was news to me) and then he proceeded to tell me that I wasn't in a relationship. "Actually I am," I replied. "Well, it's not serious," he countered. "Er, well, I'm getting married next month," I answered feeling thoroughly irritated. "Oh no you won't," he said firmly. What a hideous thing to say to someone. I walked away thinking it was utterly ridiculous but, over the next few days, it started to prey on my mind. Why wouldn't we get married? Would I have an accident? Would Adrian, my partner, have an accident? Would there be a death in the family? Although rationally I knew the man was hopeless (after all I'm certainly no nurse), my subconscious went into alarm mode. Needless to say, we got married without a hitch, but the weeks before the wedding contained one more stress factor I really didn't need.

So, be wary. But don't let that put you off exploring what can be very useful tools for understanding your psyche. Just be careful that you don't end up relying on them too much. Some people badger oracles incessantly, trying to get the answer they want. That is pointless. Used properly, an oracle is a means of stilling your mind and allowing maybe your subconscious or super-conscious a chance to have a say. Often the answers can be very revealing—if you are prepared to listen with open ears.

Which oracle you choose is up to you. You may well be drawn to a particular pack of tarot cards or feel a kinship with the runes. Trust your intuition. If you are in any doubt at all I would always recommend the I Ching, which is not really a system of divination at all, more the ultimate self-help tool. Wise and gentle, it has none of the negative connotations surrounding tarot and no weird images that could possibly frighten you.

THE I CHING: A WISE FRIEND

The *I Ching* is one of the oldest books in the world, yet the advice it offers strikes straight to the heart of most modern dilemmas. The *I Ching* or *Book of Changes* (which dates back to at least 3000 B.C.) is a personal guidebook on how best to handle the complexities of life, giving precise instructions on how to deal most effectively with your career, your relationships, your family, your health. If you are uncertain which path to take, what action to follow, ask the I Ching. It will tell you how to act, when to act or when simply to keep your head down and do nothing. If you're at all indecisive, the I Ching could be your greatest ally—it truly is the great decision-maker.

The I Ching is often mistakenly represented as a form of divination, but in reality it is perhaps the first self-help manual. The process is very straightforward, based on throwing coins and noting which way they fall. You shake three coins of the same denomination in your cupped hand and let them fall onto a flat surface. You will receive one of four possible combinations: three tails, three heads, two tails and one head or two heads and one tail. Each combination is represented by a broken or unbroken line; three tails or three heads give rise to what are known as "moving" lines which are marked accordingly. It sounds complicated but the process soon becomes second nature. It may seem like little more than fortune-telling but most people who try the I Ching soon realize it is far more complex: the text doesn't tell you what will happen but rather advises you on the best way to maximize the potential of the current situation. It won't promise tall dark strangers or presage a sudden windfall on the lottery. In fact it comes across not as a soothsayer but more like a sage grandparent, offering cogent (and not always welcome) common-sense advice.

I have used the I Ching for about fifteen years and have found it uncannily accurate. Once when I was house-hunting I decided to throw the coins to check a flat I was considering. The oracle expressed deep disquiet telling me in no uncertain terms to beware of a "hidden pool of dark water." This seemed a little dramatic but, on a return visit, I moved a bed and discovered just that—a dark puddle of water created by seepage.

I Ching expert Sarah Dening showed no surprise at my experi-

ence. As a Jungian psychotherapist she has used the I Ching in
her practice for many years. She is also the author of *The Everyday I Ching.* There have been many translations and commentaries of the Chinese text over the years, most of them complex
and often confusing. *The Everyday I Ching,* however, offers an
ideal starting point, giving clear concise instructions on how to
use the oracle and answers couched in everyday language while
still remaining true to the original intent of the I Ching. Once
you're familiar with it you will probably want to obtain a copy
of the larger, more complex, commentaries. Rest assured that the
I Ching can become a lifetime's study. Many people use it as a
basis for their whole personal philosophy.

"The I Ching is remarkably accurate if you use it properly and
respectfully," says Dening. "Use it well and it will enhance your
life as though it were a wise and trusted friend." She explains
that the I Ching predates acupuncture and the ancient exercise
systems of t'ai chi and chi kung; it is older still than the increasingly popular science of feng shui which we discussed last
month. In fact, the I Ching is the foundation on which all elements of Chinese philosophy and science are based. Acupuncture
clears away blockages in the body by allowing the vital energy,
or *chi,* to circulate freely and easily. Feng shui does the same in
the outer environment by allowing a clear energy flow around
the home and workplace. Similarly, the I Ching advises you on
the right actions and the right timing to allow yourself to move
freely and easily through life itself, to "get into the flow."

It might sound rather vague and "New Age" but the I Ching
is anything but. It was used for centuries by Chinese rulers who
wanted to govern well and, as Sarah Dening says, "It is very
strategic, quite political almost—and highly pragmatic." In America,
she points out, it is often consulted for business purposes and
she says, with a smile, that it wouldn't do prime ministers and
presidents any harm to consult it from time to time.

However, most of Dening's clients are not concerned with affairs of state. One came because she had been offered a five-
year contract at work but felt uneasy about accepting it. The I
Ching advised against it, promising that something better was
around the corner. Against all practical considerations, she re-
jected the offer and went on holiday to take her mind off her
decision. On the beach she made friends with a couple who

turned out to have wide connections in the field in which she had always wanted to work. Now she has a new and very rewarding career.

Another woman was anxious about her marriage. Her husband had a very high-powered job and she felt she was neglected and unappreciated. She retaliated with moods and arguments and the relationship was floundering. The I Ching reprimanded her to stop "making dramas" and not to imagine problems that didn't exist. "She was stunned," recalls Dening. "She just sat there and nodded. But she took the advice seriously and stopped criticizing and demanding attention and, in turn, her husband began to relax and the whole situation turned around."

But how can simply throwing coins come up with such precise and accurate advice? "Nobody really knows how it works," admits Dening. "It's certainly uncanny, and yet I don't believe there's anything magical or mystical about it." She thinks most likely the I Ching connects us to the unconscious part of our brain, the intuitive side. "It seems to act as a bridge between you and your deep intuitive knowledge. Somewhere deep inside you really know the answer to the question, it's just hidden from conscious thought. I can't prove it but I think it allows you access to right brain information that allows you to see the whole picture."

To get the best out of the I Ching you have to phrase your question very clearly and precisely. Sarah Dening finds that often the simple process of focusing on the problem helps to straighten it out. She often sees people for a one-off session when they feel stuck in a situation or can't make up their minds which course of action to take. "Often simply talking about it can help," she says, "and sometimes the answer appears as they formulate the question." One thing the I Ching will not stand is idle or foolish questions, or being asked the same question over and over again in the hopes of a more palatable answer. Ten to one the flippant questioner will end up with the hexagram which in Sarah Dening's book is called Inexperience: "Advice is only useful if you are prepared to listen," it warns. "It may be you already knew the answer or, as so often happens, you have already consulted the I Ching on this point. The answer you received was not the one you wanted and so you keep on asking in the hope of being given something more to your liking." This, it says quite brusquely, is not acceptable. Reading it makes you feel like a naughty child.

On the whole, however, the I Ching is gentle, wise and kind. Used properly it can become a valuable tool, not just for negotiating the pitfalls of life, but for self-development and growth. C. G. Jung, the famous psychotherapist who was a great advocate of the I Ching, believed that it would help you to discover your true essence. "Jung said that we come into life with an essential blueprint of what we are," says Sarah Dening, "and that all psychotherapy and growth was about finding your way back to the essential self. He said it was the point at which you were touched by the divine."

However it works, the I Ching has a profound effect on everyone who uses it. It's like tapping in to an infinitely wise, infinitely loving source of knowledge. And yes, at times it does feel like talking to something close to divine.

ASTROLOGY AND KI-OLOGY: THE CARD FATE HANDS YOU?

Astrology is hugely popular. There is hardly a paper or popular magazine which does not carry horoscopes. People buy hoards of books telling them whether, as a Cancerian, they will get on with their Piscean husband or how to prevent rows with their Leo or Scorpio child and spend small fortunes calling up telephone astrological services. However, astrology, like most things in life, is only as accurate and as good as the person who is practicing it. Certainly the horoscopes appearing in the paper or on the phone lines will hardly be precise enough to offer any real advice. However, a really good astrologer can draw you up a personal chart and give practical advice which can help in all areas of life.

As with divination and oracle-consulting, astrology has been debased and turned into a bit of a giggle. But there is little doubt that good astrologers can see which influences will hold sway over us in our lives, and a professional and ethical astrologer can give good advice on how best to manage difficult aspects or capitalize on the good. Some astrologers now combine their work with professional counseling which is something I have not personally experienced. However, if it does appeal and you can find someone who can satisfy you that they are suitably qualified in both areas, then it may well prove very valuable.

While astrology is very well-known, almost too well-known for its own good, there is another system which seems to have equally accurate results but which has mainly avoided astrology's widespread appeal in the West. Once again, we have the Chinese to thank. Nine Star Ki or ki-ology has been used by them for millennia. Now it is beginning to be practiced in the West and is well worth investigating if you fancy an alternative to Western astrology.

A ki-ologist can interpret the great imponderables of life. They can explain such mysteries as why, when you patently adore your family, you are always at each other's throats. Or why everything has gone horribly wrong since you took that wonderful new job. "Luck is not random," insists Takashi Yoshikawa, an acknowledged master of the science. "It is the outcome of moving harmoniously with the laws of nature." Ki-ology has its roots in ancient China and follows the same philosophy that guides the I Ching. It evolved centuries ago over a long period of careful and precise observation of nature. The ancient Chinese recognized that not only was there a fundamental duality in nature (which they called *yin* and *yang:* negative and positive, female and male) but that vital energy (*chi* or *ki*) expressed itself in five different ways—Wood, Fire, Earth, Metal and Water (as discussed in the introduction to this book). The ancients watched the unfolding of the yearly cycle in nature and gradually came to realize that the same cycle was governing their own lives as well. However, not everyone was at the same place in the cycle: each person seemed to have an individual pattern determined by their date of birth. Such were the origins of ki-ology and, over time, the system became even more refined. The five elements became subdivided into nine numbers and by using a quick set of calculations, ki-ologists can take your birthdate and from it uncover the three numbers which hold the key to understanding how the elements shape your life.

"The energies combine and interact in different patterns," says Takashi. "They are always changing, yet they repeat according to certain cycles. These cycles can be traced in charts that reveal their patterns and show how the ki-energies can be used to our best advantage." By comparing an individual's energy pattern with the energy pattern of the year, ki-ologists are able to make uncanny and highly precise predictions. Takashi predicted the outcome of the Bush/Clinton election and warned of problems in the marriages of Princess Diana and Prince Charles, the Duke and Duchess of York, even Madonna and Sean Penn.

Work with the elements, and life will run smoothly and harmoniously; buck the tide, and mere existence can seem like a permanent struggle. "Natural laws control our lives," says Takashi. "So if you understand the natural laws, you can make life much happier: decisions about travel, the home, marriage, getting a job, making an investment are all easier."

In Japan many top businesspeople won't sign a contract or make a large investment without consulting Takashi. In the States he is in constant demand from film and music stars. But in the UK few people have even heard of ki-ology and there are only a meager handful of ki-ologists. However, Simon Brown, who was taught by Takashi, believes the situation will soon change. "In five years time, ki-ology will be quite commonplace," he predicts. "People will use it because, quite simply, it works." Simon regularly advises pop singers on everything from which producers to work with to when to release a single; actors on which projects will pan out best. Other clients use him almost as a cosmic dating agency, phoning in to check the numbers of people they meet to see whether the relationship is worth pursuing.

Quite fascinated, I asked Simon to check my ki-numbers. He ran through a swift calculation in his head, consulted a book and then announced that my numbers were 5, 1, 9. The first number is the key number, our basic nature. The third shows how we appear to other people and the middle number shows our emotions. He proceeded to draw a pretty accurate character sketch. Then he checked my husband's numbers to see if we are compatible. I held my breath and waited for the verdict but luckily our energies are quite happy with each other. "He needs to give you space and you have to be careful not to hurt his dignity," says Simon, "but if you can keep that in mind you should be fine."

He feels that all relationships could do with a little ki-scrutiny. "Ki-ology can give a lot of clues as to why relationships aren't working well. It is totally objective, like holding a mirror up to your relationship. I find it works perfectly for all sorts of relation-

ships—romantic, work, family. It helps you understand why people work in certain ways." He cites the example of a woman
who had always felt she was the black sheep of the family. Her
parents and brother had always seemed to exclude her in a subtle
way and, over the years, it had undermined her self-esteem and
she had piled on excess weight. A ki-ology consultation revealed
that the rest of her family shared the same middle number, indicating that they communicated on precisely the same wavelength.
As an opposing number, she wasn't being deliberately excluded:
she just didn't speak the same language. Understanding this made
all the difference and allowed her to get over the feeling that
she was in the wrong. She stopped blaming herself for their
disagreements.

A detailed consultation with a ki-ologist can provide you not
only with a good insight into your character but also with a list
of auspicious dates and, equally, a guide to the best directions
in which to travel. It sounds crazy but apparently the very route
you take to work could be affecting your career. And moving
house in an inauspicious direction could completely stagnate
your work opportunities and even scupper your sex life. It all
appears distinctly perilous; rather like running blindfolded along
a cliff top. One move in the wrong direction and you're pitched
into disaster. "It's not as drastic as that," soothes Simon Brown.
"Many people follow Nine Star Ki guidelines almost by instinct."

Given the choice, I'd rather have an insider's tip at the hand
fate holds for me. And while, like feng shui consultants, consulta-
tions are very expensive, those who rely on ki-ology to clinch
their million-pound deals or simply save their marriages would
say the advice is priceless.

COULD YOU BE PSYCHIC? DISCOVERING THE HIDDEN PART OF YOUR MIND

Halloween wouldn't be Halloween without tales of ghosts and
apparitions; of weird and bizarre happenings. There's nothing
more spine-chillingly fun than sitting around a glowing fire with
candles the only other source of light and telling true-life ghost
tales. Almost everyone has a personal ghost story—whether it
happened to them, to a friend or to the inevitable "friend of a

friend." Some people appear to be naturally psychic. Certainly most children seem to be able to see things not visible to the naked adult eye. I swear I saw the ghost of my cat when I was very small; and heard the ghost of my grandfather and smelt his tobacco. I also remember my nephew when he was very young telling us that there was a man lying on my grandmother's bed. My mother and I were alarmed, to say the least, but when we looked in the room there was no one there. However, the child could clearly see someone who made him very nervous. Needless to say, it made us pretty nervous too.

I haven't seen any ghosts since then but I would never dismiss the paranormal. There is simply too much in the world we do not properly understand yet to say with certainty that such things as ghosts and ESP and telekinesis and so forth just don't exist. And now there are an increasing number of DIY psychic courses appearing all over the UK which claim that learning to be psychic can help you in all areas of your life. Furthermore, they promise that virtually anyone can learn how to do it.

ESP, dowsing, telepathy, clairvoyance—terms that used to be met with a howl of derision—are now being reassessed. The psychic realm is growing in popularity by the minute, and it's no longer solely the province of elderly ladies peering into tea cups or New Age mystics touting tarot cards. In America, hard-nosed businesspeople are calling on the services of professional psychics to help them make the right decisions and recruit the best staff. Scientists who for years have scorned psychic phenomena as incompatible with the laws of physics are begrudgingly starting to concede that it might just be their knowledge of physics which needs to be reconsidered rather than the phenomena.

But can mastering ESP really prove of practical help in your life? Isn't it little more than yet another magic trick to amuse guests at parties? Not so, insists Richard Lawrence, author of *Unlock Your Psychic Powers* and an expert in the field. "ESP can be very practical," he says. "Having a developed intuition can help you in every area of your life—from making decisions on the family holiday to working out a better way to health." It could even perk up your love life. As Lawrence points out, "You might have a strong intuition to go to a particular party and end up meeting the person you marry."

As someone who traipsed to a decade of parties, intuiting

(quite erroneously) that I'd bump into Prince Charming I was
skeptical, to say the least. But Lawrence was unfazed by my
caution. As European secretary of The Aetherius Society, which
runs dozens of courses in DIY ESP, he has witnessed hundreds of
skeptics transform into fully fledged psychics. I challenged him to
turn me clairvoyant. "Let's start with something easy—dowsing," he
advised. I held a thin string with a light wooden pendulum between thumb, forefinger and index finger and Lawrence instructed me to ask a question to which I knew the answer. "Is
this carpet green?" I queried and, before long, the pendulum
started to swing quite independently and quite distinctly in a
clockwise circle. At first the feeling is quite unnerving, almost
spooky, but it quickly seems quite natural.

Having ascertained that the pendulum would swing clockwise
for yes and counterclockwise for no, we moved on. Lawrence
laid out a selection of food items in front of me and asked me
to concentrate on health. The pendulum veered approvingly
toward the olive oil but disliked the coffee, lemon and eggs
(looping grumpily around in a circle). All perfectly accurate: I'm
pretty intolerant of citrus fruits, coffee and eggs. But then this
was information I already knew, so perhaps I was influencing
the pendulum. Even so, how was the darn thing moving in the
first place?

We moved on to psychometry—picking up information from
an inanimate object. Handing me his wedding ring, Lawrence
asked me to relax, close my eyes and focus on the ring. "Watch
and see what happens," he advised. My first impression was of
a house with a stream at the bottom of the garden with a large
labrador. Was this where he lived? "No, but I've stayed somewhere like that." Not good enough. Next up was an image of
chimneys and a high-walled garden. Much better—Lawrence has
a roof garden surrounded by chimneys. I scored with images of
mountains (Lawrence has been up several recently) and a striped
golf umbrella (he plays golf and has one), but still I wasn't sure.
After all, I only had his word for it. Then I "saw" a stark room
containing a massage couch. There were posters on the walls
and no windows, making it dark. Lawrence was ecstatic. "Come
downstairs," he instructed, leading me down into a basement
room which was curiously similar—pretty bare, pictures on the
walls and a massage couch. It was very close but not quite the

same, I complained. "You won't get every single detail to begin with," he explained patiently.

Lawrence believes everyone can become psychic with a little training and solid persistence. And he insists there is nothing "magic" or "occult" about it at all. "People talk about having a sixth sense," he said. "Well, what I'd say is that there are five extensions to our five senses—psychic sight, hearing, smell, touch and taste. It's a case of extending your senses, learning to listen to your feelings, to your hunches."

Don't, however, think you can toss aside your reliance on more practical, intellectual methods overnight. ESP takes time and training before it becomes focused enough to trust implicitly. And although Lawrence insists that psychism is "certainly safer than driving a car," there are, he warns, some possible pitfalls. "You have to recognize that you can make mistakes and you do need a sense of humor," he says. "A big danger is to think that every single impression is infallible. Some trainee psychics get the impression of water and think that London is about to flood when all it meant was that the bath might overflow."

Above all, he is dogmatic that there is no implacable fate that rules our lives and is appalled that professional psychics can sometimes make people feel trapped in the web of predestination. "Fatalism gives the idea of a destiny out of control and that's wrong. The whole point of this is to control your destiny more." He insists that a good psychic should be able to help you get more out of life, pointing out areas of difficulty and pinpointing times of good fortune, enabling you to maximize your potential and minimize your risks. "It would be irresponsible to say to someone, 'if you travel by car, you'll die' but you could suggest that they take particular care while driving, have the car checked out and so on. You could save people from accidents." He was horrified by my tale of the tarot card reader saying I wouldn't get married.

Common sense is the order of the day. "Psychic abilities are just another tool at your disposal," says Lawrence. "Everybody should use them in their life. Not as a be-all and end-all, but as another valuable attribute."

Becoming Psychic

Psychometry is one of the easiest psychic skills to acquire. These are Richard Lawrence's guidelines:

1. Choose an item that is always worn by the person, for example, a wedding ring, watch, necklace.
2. Sit upright in a hard-backed chair. Remove your own watch and any rings.
3. Relax your shoulders, shut your eyes and start to breathe slowly and deeply.
4. Pick up the item and hold it between the thumb, forefinger and middle finger of your dominant hand.
5. Keep calm and quiet and wait to see what images or thoughts come into your mind.
6. You need to differentiate between imagination and psychism. When something comes into your mind, let it float away and see if something else comes in its place. Wait until an image or thought stays.
7. Try to find more detail about a scene. Are they any people there? Are they saying anything? Ask questions.
8. Do you have any impressions about the person? Any gut feelings or hunches?
9. Check each thought with the person whose item you are holding. Ask for feedback.
10. Don't worry if you are not accurate all or any of the time. Keep practicing.

November

November can be a bleak month. It's the forerunner to winter but without any of its delights, or so it seems. Nowadays November becomes almost lost in the early preparations for Christmas that take over the world. Christmas decorations arrive rather implausibly in the streets and the Christmas editions of magazines arrive at the beginning of November—a full six weeks before the event itself. And yet November has its own charms, a softer quieter energy than October—the start of the gentle slumber into winter. We are firmly into the Frost Time in the Native American calendar and fast approaching the Long Nights Time.

Guy Fawkes night kicks November off to a fiery start with its bonfires and fireworks and there are plenty of celebrations around the country to cheer up the first weeks of the month. These are continuations of the old Samhain/Halloween rituals and are linked to the old pagan fire festivals. Interestingly, Armistice Day falls within this period too, on November 11—a time for recollection and remembrance of those who died in the Wars and naturally allied to this time of the year when we are thinking about death and the past.

November shouldn't be a hectic month spent running around trying to sort out Christmas early. It is really a period during which we make our final preparations for winter and start to turn our thoughts inward. Marian Green, an expert on folk traditions and their inner meanings, talks about this time in the year as being one of revelation. Just as the fields are now stripped and bare, so we start the process of revealing our own emotions, minds and souls; we too can transform and open up. In the ancient times this strange period was a lull, an inbetween time: the old year had died and was waiting to be reborn. Meanwhile, we wait and watch.

I always feel as if we should put some effort into making November special in some way, to find small ways of making life a little brighter. One suggestion which always seems to work quite well is designating one day of the week as a Special Day. Ask yourself which day of the week seems the most dreary or dragging (most people seem to choose Monday) and then make a commitment to always doing something to make it special.

I hated Mondays toward the end of my time of living in London. Generally, we would have spent the weekend away in the country and then it was back through the traffic jams to work, unfriendly people, crowded tubes and noisy neighbors. For some people it might be quite the opposite, or it might be Wednesday you dislike, or Friday—whatever. The point is to give yourself a little lift whenever you feel the most low. That might involve cooking a special meal, going out to eat, spending an evening at the cinema or going to a gallery at lunchtime. It might mean having a warm, sweet-scented bath and retiring to your bed for the evening. I would firmly suggest some kind of massage as a supreme mood-elevator. Or treat yourself to a luxurious steam bath or a sauna. Or, even better, book in to a health farm or spa or a day and allow yourself to be totally pampered.

Such measures will also help you relax. More than ever at this time of year you need to keep calm and in control. It can be tough. But if you start to get your stress levels under control now, you will find December and Christmas much easier to handle. Stress is a common buzzword nowadays and generally banded about without much thought. But, if we want to keep happy and healthy we all, without exception, need to take stress very seriously. This is a good time to take a long hard look at understanding—and beating—stress.

Stress: The Penalty for Being Superpeople

Stress is a fact of life. Whether it is superhuman deadlines at work, the hassle of the morning commute or babies who just won't stop crying, there are few people who escape the symptoms of stress. Yet, according to doctors, stress can kill. Under stress, the body produces the hormones cortisol and adrenaline which cause changes in heart rate, blood pressure and metabolism to prepare the body for flight or fight. In normal life we can hardly run away from the situation or punch the person who is causing us anxiety so the body does not get rid of the excess hormones, resulting in unproductive or harmful stress.

Untreated, long-term continual stress can result in depression, anxiety, palpitations, ulcers, headaches or irregularities in the menstrual cycle. Allergic reactions can even be stress-triggered. Fortunately doctors *are* starting to become more sympathetic toward the problem. Whereas the old tendency was to dismiss the question entirely or fob the patient off with tranquillizers, GPs are now suggesting self-help techniques such as deep breathing and relaxation, hypnotherapy and meditation to teach them how to deal with the condition.

Yet many people feel they have no right to be stressed and dismiss the whole idea. They argue that we never used to have all this stress: in the "old days" we just got on with life and didn't waste time complaining about intangible problems like stress. Well, it may well seem like that, but do remember that we no longer live in the world of yesteryear. We are living in a world which is changing faster than ever before. Just think that there are people alive who grew up without air travel, without television, without computers, without superstores and convenience foods. Life was totally different. Not to say that there weren't stressful factors—certainly poverty was far more prevalent than now, and life could be excessively hard. Yet the sheer speed of life wasn't there. Nowadays we are all jugglers, balancing home and career in ways our ancestors simply couldn't have considered. The causes of modern stress are myriad. But how do you deal with it?

The key to combating stress is by realizing what pushes your buttons, what causes you stress. Is it just odd occasions or do you have a deep-seated problem with stress?

SHOCK TACTICS FOR SHORT-TERM STRESS

These tactics can be useful for occasions when you need immediate relief for tension and stress:

1. Don't fly for the coffee machine or reach for a Coke—caffeine merely exacerbates your stress mechanisms. Drink a long, cool glass of water or orange juice instead. Then get up, walk or jog around outside in the fresh air for a few minutes. At the very least get up and stretch—it gets the oxygen moving around your body, gives you fresh energy and stops rising panic.
2. Vent your spleen. If it's feasible, yelling your head off is a wonderful way of getting the stress out (I regularly scream like a banshee while belting along the motorway). Or invest in a punching bag for the office/home wherever, and give it a good thump or six. I've recently taken up Boxercise which is a circuit-training class based on boxing training. We get to punch and pummel all kinds of punch bags—everyone there insists it helps them get rid of stress.
3. Pratice constructive vandalism: beat the hell out of bubble wrap. It sounds acutely weird but American professor of psychology Dr. Kathleen Dillon has proved that popping bubble wrap (apparently the big bubbles work best) dispels pent-up nervous energy and muscle tension. She also points out that unlike many other forms of stressbusting, bubble-popping requires no instruction and no practice.

MID-TERM STRESS STRATEGIES

If you regularly find yourself at boiling point, it's time to adopt some longer-term self-preservation techniques.

1. Adopt a good mood diet. Doctors have always recommended regular meals to combat stress, but now they know that the actual foods we eat can affect our mental state. Depression, anxiety, an inability to concentrate, panic attacks, mood swings, forgetfulness and lethargy—all symp-

toms of stress—can be triggered by sensitivity to food. The new anti-stress diet is high in fruit, vegetables, pulses, nuts and grains—very similar to the sensible eating plan introduced at the beginning of this book. In their book, *Superfoods,* Michael van Straten and Barbara Griggs recommend grapes, millet, wheatgerm, brewer's yeast, oats, molasses and buckwheat as the latest anti-stress superfoods. Foods to avoid include all refined carbohydrates, sugar, tea and coffee, sweetened commercial drinks and excess bran. Hopefully, this will already be the way you are eating. If not, go back to the early chapters on healthy eating and consider changing your eating habits.

2. Exercise—strenuously. A good tough aerobic workout can release stress like virtually nothing else. Sports psychologist Christopher Connolly explains that when the body cannot rid itself of the excess hormones generated by stress it causes a harmful state in which the mind and body are permanently aroused. "If you're stuck in this twilight zone, you need to kick yourself into a state of pure physical arousal rather than pure mental arousal," he advises. "Then you can swing back into the state we know as rest."

3. Float. I enthused about floating in my first book, *Supertherapies,* and I still think it can be absolutely wonderful, so if you haven't yet tried it, do have a go. Regular floating in the equivalent of an isolation tank is one of the best stress-busters going. Not only does it relieve stress but it also enhances creativity, decision making and problem solving, so it is often used by high-flying businesspeople and creative souls. One of the frequent criticisms of stress-busting techniques is that they take up too much valuable time. "I'd love to do meditation or yoga," says a very stressed friend of mine. "But I just don't have the time." Well, floating could save you time in the long run. The ideas you come up with or the creative solutions to sticky problems might well save you hours in the normal world.

DEEP DARK STRESS: LONG-TERM SOLUTIONS

1. Delegate. You're not superman or superwoman. You can't do absolutely everything and, believe it or not, the world won't fall apart if you say no occasionally. Stress-management counselors all recommend taking stock of your life and deciding what's important and what can go by the wayside. Write a list of what causes you stress and see if there is anything that you can drop or delegate.
2. Meditate. Researchers have found that meditation reduces hypertension, serum cholesterol and blood cortisol which is related to stress in the body. Meditators see their doctors less and spend seventy percent fewer days in hospital than other people. Anxiety, depression and irritability all decrease while memory improves and reaction times become faster. Meditators, it appears, have more stamina, a happier disposition and even enjoy better relationships than the rest of us. Why wait? There are around sixty teaching centers around the UK where you can learn TM (transcendental meditation)—the easiest form for Westerners.
3. Practice mental circuit training. If meditation seems too far-out and mystical, follow the example of cosmonauts and astronauts, airline pilots and Olympic sportsmen, and learn autogenic training. It's recognized as one of the finest stress-busters in the Western world and, not only will it give you instant stress relief wherever and whenever you need it, it will also bring down blood pressure and cholesterol, relieve insomnia and ease migraine. It is easy to learn. A short course will set you up for life and after that you need only spend a few minutes a day on the exercises—or use them when you feel yourself getting severely stressed.

And, if after trying these strategies you still find stress is ruling your life then seek expert help. Try your GP first. He or she may be able to put you in touch with a psychologist specializing in stress management. Otherwise, the psychological associations or your natural health center should be able to put you in touch with someone who can help. If, however, you fancy something completely different take a look at Quindo.

Quindo: Banishing Stress and Boosting Assertiveness

Khaleghl Quinn has evolved an anti-stress system for the twenty-first century. A clinical psychologist and martial arts master, she has selected the essentials from various ancient practices and fused them with modern psychological and physiological research to produce Quindo, a streamlined system designed to beat stress and increase vitality; to increase self-confidence and give people back control of their lives.

"Quindo concentrates on five principles," explains Quinn, who has spent over twenty-six years developing the system. "Awareness, strength, confidence, safety and happiness. All the techniques we use work on these very basic qualities." The five qualities, she says, are the linchpin to well being. "When I was a psychologist the same words kept coming from my clients like a broken record: 'If only I were more confident'; 'If only I felt happier'; 'If only I had more strength.' "

Quinn had found her own answers through the Eastern martial arts and the ancient exercise and meditation system of chi kung; for many years she taught these principles, with good results. However, she found that many people were put off by the esoteric nature of chi kung or the very idea of martial arts. So she extracted the key elements of the ancient paths, pulled them together and developed an accessible modern system that would suit everyone. Now she offers Quindo in classes or individual sessions to everyone from young children to corporate giants, from housewives to physiotherapists.

A ninety-minute Quindo class packs in all aspects of Quinn's philosophy. A swift five-minute warm-up exercise from kung fu gets all the muscle groups of the body working and imparts an instant jolt of energy. Based on the principles of Tibetan and Chinese medicine, it dispatches the body's vital energy, *chi,* to race through all the meridians, or energy channels. Then she moves seamlessly on to personal safety, teaching simple effective techniques to put you back in touch with your own power. The aim is not aggression but assertion, learning how to stand your ground or wriggle out of trouble.

It's not all physical moves either: Quinn aims to improve your powers of intuition and awareness, learning how to see problems arising and avert them before they become unpleasant. Then she shifts the emphasis to tranquility training, instructing on how to create balance in your life, how to calm yourself and broaden your perspectives. The final element is de-stressing, exercises you can perform either standing or lying on the ground to promote deep relaxation and revitalization.

"It's very simple and down to earth," says Quinn, "but you're working with some very powerful concepts and techniques. They've been made simple without destroying their integrity." People who take the courses claim Quindo gives them more confidence and a greater feeling of belonging in the world; it removes much of the fear and uncertainty. It works wonders on people who are inherently shy and nervous. "The key is not being hooked into the bully/victim syndrome," says Quinn. "We want to be confident people with many resources at our finger-tips. Then you don't need to put people down, you take your own power." It's clear to see why Quindo works so well with children. Bullied children become poised leaders; shy children start making friends; parents are thrilled to see their sons and daughters become more confident; teachers are astounded to see marks improve. Quinn points out that the whole world is like a giant playground: there are always the bullies and the victims, even in families and large corporations. Quindo evens out your chances in a difficult world.

I have tried Quinn's classes in the past and found them excellent: well-planned and effective. However, this time I wanted to sample her new Quindo clinic where you receive one-to-one treatment to achieve "energy, vitality, serenity." The first step was filling in an in-depth questionnaire on my life. In addition, I had to mark on a drawing of the human frame where I felt I held stress: by the time I had finished you could hardly see the original drawing. "In fact the only things that actually *cause* stress are traumatic injury or pollutants," instructs Quinn. "Everything else is merely a contributing factor. When you realize that, it puts you back into a controlling position. The purpose here is to gently educate your mind and body to react in a healthy balanced way to stressful situations and to transform stress into vitality. We don't want to get rid of stress because it's an energy, but if we change it, it can work for you. It's all about transformation."

Quinn's clinical psychology background gives her a fondness for quantifying and measuring. She plots progress on an array of graphs so you can watch how your stress drops and your vitality increases over the weeks. She also employs a perception exercise. "Choose an object in the room," she requested. I picked a ceramic model of a waterfall on her desk. "Now describe it to me in detail." I picked out the colors and the material. She wanted to know how intense the colors appeared to me and how I knew it was three-dimensional. Then she instructed me to raise my right arm in front of my nose and to slowly swing it round toward my right ear, all the time focusing on the waterfall in front. I had to stop at the point where I could no longer see my fingers (just around my ear). Then I repeated the maneuver on the other side. The purpose of the exercise, she said, would become clear after the session.

We moved swiftly on to energizing the body, swinging arms in swooping movements from side to side and then to breathing techniques. The deep anti-stress breathing comes from chi kung: Quinn taught me to breathe from my abdomen right up through my chest, filling and emptying my lungs to a much fuller capacity than normal. Then she moved me onto the couch. Fully clothed, except for shoes and jewelry, I was tucked up in blankets like a small child. Quinn worked over my whole body, moving from back to front, feet to head, using a combination of rubbing and gentle acupressure. To be honest, I can't recall the whole sequence because within about five minutes I was so deeply relaxed that I think I must have fallen half-asleep. When she called me back I felt as if I had slept for eight clear hours: alert, refreshed and amazingly calm.

But the session hadn't finished—quite. Once more, Quinn asked me to focus on the waterfall and describe it again. I'm not sure whether it was because the sun had come out but the whole object seemed clearer and brighter, more focused and with greater contrasts in color and depth. When I repeated the arm exercise, I found to my surprise that I could still "see" my fingers when they had disappeared behind my ears. "You have moved a good few degrees back," confirmed Quinn. "It's because when you are more relaxed, more oxygen reaches your optic nerve and the cells fire with more ease." The exercise isn't just to prove how effective the treatment is; like everything in the Quindo system its aim is to expand your horizons.

"As children we are taught to see just what is in front of us and it shortens our imagination," she says. "Once you realize you can see beyond that, it allows you to perceive life in more detail. It's easy to say an object is 3-D but when you're facing a problem you often don't realize you are approaching it in a flat way."

True masters of Quindo can expand their perceptions to 360 degrees—they develop "eyes in the back of their heads." In a tough and ruthless world, that could prove an invaluable tool. In fact turning stress into vitality the Quindo way could become an essential alchemy for survival and happiness in the next century.

Learning to deal with stress is a big task and one which cannot be "cured" in a single month. But make a start, pick up some good habits and then keep a beady eye on your stress levels throughout the whole of the year.

As November continues, the focus turns further inward. In SEPTEMBER and OCTOBER we looked at ways of working with the energy of the year, finding how to best move and act. Now it's time to focus on our inner selves. There are two quite delightful ways of doing this. The first is art therapy, a way of tapping quite deep into your psyche and soul; the second looks at how an understanding of our dreams can illuminate our waking life. Both fit perfectly into the pervading mood of this time of the year and the month's focus—revelation, opening up and transformation.

Art Therapy: Unleashing the Inner Artist

When we were children we used to paint and draw with pleasure and delight. For a few short blissful years we could do no wrong with our paints and crayons; we were free to explore, imagine and create. Then we began to be taught what was "good" and "bad" in art: those of us who were "good" at art started trying to perfect our skills, while those of us who were not "artistic" simply threw away our paintbrushes. And that, say art therapists, is a crying shame. Uninhibited art, they explain, has the power to heal: it offers a clear, straightforward route to the unconscious, to the hidden depths of our psyche. Rediscover the joy of art and you could put yourself back in touch with repressed emotions and long-buried hurts. You could even start up a conversation with your very soul.

Art therapy is most definitely *not* about painting or drawing "properly." The aim is not to make pretty or life-like pictures but rather to let go of any expectations and simply see what happens. Art therapy is like a key to a secret language of the psyche. Paint and you could discover different sides to your personality; you could gain confidence and self-esteem; you might even find quite physical ailments disappear when you allow yourself a creative outlet.

Art has been used as a therapeutic tool for many years. Back in 1810 a German psychiatrist, Johann Christian Reill, positively encouraged his patients to paint. His colleagues thought it was a way of diverting them from their problems, but he insisted it was rather an attempt to put them in touch with their "passions," their inner desires, hurts and fears. Since that time many psychiatrists and psychoanalysts have discovered that when people paint freely they are able to express feelings and give a form to fears and terrors on paper that they are quite unable to express in words. Art as therapy is, quite simply, a direct way of communicating with the unconscious.

Since those early days, art therapy has become well established in the NHS in Britain where it is often used to help those who are mentally or terminally ill, people who have been abused or who are addicted to drugs. It can be a wonderful tool to communicate with children with special needs and adults who find it difficult to talk about their feelings. But it is also becoming increasingly popular amongst people with less pressing needs. Workshops are springing up around the country and more art therapists are starting to work with individuals on a private basis. Some people simply enjoy painting without the pressure of having to produce a masterpiece; others find it a wonderful way to relax. Yet more regard it as a serious tool for sorting out their lives: a way to look at problems or fears in a safe, controlled environment. Everyone, it appears, can benefit from holding a paintbrush and splashing paint.

I haven't painted since I left school and so it was with a certain amount of trepidation that I made my way to The Pelican Center, a rambling medieval house in a small Somerset village which hosts a weekly art therapy group plus frequent residential weekend workshops. About twenty of us gathered, plied with coffee, in a comfortable room full of armchairs. Michael Edwards, a Jungian analyst and art therapist who was running the weekend, immediately put the most paint-phobic at ease. "I'm not asking for any skills," he insisted. "You can't make a mistake; you simply can't do it wrong. Nobody has to know what your pictures are or mean—you are only answerable to yourself."

Although many art therapists will allow you a totally free rein, to paint whatever you choose, he had chosen the fairytale of Sleeping Beauty as a rough theme for the weekend. For some time we discussed the symbols and themes of the tale. "Fairytales pick up the deep truths of life," he explained. "However painful, uncomfortable and impossible they may be, they touch the deep roots of life." We talked about the many versions of this ancient tale, including its less well-known and vastly more sinister versions (full of child-eating ogres and grisly suicides) that Disney carefully chose to ignore. Then it was time to paint.

The art studio with its smell of paints and crayons brought back a flood of schooltime memories. "Find a comfortable place," urged Edwards. "You might want to hide in a corner—that's fine. Sit and think quietly before you begin and let the story work on you. See what comes up. It might dimly connect to your life; you might just enjoy the images. Let them come."

I sat and stared at my blank sheet of paper with something approaching horror: it felt like looking at an exam paper and not knowing any of the answers. Then, slowly, I started tentatively to paint. It began as a representation of Sleeping Beauty asleep amidst the briars. Then I found the paints I chose getting darker and darker, the paint strokes more and more harsh. "She's not asleep, she's dead," I found myself thinking and almost burst into tears as thoughts of my grandmother's recent death came flooding back into my mind. Fear, sorrow, pain, hurt, a bleak sense of mortality all poured out onto the paper. As if by sixth sense, Michael Edwards appeared at my shoulder and talked quietly and calmly before urging me to start painting again on a fresh sheet.

At the end of the day we all paused and assessed our work. "Try talking to your pictures," urged Edwards to the group. "You might write a commentary or simply scribble a letter to your painting. Ask it questions: it might answer. I know it sounds nuts but it does seem to work." "My picture said I needed a rest," laughed one woman and added, "I think I'll take its advice." Another said, "I felt my picture had no point to it but then I thought why does everything have to have a point? I decided I could have time in my week where there didn't have to be a point." Some people chose not to say a word—nobody was pushed.

"Art leads people gently into their psyches," says Edwards. "Sometimes distressing things come up, but somehow they can be contained by the paper. You might feel at the mercy of a nightmare or a fantasy, but by putting it in a picture it becomes objectified. And you always have a choice, you can put that unconscious world, however distressing, away in a drawer." In other words, art can give you back an element of control over your unconscious mind.

Edwards is loath to claim the miraculous for his therapy but sometimes, he grudgingly admits, people even find physical problems disappear. One woman had suffered for years from a frozen shoulder: once she started painting, the shoulder cleared up almost instantly. "You can't count on it, but yes it does happen," he says. "I wouldn't say come to art therapy and get rid of your rheumatism but it does happen."

But most people don't seek out art therapy as a cure for physical aches and pains. Rather they see it as a journey into the recesses of their own minds. And like a voyage over uncharted seas, no one quite knows what they will find. It might be frightening, full of terrors or it might uncover hidden strengths and talents, new resources and strategies. Quite likely it will do both. I left the Pelican Center with an armful of paintings, feeling very small, sad and vulnerable. As I drove home I quietly grizzled, realizing that I still had not given myself permission to fully grieve. Back in the safety of my own kitchen, I allowed myself to let go and really cry. I sobbed for about three hours and emerged with red-rimmed eyes and a mascara-smudged face. From the outside I looked terrible but inside I felt 100 percent better.

STARTING TO PAINT FREELY

To get a feel for art therapy try this exercise. The object is to paint your life—from beginning to end.

• Take a large piece of paper and any art materials you choose (paints, crayons, felt-tip pens). Imagine that the paper represents your whole life: the beginning, the now, the future and the end.
• Sit quietly for a few moments and then fill it as you choose. Don't expect anything or try to draw "properly"; use whatever symbols or images you feel appropriate. You might choose to depict events in your life or simply choose different colors to represent different parts of your life or feelings.
• When you have finished, be aware of how you feel, both in your mind and body. What is your painting saying: does it show more about how you think or how you feel about your life? What are the themes and questions in it?
• Don't throw it away afterward. Keep it and look at it from time to time to see if any new insights appear.

FREE YOUR INNER ARTIST

Fiona Arrigo who originated Stop the World also has a lovely exercise to free your inner artist and to see how you feel about yourself. She has people lie on the floor and then someone draws around their outline on large sheets of paper. You can adopt whichever posture feels right. Then you can decorate your "self" figure with whatever comes to mind and hand. It doesn't have to be paint or crayons—you could use wool or string or leaves. Fiona also suggests following something rather like the treasure map exercise we looked at in MARCH—cutting out images and words that seem appropriate from magazines and papers and sticking them on the figure. When you have finished, pin the figure up on the wall and look at it from a distance. What comes to mind? What does it tell you about yourself?

If you have children, they generally love doing this exercise, and they will enjoy it even more if you are doing your own "self-portrait" at the same time.

The Mystery of the Night: Working with Your Dreams

The other great tool for unraveling your psyche lies in your dreams. Sarah Dening, the Jungian psychotherapist and I Ching expert, uses dreams frequently in her work. She finds that by working out the hidden meanings of dreams, messages from the unconscious mind, she can help her clients quite literally change their lives. Take the example of the accountant who became an astrologer; the physiotherapist who transformed into a writer; the high-powered businesswoman who merrily swapped board meetings for nappies; the battered women who now have bliss-fully happy marriages. All of them put such dramatic life changes down to their dreams.

"Dreams are the way your unconscious uses to speak to you," Dening explains, but points out that most of us ignore these messages from the night. It's a pity, she says, because our con-scious minds are so overloaded with all the practical considera-tions, fears and conventions of everyday life that they often can't see the woods for the trees. However, our unconscious, free of such constrictions, generally knows precisely what we really need. Learn to listen to your unconscious and it could help make your waking life much more fulfilling: your relationships should improve; your career could change; it could even help your health.

We spend a third of our lives asleep and, even though you may not remember your dreams, there is no doubt that we all, without exception, dream every night. So it's curious that so few people bother to consult the oracle in their own heads. It's not even as if the concept of dreamworking were anything new. The Old Testament is full of references to prophetic dreams, while in ancient Greece people would regularly spend a therapeutic night in a Temple of Sleep where they believed the god of the temple would send healing dreams. Native Americans have used the power of dreaming for centuries—they would regard ignoring a dream as sheer stupidity.

In the West, however, dreaming has been very much marginalized for centuries, dismissed as either florid imagination or simply the mind's way of rubbishing the detritus of the day. It wasn't until Sigmund Freud started investigating dreams that these pyrotechnics of the night started to be taken seriously. But even Freud saw dreams simply as repositories for all that lies repressed in human nature. It was left to Carl Jung to really map the dream world, and it is Jung that most modern dream therapists follow when they travel into the land of night.

The techniques of modern dream therapy are actually quite simple, but it takes time and effort to learn how to decipher their unfamiliar language. Dening usually sees people for between eighteen months to three years, generally once a week. But you can learn a lot from a dream workshop and can easily apply the principles to become your own sleep sleuth. The first thing Dening warns against is simple, blanket interpretations. "You can't just run to a dream dictionary and look up a symbol in your dream," she insists. "You have to look at your personal associations. Nothing is written in stone." If you have a particularly vivid dream, she suggests you pick out the major symbol in it (say the sea, a lion, your old school) and write down everything it reminds you of. Often quite surprising insights can appear and frequently the symbol will draw into your conscious mind long-forgotten incidents from the past.

The second technique she teaches is learning how to "dream your dream on." "It's what Jung called active imagination," she explains. Basically it involves going back into your dream from a waking state and trying to find out more about the situation and characters within it. To get in the right frame of mind, she suggests you find a quiet, dark place where you won't be disturbed and let yourself deeply relax. Then start to imagine your dream in all its detail, not just visually but with all your senses, hearing the sounds, accessing the feeling in your body. There might be a character in the dream you want to question. If so, she says, simply ask the character if it would like to talk to you and then wait for the answer. "The whole art is the ability to wait," says Dening. "You have to have patience to wait for the answer and not rush to put something in. You will get a sense of when it's coming and it won't just be something your conscious mind is making up."

Generally, the people you meet in dreams will tend to be different aspects of yourself, often those repressed in waking life. One powerful aspect that often comes up is the "shadow," a dream character which normally manifests as someone of the same sex as yourself. Jung said it represents all the things about ourselves that we find unacceptable and so try to repress. Hence, if anger wasn't acceptable in your family as you grew up, your shadow might appear as an angry or violent man or woman. Dening says that if you can talk to your shadow and get on good terms, it will allow you to express your anger appropriately without flying off the handle. "Ruthlessness is another common one for women," she says, "because lots of little girls aren't allowed to be ruthless. Or if your mother wanted you to be a nice dainty little girl, you might well have a tomboyish or violent shadow. One woman had a cowgirl with a gun—everything that wasn't acceptable in her family."

To begin with, your dreams can often seem obtuse or simply meaningless, but with patience and perseverance you can arrive at quite profound realizations. One of Dening's clients, a high-powered business executive, kept having dreams of a rather bullying man pushing her to do impossible things, like driving up a cliff face. She came to realize that she was being driven by her masculine, ambitious side without stopping to ask what her emotions really wanted. When she worked with her dreams she realized that what she really needed to do was to give up work and bring up her children. She's now a full-time mother and blissfully happy.

Everyone can benefit from dream therapy, says Dening. "It sounds corny but it really can help people fulfill more of their potential. It's particularly useful for people who feel "stuck" in their lives, for those who have problematic relationships or who don't know which way to turn career-wise. It also inevitably tends to unleash your creativity." And don't forget that, just like in the

Bible, dreams can still sometimes be prophetic. Look at the woman who took her lottery numbers from a dream—she won thousands. If that's a case of the unconscious at work, we all need to do some night research. Who knows, your dreams just might come true.

DREAMWORKING

Recalling Your Dreams

But what if you never remember your dreams? Another dream expert, Lucy Goodison, author of *The Dreams of Women*, admits there is no one infallible way to remember dreams. "Some people find that simply saying aloud before sleep that they want to remember their dreams has helped," she says. "Some ask for a dream on a particular topic. Others meditate. Others just wait and see what happens." There are a few things which seem to help universally:

• On waking it can help to stay lying still in your sleeping body position to recall your dream.

• Try saying it aloud or telling someone else your dreams as you wake.

• Having a "dreambook" or journal by your bed to write in as soon as you open your eyes can be a very useful way of capturing a dream. Sometimes rewriting and rereading dreams can add to understanding them. Equally, if you prefer, draw an image that sums up your dream.

• Sometimes a simple ritual before sleep, like spending ten minutes gazing at a candle or into a glass of water, burning aromatic herbs or dancing to a favorite piece of music can help lead us into dreams.

Exploring Dreams, Talking to Your Dreams

In *The Dreams of Women* Lucy Goodison covers all the major techniques for working with dreams. And she suggests ways of working on your own, with a friend or in groups. The following offer some starting points:

Gestalt therapy: One technique she suggests is similar to Sarah Dening's suggestion about continuing your dream. This, however, comes from Gestalt therapy and is called "talking to your dreams." "Use two chairs or two cushions," she explains. "Sit yourself on one and imagine your dreams are on the other. Try speaking to your dreams, telling them how much you want to remember them. You may feel silly at first, but persevere as it can be very illuminating," she urges. "Then switch seats and speak as if you were the dreams replying. Say whatever comes into your mind, without censoring or getting embarrassed. Give the dreams a voice, let them describe themselves and tell what would help them to surface. You may be surprised at what comes up."

Painting: A creative way to start exploring dreams is through painting or drawing them. It's also a nice way to incorporate the art therapy we've just been discussing into dreamwork. It may be a literal picture of what happened in the dream or it may be more of an expression of the mood of the dream through shape and color. Don't ask other people to "interpret" your painting, although it can be helpful to discuss it with someone else. Ask them what they notice about it.

Visualization: If a dream ends on an uncertain or disconcerting note, try continuing it in waking time. Relax and do some deep comfortable breathing and then imagine yourself back in your dream. What would happen next? One woman ended her dream by digging under the earth and finding red letters spelling her name. When she "continued" the dream, she went back and carried on digging. She found a starving, pathetic kitten which she felt was a part of her which had been buried. From this point, says Goodison, she could try drawing the kitten or asking it what it needs using the Gestalt technique.

What Do Our Dreams Mean?

Although most dream "dictionaries" are too general to be of use, Sarah Dening says that there are some very common images that arise in dreams which can usually have a ready interpretation for the majority of people.

The Queen A very common dream which, for a woman, usually represents her own sovereignty and power. For a man, it tends to represent his ability to deal with the feminine side of his nature.

Rock Stars and Film Stars These generally represent the hero, excitement, creativity. Dreaming about a star means you want to project the part of you that craves attention and the center stage.

Babies Babies represent new life of all kinds. These dreams often occur when a person needs to develop other sides of themselves, often when their children have grown up and left home.

Going to the Toilet in Public These are very common dreams, particularly in repressed Britain. Urinating in public represents spontaneous self-expression, while defecating generally represents your creativity. It usually means you haven't found your true way of expressing yourself.

Being Naked in the Street Another common dream which classically means a fear of revealing who you really are. Usually it will suggest that you need to reveal more of your true personality.

Being Chased Dening says that usually whatever or whoever is chasing you is a part of yourself that wants to make contact with you. Animals can represent your instinctual nature—you are leading too cerebral a life.

WINTER

The Season of the Soul

KEY FOCUS
Finding your inner self; making peace with your soul.

SECONDARY FOCUS
Consolidating this year; looking forward to the next.

TASKS
Becoming mindful; seeking your spirituality; investigating the past;
gaining a positive attitude toward the future.

QUESTIONS
Who am I? Am I really living life as me? What do I need to sort
out from my past? What prevents me from being at peace?
What do I want from my future?

CHALLENGES
Make Christmas stress-free; jump off the world for a week; allow yourself
time; give yourself permission not to be bright and cheery all the
time; trust in your healing powers; grant yourself happiness.

FESTIVALS AND CELEBRATIONS
Christmas/Yuletide; New Year; Imbolc/Candlemas.

Few people would claim that winter is their favorite season. The bright leaves of autumn have all fallen, while the new growth of spring seems a world away. It is a quiet time, a resting time, when nature withdraws in on itself and waits, slumbering. If we are sensible, we will follow nature's example and use winter as a reflective pause, a time to think about our lives, a time to replenish our energy reserves. It's a season to curl up by a fire with a good book, some quiet music or merely to sit musing, staring into the flames. Winter naturally makes us more contemplative and less outgoing. The days are shorter, there is less light and the weather is often inhospitable: shrouding fog, endless rain, beautiful but chilly snow, cruel frosts and ice. No one feels on top of the world, especially when you are getting up in darkness and going home in darkness again after a long day's work. It's no wonder we often get more depressed and low in the winter months.

Christmas of course brightens up the world throughout December, with gleaming lights, cheery greenery and steaming cups of mulled wine. The prospect of parties and presents keeps most people happy, although undoubtedly harassed as well. Then New

Year arrives with more festivities, more feasts, more fun. And
then? Nothing. We are left stranded in the dark gloom of January
with months still to go before the fresh upsurge of spring. Small
surprise that the ancients used to go to such great lengths to
persuade their gods to bring back life and growth and the sun
in spring. In the depths of winter it must have seemed as though
they had been abandoned forever in a harsh, cold, unforgiving
world.

Yet, although winter may seem bleak it is no less important
than any other season. In fact, in many ways, it can be the time
of year when we can do the most important inner work. It is a
season when the body takes backstage to a degree. Although we
often associate winter with colds, coughs and other ailments, it
is not necessarily a fact of life that you have to be ill during
winter. If you have taken care of your body throughout the year,
eating well, exercising well and building up your immune system,
then there is no reason for it to get sick. If you have strengthened
your system in the run-up to winter, you should be resistant to
most bugs. And, if you *do* get the stray cold or flu, then it is no
bad thing. Unless you are very weak, a cold won't do your system
any harm at all. In fact it will do you positive good, giving your
body a chance to test out and build up its defenses. So, if you
do fall ill, don't look on it as a nuisance but rather as a sign that
your body simply happens to be running a little below par and
needs a rest.

In these frenetic days we stumble into work or on chores when
we are almost dropping with tiredness and sickness. It's madness.
The best thing to do if you are feeling ill is to wrap up warm
and take to your bed in good old-fashioned style. A couple of
days of rest with comforting, sickbed food and soothing drinks
will probably sort you out. However, if you stagger on with
normal life, your cold might get worse and deepen, perhaps even
turning into something more serious like a chest infection. Then
you could end up on antibiotics and perhaps have to take a
week or more off work. Is it really worth it? The other point that
we tend to forget or ignore is that when we stoically battle on
with normal life with a cold or flu we are most likely to pass it
on to our work colleagues, our friends, the people we bump
into on the bus, the train or the shops. Keep your cold to yourself

and keep to your bed in the warm is my advice and weary, overworked GPs would, I'm quite sure, agree.

The Season of Water and the Evil Cold

In the Chinese system winter is a season of extreme *yin* energy: energy is being condensed, conserved and stored before the explosion of spring. They link this to water, an element they consider to be highly concentrated and full of hidden potential. In the body, water rules some of our most mysterious functions: our hormones, the lymphatic system and the essential enzymes. It also controls the bladder and the kidneys, all our bones (including the marrow, our teeth, our skulls and the spine), the sex organs, and our ears and hearing. A strange combination, but all in some way connected with mysterious fluids.

The Chinese consider the bladder to be the seat of the emotions in the body, while the kidneys are said to store the energy of the life force itself and are seen as relating to the whole cycle of transformation—from birth to life and on to death. More links with this mysterious, soul-seeking aspect of winter. Willpower is also said to come from the kidneys and so, if you lack willpower or ambition, a Chinese physician would look to see if you have a water imbalance. Other symptoms of water imbalance can include fears and phobias, general states of anxiety and negativity, a feeling of constant pessimism, right down to states of severe paranoia.

The "evil" of winter is, not surprisingly, that of cold. When cold enters the body, it can create chills and fevers, headaches and the sensation of feeling "aches and pains all over." If cold settles in the intestines, it can cause diarrhea, abdominal pains and cramps and excessive flatus and flatulence. The evil of cold also appears when you feel chilled and cold in your extremities— your hands and feet, and especially the tip of your nose all feel like ice. So it's well worth aiming to keep cold evil at bay throughout the bitter days of winter.

It sounds like the kind of advice you were given as a child, but really and truly the best thing you can do is to wrap up well and keep yourself warm. How many of us nowadays work in cocoons of centrally heated offices and homes? We spend winter days wandering around in shirt-sleeves while outside the elements roar. Then, when it comes time to step out into the rain and cold—or even sleet and snow—we don't bother to put on extra clothes as we race to our heated cars and the warm press of bodies on public transport. The easiest way to throw your body out of balance is to fling it from one extreme to another— from extreme warmth to extreme cold and vice versa. Follow grandma's pleas and wear a vest, an extra sweater, a warm hat, cozy socks and boots and gloves.

The Winter Diet: Fortifying and Strengthening

To avoid the evil of cold, you need a diet that produces more heat in the body. Obviously, if you already have too much internal heat (an imbalanced *pitta*), you would need something more subtle and should consult an expert. However, the general guidelines suggest that we eat more carbohydrate and protein in the winter—we need to keep warm. We also need to watch that we don't eat too much and put on excess weight—it's very easy to do, especially with Christmas and the miserable weather. We exercise less, eat more and pile on the pounds.

It's quite natural to put on a few pounds over the winter—we need a little more bulk to keep warm and it can easily be shed as spring approaches. But be wary about putting on too much. Christmas offers one temptation after another. I'm not saying you have to deny yourself; that wouldn't be natural and would only make you feel resentful and dispirited (hardly the atmosphere of Christmas). Just be aware of what you are eating; indulge but indulge moderately. Buffet food looks innocent enough but is usually laden with fat and empty calories (the ones that pile on the weight but don't do your body any good); nuts, dates and figs are nutritious and healthy but don't overdo them as, again, they are high in calories. Chocolates, sweets, Turkish delight, sugar jellies, mince pies, Christmas cake, Christmas pudding all sit around as perfect temptation. Have the odd one or two, but don't eat the box or devour the whole cake!

Christmas aside, the perfect winter diet—as with all the seasons—takes it cue from nature and uses the foods that are freshly available, local and seasonal. This is the time that the root vegetables really come into their own, and they can form the basis of delicious soups and stews, made tastier with herbs or with a little meat added for flavor. Make sure you get your greens as well: there are plenty of winter greens, cabbages, cauliflowers, leeks and sprouts around. And bulk up everything you cook with onions and garlic, the great natural purifiers and strengtheners. The other winter staples are the cooked wholegrains and pulses. Make the most of millet and buckwheat, red aduki beans, green mung beans, black beans and orange, yellow or green lentils. They all add color and nutrition to simple but tasty food.

There is less choice of fruit now: apples and pears are still available, but it's worth bulking them out by cheating a little and eating the not exactly local oranges, satsumas and kiwi fruits for their vast stores of vitamins. Be careful that you don't give up on fruit altogether. If you don't like eating fruit in winter, try extracting the juice and then gently warming it (don't allow it to boil). You can add a little honey and some spices for a warming delicious and nutritious drink. Or eat your fruit gently stewed— just remember not to overcook it or you will lose all the goodness.

Generally speaking, this is the time of year when most people can handle heavier, richer food. As with autumn, you can deal with a little more dairy produce at this time of year—the ayurvedic physicians say that the extra fat will help you digest the winter diet and lubricate the body, preventing it from getting stiff. But follow your instincts. Remember, if you feel you might be allergic to dairy, avoid it. Or try sheep's, goat's or soya produce. If you can take milk, this is a time of the year when hot milky drinks can be very soothing and warming. You can add a few spices (cinnamon is lovely) to warm it even further. And although the scientists can find no real reason why a hot milky drink should help send us to sleep at night, it still seems to work. Maybe they just haven't found the answer yet or maybe it's all in the mind. Who cares? If it works, use it.

Again, we can generally take more meat at this time of year

as well. Remember, the key is to use it as a flavorer and taste-enhancer rather than relying on it to provide all the meal. In other words, have a few pieces of meat to flavor a vegetable and bean stew rather than a slab of steak garnished with a few peas. Even a little red meat, usually abhorred by nutritionists, can be beneficial at this time of year according to the Chinese doctors. Red meat is a great building and fortifying food which tonifies the blood and stimulates the heart and skin. As always, stick to organic meat if possible and always lean cuts. But don't overdo it—too much red meat can overstimulate your system and can be bad for your heart, blood vessels and kidneys.

In the ayurvedic system winter is the season of *kapha*. *Kapha* builds and strengthens; it provides solidity and bulk. So not surprisingly, Ayurveda allows us to eat heavier foods in the winter. In fact, Ayurveda states very clearly that, of all the seasons, this is the one in which you need to eat more food. So don't be tempted to try crash diets before Christmas or to lose a few pounds with a short fast so you can squeeze into a party dress; your body won't like it and will probably repay you with a dose of flu or some other bug.

Both the ayurvedic and Tibetan traditions say that the tastes of food to look out for in winter are predominantly sweet, sour and salty. And they both, rather delightfully, warn against staying in houses that "let in breezes." While few of us probably live in houses the Tibetans describe as "a shack of boards," you can get the picture—stay out of draughts and keep yourself warm and cozy. In particular, say the ayurvedic texts, you should keep your bedroom warm with plenty of cocooning blankets on the bed. In fact, Ayurveda seems to see winter as a time for indulgence: it advises that you can healthily indulge in sex as often as you choose and can drink wine and other alcoholic beverages to a greater degree, although still not to excess, of course.

Winter Tonics

There are a few tricks in the herbal medicine cabinet to deal with coughs and colds should they arise—and a fair few to stave them off in the first place. Many of these cures are quite literally on our back doorsteps—in the garden or out in the countryside—so make the most of them.

BANISH COLDS

Wild rosehips abound during the autumn and early days of winter—pick them (best after the second frost but before the birds get a chance to eat them all) and use them as a cold-banishing tonic, packed with vitamin C. If you have an abundance of rosehips, you could make rosehip syrup as did all wisewomen and good housekeepers of old. If not, try a simple tonic drink. The famous herbalist Culpeper said that rosehips are "grateful to the taste and a considerable restorative, fitly given to the consumptive person, the conserve being proper in all distempers of the breast and in coughs and tickling rheums. It has a binding effect and helps digestion." In all, a wonderful free tonic.

Rosehip Syrup
Crush around 450 g of rosehips and put them into a pan containing 900 ml of boiling water. Bring them back to the boil and then turn off the heat and allow them to stand for around twenty minutes. Strain (preferably through muslin), and then put the fruit, which will now be pappy and mashed, into around 300 ml of fresh boiling water. Once again, allow to stand for a further twenty minutes and then strain again.

Mix the two sets of strained juices together and return to the pan. Boil on a low but steady heat until the juice has reduced down to around 600 ml. It will be syrupy by now. Allow to cool, sweeten to taste with wild honey and bottle in sterilized bottles as you would with any preserve.

Rosehip Tonic Drink
Simply chop up two teaspoons of rosehips and add them to around 300 ml of boiling water. Allow to steep for fifteen minutes and then strain and sweeten with honey to taste. You can make larger quantities and keep in the fridge for up to three days. It tastes lovely too.

OLD-FASHIONED COUGH CURES

Many of the oldest and simplest remedies are the best, particularly when it comes to battling with irritating coughs. Modern cough mixtures often have side effects. These powerful alternatives have none, except to build up your system further to prevent more outbreaks. Try them and see.

Garlic Syrup
This is so easy to make and surprisingly effective. Although it sounds disgusting, it's actually quite pleasant and very soothing. Simply put four or five plump freshly peeled cloves of garlic into a sterilized jar along with four tablespoons of clear, runny honey (always try to get organic cold-pressed honey). Leave it to stand in a warm place (an airing cupboard or near the cooker) for two or three hours. Take a teaspoon to ease coughs.

Onion Syrup
Another old and curiously effective soother which loosens phlegm and eases bronchial coughs. Cut up six large onions (preferably organic, some recipes also insist on white onions) and place them in a *bain-marie* (a bowl sitting inside a saucepan of gently boiling water) along with 150–200 ml of clear runny honey (cold-pressed, as before). Cover and cook very slowly for around two hours. Strain and take warm at regular intervals.

Cabbage and/or Leek Water
Strange but true, the water that you have cooked cabbage or leeks in has been used for centuries as a cure for catarrhal infections, coughs and bronchitis. Drink it warm both morning and night—and don't worry, it just tastes like very thin soup.

EASING WINTER ACHES AND PAINS

There are numerous remedies aimed at easing rheumatism and arthritis, and to find something truly effective you would be best advised to see a qualified medical herbalist or naturopath who have very good results with these conditions. However, the following are worth a try—they certainly won't do you any harm.

Rosemary Poultice

You need around two cupfuls of fresh rosemary and three cups of brandy. Steep the combination for a week and then strain. Apply the liquid as a poultice on the painful joints. An alternative is to grind black mustard seeds with equal amounts of vegetable shortening and use as a rub on the affected joints.

Cabbage, Onions and Celery

The water that cabbage has been cooked in also eases joint pain. Onions are very helpful too, as is celery—try either the juice or make warming soups.

Soothing Baths

Baths can be very soothing and relaxing. Epsom salts have long been used to help rheumatic aches and pains: put a good handful or a cupful in a warm bath. You could add a few drops of any or a choice of the following oils: lavender, pine, juniper, rosemary.

Warning: Don't use Epsom salts if you have high blood pressure.

Sweet and Spicy Scents for Winter

Aromatherapy comes into its own in winter. Lovely at all times of the year, it turns highly therapeutic in the season of colds and low spirits. There are many good books on aromatherapy now available (see the back of this book for details) and so I would suggest you buy one and experiment to find which oils and recipes particularly suit you.

However, I would beg you, as always, to be very respectful of essential oils. They are powerful and, if handled incorrectly, can do far more harm than good. Always buy absolutely pure, preferably organic, oils and only use the precise amount of drops given in a recipe. Any more and you could irritate your skin or even cause toxicity. Pregnant women in particular need to be very careful. If in any doubt, I would always consult a professional practitioner. Don't let this put you off using aromatherapy. Just treat it as you would a medicine given you by a doctor—

you wouldn't take three antibiotics when the bottle said one, would you?

BATTLING BUGS

Many of the essential oils have remarkable antiviral and antibacterial powers. They smell lovely but also pack a punch. Any of the following will work wonders: tea tree; lavender; cinnamon; clove; pine; lemon; geranium; bergamot; melissa. Use your favorite or a combination in oil burners, in the bath, or added to water in a plant mister. Cinnamon, clove and pine make a lovely Christmassy room spray and will protect you from all those people carrying their colds with them. An aromatherapist I met recently recommended a new oil called Ravensara which is apparently an incredible antiviral and antiseptic. It sounds well worth investigating.

If you feel you have a cold coming on, the best thing to do is to retreat to a warm bath spiced with five drops of tea tree oil and three of black pepper. Soak and breathe in the scent. Then keep tea tree oil scenting your bedroom throughout the night: use a burner until you want to sleep, then (for safety's sake) switch to a bowl of hot water by the bed with a few more drops added. Or put a few drops on a handkerchief or tissue and keep it by your pillow to sniff through the night. You can also use five drops of tea tree plus the same quantities of two other of the antiviral oils given above to 30 ml of almond oil and use it as a massage. It will help you relax and, hopefully, you will wake up the next morning feeling well and healthy.

STRESS-BUSTERS

Aromatherapy is an amazing stress-buster. In the run-up to Christmas or any busy period I think everyone should give themselves a prescription for a professional aromatherapy massage. If you can't manage it, at least treat yourself to some of these oils at home. There are very many different oils for all kinds of stress. The main stress-fighters include: lavender; lemon; bergamot; geranium; sandalwood; vetiver; ylang-ylang; clary sage; grapefruit; mandarin; neroli; marjoram; melissa. Use whichever you particularly like (they all mix quite well together) and blend them into a massage oil: use no more than ten drops each of a maximum of three oils in 30 ml of base oil (e.g., sweet almond). Or pop a couple of drops of two or three oils in your bath and have a long soak. Or, again, use them in vaporizers or burners.

DEPRESSION

We all get depressed from time to time and often it gets worse in the winter. If it happens occasionally, don't worry about it— it is a bit like the way a cold hits your body when it wants a rest. It often seems that depression can hit when our minds want a rest. We just shut off for a while. Remember also, particularly at this time of year, that alcohol can trigger depression very easily. If you wake up after a party feeling not only hung over but also blue, don't be surprised. The depression may linger long after the physical symptoms have gone. However, if depression is severe or continues too long it can be very debilitating and distressing and it needs attention. Some people who suffer severe depression have thyroid problems, so it's worth checking it out with your doctor. Depression can also be caused by emotional problems or psychological trauma. If you feel this is the case (particularly if your depression started after a particular event) then it would be wise to visit a psychotherapist or counselor.

However, if your depression is low-key—a kind of low winter blues—then do try the following oils which are all used by aromatherapists for the treatment of depression. The citrus oils are very uplifting: lemon, orange, grapefruit, mandarin. And so too are clary sage, marjoram, lavender, petit grain, neroli, rose, ylang-ylang, jasmine, bergamot and Roman chamomile. Try blending lavender, bergamot and clary sage or geranium, lavender and petit grain. As before, mix with a base oil for massage, or use in the bath or around the room.

Another gentle cure for the blues and low-level depression comes from medical herbalist Andrew Chevallier, president of the National Institute of Medical Herbalists. He recommends taking St. John's Wort (also known as *Hypericum*) as a gentle, nonaddictive, without side effects antidepressant. A medical herbalist can make you up a tincture or there is an over-the-counter preparation called Kira, which contains the correct dosage of the herb. Don't expect instant effects—herbs act slowly and gently—but it could be a life-saver if you find the winter blues too much to bear.

Exercise and Winter

It's hard, isn't it? The days are short and it's cold outside. The gym beckons but you would much rather snuggle up in front of the television. However, do try to keep exercising throughout the winter. There are several quite compelling reasons. Firstly, the exercise will keep your body in tip-top condition so it can more easily fight the bugs. Secondly, it will help you win the battle of the winter weight gain. Thirdly, aerobic exercise has been proven to help fight depression, so if you suffer from the winter blues, it's well worth continuing the fitness program you started earlier in the year. And, last but not least, just think what happens when you stop exercising.

It only takes three to six weeks to lose your hard-won fitness level. First to go are the mental benefits—the good moods and the enhanced feeling of well-being. Heart and lung fitness follow close behind, with cardiovascular fitness dropping most rapidly in the first weeks after you stop. Then muscles start to stiffen from disuse and joints can feel creaky. And, of course, if you continue to eat the same diet as when you were exercising, you are likely to put on weight as well. Is it worth it? Once you start exercising again, it will take you between eight and ten weeks to regain your former fitness level. Don't let all the hard work of the past year go to waste.

The key is to give yourself extra motivation and maybe to adjust your exercise and workout regime to make it more palatable in the cold weather. You might simply adore racing around in the freezing cold (I always watch rugby players with complete and utter stupefaction). But for many of us the exercise we loved earlier in the year somehow isn't quite so appealing now. For example, the lovely cool pool you dived into in the hot summer won't be so inviting now when the frost is on the ground. The brisk morning walk or run won't be so much fun in the pitch dark as it was in the glorious early mornings of spring and autumn (and it might not be very safe either). So think of other things to keep you active and fluid. As with autumn, team or pairs sports can be fun—why not learn something new?

Providing your gym isn't an icy barn, this is an excellent time of the year to work with weights. Remember this is *kapha* time with its emphasis on structure, solidity and strength—the perfect time to start a strengthening program. Many people are put off the idea of weight-training because they imagine gyms are full of Mr. Universe-type muscle-bound jocks. Men are put off because they feel they won't measure up, and women are put off by the idea either of being surrounded by testosterone or of ending up looking much like the blokes. The image isn't quite accurate nowadays. Although there are still gyms which cater predominantly for body-builders, it's normally pretty easy to figure them out. But most gyms nowadays are keen to foster an image that invites everyone in. At my gym in Somerset you could not see a wider variety of people. From lithe teenagers to more solid seventy-somethings, from overweight businessmen to new mothers, we are all ages, all shapes and all sizes.

A good gym will run a solid assessment and work out a program that suits you. You don't have to build vast muscles—you can use weights simply to strengthen and tone your body. All programs should include a good amount of aerobic work so that you will be helping your cardiovascular system as well—not to mention trimming weight. Although muscle weighs heavier than fat, the better your muscle/fat ratio, the more effectively you will burn fat. And another benefit of befriending your gym in winter is that you can walk or run on the treadmills, march up the stepping machines, cycle on the bikes and row on the rowers without getting cold, wet or muddy. Just to complete the picture, there is absolutely nothing to beat the feeling after a good workout. Your whole body feels alive and your mood will undoubtedly be up. A lovely warm shower (use some nice invigorating essential oils) followed by a brisk rub-down, and you are feeling on top of the world. However, it is not a good idea to continue vigorous exercise while ill. So if you succumb to a cold or flu (and particularly if it goes down onto your chest) it is sensible to take a break from exercise until you have recovered.

Make an effort at the weekend to get out, if the weather permits. Put on warm clothes (remember hats and mittens) and wellies and go for a good brisk walk. If it snows, take the opportunity to flit back to childhood. Get out there and build snowmen with the kids (or without), throw snowballs, go tobogganing. It's not strictly exercise, but it's great fun, a brilliant stress-reliever and it also puts you right in touch with the heart of the season. We often miss the strange beauty of winter tucked away in our houses. We don't see the delicacy of spiders' webs touched by frost; of gleaming hips and haws; of skeleton trees; of frozen puddles crazed with abstract markings and icy, rock-hard fields. Just keep wrapped up and explore.

A Dose of Light: Keeping Spirits Bright

One of the things most people dislike about winter is the lack of light, particularly sunlight. They look forward to spring and the return of the sun when the whole world seems to smile once more. When the sun comes out spirits lift and energy levels bubble higher, even our health seems to improve—it's as if someone had waved a miraculous wand. It may seem like magic, but the effect is certainly not merely in our minds. Research now clearly shows that pure, clear sunlight can have measurable, highly beneficial, effects on our health, both physiological and psychological.

"We spend more and more of our time indoors," says Dr. Damien Downing, author of *Day Light Robbery* and the leading UK exponent of the healing power of light. "The only time we see the sun is when we follow outdoor pursuits such as sport or gardening or go on holiday."

It's a change that has come about over the last couple of hundred years with the shift from working on the land to working in factories and offices. An office may be warmer, and drier and more comfortable than the common British field but it is certainly darker. Dr. Downing points out that our offices are lit at between two hundred and one thousand lux (the measurement for light) when, in reality, we need levels around ten times brighter. "We keep ourselves for most of our lives in perpetual twilight," he says. "Nowadays we live, without realizing it, in self-imposed dungeons."

The most common result is the well-documented syndrome of SAD (seasonal affective disorder), but Downing reckons this is the tip of the iceberg: around sixty percent of the population suffer in a less dramatic way. Lack of light can cause depression and lethargy, disturbed sleep patterns and plummeting energy levels. Our metabolism can suffer, so can our hormone levels. Even conditions like osteoporosis and asthma worsen without regular doses of light. It's bad enough for pale-skinned Celts who have spent thousands of years adapting to deal with the low levels of sunlight in this country but dark-skinned people fare particularly badly. Dr. Downing says we are now seeing the reoccurrence of rickets in some black children—not because their diets are deficient but simply because they are not getting enough daylight.

But, short of turning back to the land, how can we boost our light levels? The answer seems to be that if we can't go out into the light, then we have to bring the light in to us. SAD sufferers have used light boxes for some years now to help their symptoms but now a new brand of light therapy has been developed which promises benefits for virtually everyone. The new light reproduces as closely as possible the pure spring light of the Northern hemisphere, the clear soft gleam that so revitalizes us body and soul. In practical terms, it's a combination of fluorescent tubes that give out the whole spectrum of wavelengths in natural daylight apart from the harmful UVB rays that can cause burning.

It is the burning, say light therapy researchers, that causes the damage—aging the skin and heightening the risk of skin cancer. Recent research has suggested that we should also be concerned about UVA rays but the risk so far seems slight. "We are in far more danger staying totally out of the light than we are by staying in it. Although obviously we must treat light with respect," says Natalie Handley who has pioneered the use of the new light therapy and now gives treatment in several clinics. "It really is the therapy of the future," she says. "We need light as we need water and sleep for our general well-being and, if better recognized, it would save the country millions in healthcare costs and less absenteeism." Both she and Dr. Downing hope that the treatment will become more widely available, and particularly that the evidence will convince doctors that the treatment could be incorporated into NHS clinics. "Not everyone does well on drugs," she says. "This is a great alternative without side effects for dealing with a host of problems."

Handley sees people with a huge cross-section of needs—some simply want to increase their energy levels; some want help with serious depression or arthritic conditions. Just twenty minutes of light therapy, she says, can lower blood pressure for up to a week and also lower blood cholesterol levels. It balances hormones and so can be used as an alternative to HRT (hormone replacement therapy) and also to help fertility (incidentally, Dr. Downing points out that sunlight can increase libido—the sun actually does make us sexier). The full-spectrum light can kill bacteria and accelerate wound healing. And, because exposure to the lights increases the production of vitamin D in the body, which in turn aids the absorption of calcium, phosphorus and magnesium, it is useful in cases of arthritis, osteoporosis and dental caries. There's still more. Because daylight suppresses the production of melatonin (which helps send us to sleep), light therapy can be used to treat sleep disorders and jet lag with great success.

In short, says Natalie Handley, there really isn't anyone who wouldn't benefit from some light therapy, especially during our dark and gloomy winters.

The day I visited Handley was the archetypical winter day: gloomy, cold, dark and wet. Summer—and sunlight—seemed a million miles away. But Handley was bright and cheerful, beaming with good health and vitality: she's a shining endorsement of her treatment. She regularly combines the light treatment with reflexology because, she explains, the combination will treat more or less anything.

First of all she took a detailed medical history from me. The lights, she promised, are totally safe and completely without side effects. In particular, she assured, they will not tan nor will they cause any damage to the skin. The case history, however, is necessary for reflexology so she can tailor the treatment to your needs. Then she invited me to take off my shoes and as much clothing as I liked and get on the couch. Any glasses or contact lenses are taken off or out because, she explains, the light can only reach the pineal gland (essential for hormonal balance) through the eyes.

The lights are mounted in a panel above the couch several feet above your body. They look much like a sunbed except that the center tubes are a beautiful shade of blue. For best effects, you keep your eyes open (although you don't have to look directly at the light) for the first twenty minutes.

The combination of the warm, clear light and the firm but soothing touch of the reflexology were, I had to agree, a delightful combination. Without the reflexology I might have become a bit bored just lying in the light, but the two together were like snoozing in the garden on a soft summer's day with your feet being cradled in a lap, gently being massaged. It was total bliss.

After an hour I slid off the couch with a broad smile. My skin felt warm and soft and a slight grumble in my lower back had been much eased. But most noticeable was the increase of energy that steadily rose throughout the day. Several hours after the treatment I felt as if I had been given a happy pill: I was bright and bubbly, several light years away from the tired, slightly gloomy person who had greeted another winter's day with a wince. I think I've seen the light.

BRIGHT IDEAS TO BRING SUNLIGHT INTO YOUR LIFE

Lightbathing, says Dr. Downing, stimulates the circulation, detoxifies the body and boosts the production of vitamin D and hormones.

• At this time of year when the danger of burning is very low, get as much natural daylight as you can. Brisk digging in the garden, dog-walking or even just walking outside in your lunch hour can help. But keep wrapped up and warm.

• As the sun gets brighter in spring and summer you need to adjust the amount of sun you take to suit your skin type. Dr. Downing insists that it is burning that causes skin cancer, not sensible exposure. As a rough guide you need to stay out for half the amount of time that you can safely be in the sun before

burning—for very fair skins that will be around ten minutes in the very bright sunlight through to an hour for very dark skins.
• Don't use creams or blocks for the periods you are lightbathing—they block out the useful UV rays. Obviously you'll need sunscreen if you are staying out for longer than these periods.
• The more of your skin that is exposed to the light the better, but don't get cold. There's no point in stripping off only to get a chill.
• Glasses, sunglasses and contact lenses all filter out the light. Wearing dark glasses all the time, says Handley, will tend to make you depressed or irritable. Use a hat instead to shield you from glare.

The Quietness of Winter: A Time for Reflection and Growth

I've called winter the season of the soul, which for many people might pose a puzzle. Nowadays we are not used to the idea of healing our souls, or even looking at them. Some people would doubt we even had a soul. Scientists might ask precisely where our soul resides and how I can prove it's there. I can't. No one can—at least, not yet.

Yet for as long as there have been records of humans thinking, there has been the concept of soul, of spirit, of an ineffable part of ourselves which has a link with something far removed from our physical and even emotional and intellectual worlds. You could call it our inner essence. Our soul is the part of us that yearns for something more than daily humdrum activity. Not for greater riches, but for a sense of peace, of fulfilment, of finding a place in the vast lonely universe. Our soul is the part of us that shivers in the cold of winter—that thinks about the immensity of eternity and quakes. It is the part that ponders the existence or lack of existence of God.

At some point in our lives, most of us think about the Big Issues—about the meaning of life, about the mystery of death, about where we figure in the endlessness of space. That is the soul. Each and every one of us has to find different ways to soothe our souls. It helps to be in work we like and value; it's a boon if our relationships are loving and caring, and it is easier if we can look on our bodies, minds, emotions and souls as one holistic whole rather than a perpetual battlefield. But there is no formula for soul-searching. I cannot give you recipes or programs that will lead you neatly to a sense of peace. That has to come from you. However, through the months of winter, I will suggest therapies and ways of looking at life that have helped other people. As with everything in this book, see if any appeal and, if so, try them. If not, ignore them and find your own way. I think we all get there in the end.

Mindfulness

One technique which seems to touch even the most prosaic people at the soul level is mindfulness. Professor Jon Kabat-Zinn has developed a program that promises peace, self-acceptance and a true sense of inner happiness to those who practice it. It is uncomplicated, inexpensive and need only take minutes a day: he calls it mindfulness.

Mindfulness is meditation brought up to date, pared of its mystical and religious connotations and honed to slot into the most frenetic Western life. The simple idea is to put people back in control of their lives, learning how to listen to their minds and bodies rather than being tossed around by the world outside. Kabat-Zinn is no lotus-seated yogi; he's a highly qualified scientist with a Ph.D. in molecular biology who runs the Stress Reduction Clinic at the University of Massachusetts Hospital.

The clinic was started in 1979 with the realization that although the hospital could treat patients with chronic physical ailments, their problems would simply come back after a period of time. Kabat-Zinn felt sure that the answer lay in teaching patients how to kick-start their own healing powers and he spent years finding the best and most straightforward method. His choice lay in Buddhist and yogic practices which he then adapted for Western consumption. The results have been impressive: he has found his form of meditation can help to clear psoriasis much faster, can relieve chronic pain and lessen feelings of anxiety and depression. He has instructed patients whose illnesses range from heart disease to ulcerative colitis, from diabetes to cancer. "We teach these people to develop an intimacy and familiarity with their own bodies and minds," he explains. "This leads to a greater confidence to learn from their symptoms and to begin to self-regulate them."

However, you don't need to be sick to benefit from mindfulness meditation. The simple techniques Kabat-Zinn outlines in his book, *Mindfulness Meditation for Everyday Life,* can help everyone live life with greater certainty and self-confidence. It can also provide some of those soul-stopping moments when you feel surrounded by the sheer bliss of living.

Kabat-Zinn points out that most of us live our lives in a state of virtual unconsciousness, constantly projecting into the future or pondering the past. "The days, the months and years quickly go by unnoticed, unused, unappreciated," he laments. "Mindfulness, however, provides a simple but powerful route for getting ourselves unstuck, back into touch with our own wisdom and vitality. It is a way to take charge of the direction and quality of our own lives. It is the direct opposite of taking life for granted."

It is certainly simple. At its very basic level, mindfulness simply involves stopping and becoming aware of the moment. The easiest way to do it is to focus on your breathing, gently letting go any stray thoughts or worries that emerge. Kabat-Zinn asks his patients to strive for forty-five minutes of mindfulness a day but stresses that even a few minutes will make a great difference. "It can be five minutes or even five seconds," he says, "but for those moments, don't try to change anything at all, just breathe and let go. Give yourself permission to allow this moment to be exactly as it is and allow yourself to be exactly as you are."

Mindfulness may be simple but it is not necessarily easy, he warns. Not only does it require effort and discipline but often the very act of stopping and listening can summon up deep emotions such as grief, sadness, anger, and fear that have been unconsciously suppressed over the years. However, Kabat-Zinn promises that not all the surprises are necessarily unpleasant. "Mindfulness can often help us to appreciate feelings such as joy, peacefulness and happiness which often go by fleetingly and unacknowledged," he comments.

Indeed, he stresses, one of the true benefits of mindfulness is that it allows people to discover what they really want in life; their true "Path with a capital P" as he put it. It allows them to let go of feelings of inadequacy and self-dislike and instead fosters feelings of self-esteem and courage. As Kabat-Zinn puts it, "Mindfulness is a road map to our radiant selves, not to the gold of a childhood innocence already past but to that of a fully developed adult. It is a way of walking along the path of life and being in harmony with things as they are."

MAKING MINDFULNESS WORK FOR YOU

• Start each day with mindfulness. Wake up a little earlier than usual and, before you even move notice your breathing, breathe consciously for a few minutes. Feel your body lying in bed and then straighten it out and stretch. Try to think of the day ahead as an adventure, filled with possibilities. Remember you can never really know what the day will hold.

• Try stopping, sitting down and becoming aware of your breathing once in a while throughout the day. It can be for five minutes or even five seconds. Just breathe and let go, allow yourself to be exactly as you are.

• Set aside a time every day to just be: five minutes would be fine, or twenty or thirty. Sit and become aware of your breath and every time your mind wanders, simply return to the breath.

• Use your mindfulness time to contemplate what you really want from life. Ask yourself questions like, "Who am I?"; "Where am I going?"; "If I could choose a path now, in which direction would I head?"; "What do I truly love?" You don't have to come up with answers, just persist in asking the questions.

• Try getting down on the floor once a day and stretching your body mindfully, if only for three or four minutes. Stay in touch with your breathing and listen to what your body has to tell you.

• Use ordinary occasions to become mindful. When you are in the shower, really feel the water on the skin rather than losing yourself in thought. When you eat, really taste your food. Notice how you feel when the phone rings.

• Practice kindness to yourself. As you sit and breathe, invite a sense of self-acceptance and cherishing to arise in your heart. If it starts to go away gently bring it back. Imagine you are being held in the arms of a loving parent, completely accepted and completely loved.

December

The trees may be bare and the world outside gray and barren but December is brightened with all the paraphernalia of Christmas—glitter and lights, gaily festooned trees, candles and crackers. When the halls are decked with boughs of holly and there's a crackling fire with chestnuts roasting in a pan, it becomes easier to forget the chill weather outside. And that's as it should be. Christmas is but the modern descendant of generations of midwinter festivals which all had the same underlying purpose: to help us through some of the darkest, gloomiest days of winter.

In the Celtic calendar Christmas becomes Yule—again a family festival, a time to gather everyone around the fire, to feel comfort in having everyone you most need in life close at hand. Pagan priestess and therapist Shan says of Yule, "It's an extended holiday for the family and the hearth. It involves little gatherings of the people we need to survive—not necessarily the people we like!" And, as to the inevitable conflicts and fights that occur within families at this time, she shrugs and says that is all part of it. In the old tradition, Yuletide saw a ritualized combat between the King of the Waning Year and the King of the New Year. Two men would strip to the waist and either fight with swords or their bare hands while the women kept up a steady beat with drums.

"Combat and conflict have their place in the scheme of things," Shan comments wisely. "People tend to think that dealing with conflict is getting rid of all aggression, all violence, but that isn't practical." Obviously uncontrolled violence is not sanctioned, but the point is that it is quite natural and healthy to feel annoyance, irritation and anger and even to show it, providing you do so in a safe and suitable way. So as you inevitably end up squabbling over who washes up after Christmas lunch or who watches what film on TV, relax and remember this is all a natural part of Christmas.

However, there are other sides to the festival too, and I'm not suggesting it's all about fisticuffs and fighting. It really is primarily the feast of the family, a time to appreciate (if you can) the people around you, to celebrate your family by giving them gifts. And, of course, for many people this is the festival of Christ, of the birth of the son of God.

Interestingly, Marian Green notes that the ancient god Mithras was also supposedly born on December 25, in a cave surrounded by a bull and a dog, a lion and a snake, said to represent the four elements of life. She points out that the whole tradition of a god born in the middle of winter is a concept that is widespread throughout the ancient religions of the world. And, while we might think our festive customs are purely Christian, apparently that's simply not the case. The greenery we hang around our homes has very early origins. It was put up to mark hospitality around the midwinter festival. The Yule log harks back to the ancient idea of the World Tree, the Tree of Life which was said to support the whole of earth, heaven and hell in Norse and Saxon mythology. And Marian Green says that the custom of decorating trees goes way back to 2,000 B.C. in Mesopotamia where beribboned branches were carried in honor of the gods and goddesses of fertility and life.

So, before you dismiss Christmas as mere marketing and hype, think about the ancient origins of the festival. And try to follow the old customs or adapt them to suit your own needs.

As there is normally so much to do in December by way of preparations for the long holiday, I haven't included too many stringent measures for this month. Instead I want to look at ways (both practical and more esoteric) to make the season truly jolly.

Coping with Christmas

We all know how wonderful Christmas *should* be, so how come it often ends up in tears before lunchtime? There's no doubt that Christmas is the most stressful time of the year. The Samaritans receive more crisis calls at Christmas than at any other time; doctors dole out more prescriptions for tranquilizers and antidepressants; psychotherapists report a boom period in the run-up to the festive season and marriage guidance offices are inundated with cries for help. It's hardly surprising. At Christmas we worry about anything that moves: about money, about the family, about what we *should* be doing and what we *shouldn't* be doing, about whether the dinner will be cooked OK, about whether we'll pile on too much weight before the New Year. Some of us worry about whether we are enjoying ourselves enough: others feel guilty about enjoying themselves too *much*. You can't win. Or can you? There *are* ways to stop the madness and regain the true spirit of Christmas. It does take a few about-turns in your traditional thinking and a degree of co-operation from those around you, but it's well worthwhile. Try the following:

1. *Be Honest with Yourself*

Ask yourself what you *really* want from Christmas. Do you love huge parties, feeling goodwill to all men, women and children, or would you rather plump for a silent night? Psychotherapist Philip Rogers is convinced the fastest route to a happy holiday is to sit down and be honest about what you want from Christmas. "All too often we ask what other people want rather than what *we* want," he says, "and if we go off to Christmas like sacrificial turkeys, like victims, then we're not very likely to enjoy it." What makes your heart sink most about Christmas (is it all the cooking, the in-laws coming to stay, sitting in front of the television all afternoon)? Figure out if there are any simple changes that would make it better or at least marginally less ghastly. If it's something you can't do anything about, like relatives you utterly loathe coming to stay, then at least admit the problem. Then you won't feel quite so resentful.

2. Plan and Prepare

We all know the scenario: it's Christmas Eve and you haven't even started your shopping. Come midnight you're stirring your presents with one hand and wrapping the pudding with the other. "If you're going to enjoy the Christmas season, plan it, make time," advises Marigold Farmer, a stress-management consultant. "It doesn't have to be a huge military operation, but you do have to pace yourself." In other words, get started at the beginning of the month—don't leave it all until the very last moment. Spread your non-perishable food shopping over the next few weeks and put in orders for your last-minute necessities (turkey, fresh vegetables, etc.) early. Make a list of what presents you're looking for before you go out.

Stress-control consultant Robert Holden also recommends buying secret "emergency" supplies: extra crackers, enough mince pies for unheralded carol singers, replacement fuses for the fairy lights, the batteries the manufacturers never include. Keep a few "surprise gifts" on hand for those cringe-inducing occasions when friends drop by with a "surprise gift" for you. Nice bath goodies (for women), prettily packaged sweets (for kids), and gift-wrapped wine or spirits (for men) will get you out of most situations. And if you don't need to use them, you've got a few early birthday presents in stock.

3. Don't Overspend

Sensible spending flies up the chimney like Santa Claus when Christmas approaches. You blithely hand over your credit card and try to forget about it until New Year when the bills and the headaches roll in. Robert Holden says try to use cash rather than credit; agree upon a money-spending pass-not and stick to it. You don't need to spend a fortune, despite what the ads tell you. Children love making decorations (remember paper chains and Blue Peter egg box and silver paper bells and advent crowns?)—the whole family could join in. Gather in armloads of greenery and spruce them up with a few brightly colored bows or baubles. It looks much more effective than a few expensive, "sophisticated" streamers. Home-made presents can be wonderful as well: get your children to make their own presents (my nephew made us simple wooden candlesticks in his woodwork class which are more treasured than anything bought). If you're not "crafty," how about buying pretty bottles and making your own herb vinegars or bath preparations? There are plenty of books which will tell you how to do it. Cut down on all that food too. You know in your heart of hearts that you always buy too much and it just gets wasted. All those chocolates and sweets do horrible things to your health and your waistline. Trim down.

4. Make Your Gifts Simple but Selective

Refuse to get sucked into the trap of buying ever bigger, better presents. Marigold Farmer points out that "Christmas is a celebration of love, not money." Absolutely, agrees Philip Rogers: "When you give someone a present, it's a symbol, a gesture of love and affection. It shouldn't matter whether it cost 50 cents or 500 dollars." Try telling that to a child who wants the latest computer or the meanest mountain bike! No difference, insists Rogers. "It's all part of the hype of Christmas—you have to break the cycle. Talk to your children about it, about the meaning of giving gifts. Say to them 'Do you really think that because I can't buy you a computer or whatever that I don't love you?' Then give yourself time to choose the right present for the right person. It may not be expensive but it *should* be thoughtful."

5. Learn to Relax

The shops are heaving; you can't find the gift you want; the Christmas pudding has burned; the turkey won't cook—Christmas seems designed to get your nerves jangling. You can't keep running off for a soothing massage or an hour's yoga. However, just fifteen seconds can bring you back to a state of calm. "Sit down and first feel your feet firmly on the floor," says Marigold Farmer. "Feel the soles of your feet and the connection of your body to your feet. Then become aware of your bottom, feel that anchor point to your chair. And then feel your breathing—just start to be aware of it. It's very simple, but it will instantly make you breathe more deeply and make you feel more connected to your body." She also recommends what she dubs "The Magic of Minimum Effort." "The more pressurized we get, the more effort we use to do things," she explains. "We find ourselves gripping the saucepan handle, ferociously stirring, which only causes more tension. Relax and just do what is required."

6. Have Reasonable Expectations

Why is it that Christmas has to be "just right," a perfect, almost fairytale holiday? Philip Rogers says it's because lots of us hold on to the feelings we had as children when Christmas was a magical time, full of wonder and delight rather than stress and cooking. Robert Holden also warns against imagining that everything has to be spot-on: "Great expectations of a 'perfect' Christmas can turn even the most trivial incident into a test, a trial and a trauma," he says. "A dud cracker, too much salt in the stuffing, a Christmas card that reads 'with love' instead of 'lots of love' can dampen a merry Christmas." Accept that things will occasionally go wrong; that meals might not start on time; that you'll get the odd dud present; that not everyone will do precisely as you expect or plan. Let go of the control panel and just allow what happens to happen.

7. Spread Goodwill

How do you feel when the dishes start piling up and everyone seems permanently glued to the sofa? Or you're left peeling mountains of vegetables while everyone is playing games? Robert Holden reckons this is how rows and resentments start. I couldn't agree more. He recommends you sit down before Christmas and work out who's going to do what. "Sort out what will need doing and share out the tasks," he urges, "the chores of cooking, carving and cleaning, for instance." Remember to thank people too: a toast to the cook can make it all worthwhile. And if you go out on Christmas day make a pact to say "Happy Christmas" to everyone you meet: it's the only day of the year you can greet complete strangers without being branded a complete lunatic.

8. Give Yourself Time

Everyone needs time on their own, even at Christmas and even if it's only for the odd half an hour. There are times when we all need to hide from the hilarity of paper hats, cans of spray string, party poppers and festive frolicking fun and games. Robert Holden advises everyone to take time out to relax, recharge and make space for their own feelings. Marigold Farmer agrees. "Pamper yourself," she urges. "Have a long, slow aromatherapy bath, go for a walk or sit quietly with a drink and just think. Whatever is right for you." She also says we should put aside time to enjoy, rather than race through, the rituals of Christmas—arranging flowers, laying the table, decorating the tree.

9. Think About Your Life

It's often easy amidst all the food and frolicking to forget that Christmas is actually a festival with a deep spiritual purpose. And even if you aren't particularly religious, Philip Rogers believes that we all need a little thoughtfulness amidst the gaiety. "Even if we aren't conscious of it, it's a time when we do start to question our lives," he says. "It's the run-up to the New Year— a time to think about the past and plan the future." It's a good opportunity to think about what we really want from life, to write down all our hopes and wishes for the New Year and to start thinking about which resolutions we will make and keep. There's a lot more to Christmas than mince pies and mistletoe.

Pagan priestess Shan suggests a lovely little ritual. "Put out all the lights," she suggests, "and just spend some quiet time in the dark, thinking about your life. Then, slowly, put the lights back on, one by one."

Handling Hangovers

In a perfect world, of course, we wouldn't even know the meaning of the word hangover. And many people would say that if you're leading a perfect, natural, healthy life you would never have such a thing because you would never touch a drop of alcohol. Well, good luck to them, but I, for one, enjoy a drink and, yes I confess, I too have been known to overdo it and wake up in the morning feeling like something very noxious. No one's perfect, everyone bar saints occasionally goes over the top, and there's no time like Christmas for those red eyes and thumping headaches. So, just in case, here's the lowdown on the best way to handle hangovers.

Scientists claim they have drugs which will sober you up in minutes and which they trust will consign the dreaded morning after the night before into the mists of memory. However, sales of such hangover-busters are still at least a fair few years away.

As it is unlikely that we will stoically give up alcohol until its arrival, how, in the meantime, can we combat the horrors of the hangover?

Medically speaking, a hangover is a combination of severe swelling of the cranial arteries linked with irritation of the gastro-intestinal tract's lining. That's almost enough in itself to put you off. The causes are basically threefold: dehydration (all alcohol makes you urinate more); a build-up of the chemical acelaldehydro (which causes flushes, nausea and headaches) and congeners (the chemicals produced during fermentation which give drinks their flavor and color).

While the most obvious way to avoid hangovers is to steer clear of alcohol altogether or at least to limit your intake to a couple of drinks, the compulsion to get, quite literally, into the Christmas spirit is too much for most of us to resist. So consider a course of damage limitation. Make sure you've had a good solid meal before you start drinking. Drink slowly and intersperse alcoholic drinks with mineral water. And watch what you drink. As a rule of thumb, brown and red drinks (red wine, bourbon, rum, brandy, etc.) have far more (in some cases up to thirty times as many) congeners as less-colored and less-flavored drinks (white wine, gin, vodka). Many people swear by a pot of "live" yogurt or even a cup of olive oil before going out on the town. Both, so their advocates insist, will keep the stomach settled and avert a hangover.

If you know you've overdone it as you stumble home, there are a few last-minute savers—if you have the presence of mind to carry them out. Above all, get as much water as possible into your system to combat the dehydration. A couple of painkillers can help too, although avoid aspirin because it can further disrupt an already sensitive stomach. Herbalist Jill Nice suggests that a bowl of onion soup eaten before sleeping will restore equilibrium but, to be honest, if you're sober enough to cook onion soup you are probably sober enough not to get a hangover. Nutritionist Patrick Holford recommends taking a good-quality multivitamin and mineral supplement, plus a vitamin B complex and 2,000 mg of vitamin C before you retire to help your body replenish the vitamins destroyed by alcohol.

But it's in the morning when we really need all the help we can get. The very best solution, doctors say, is simply to turn over and sleep it off but, if you're faced with the office or a houseful of needy children, it's not that simple. Most commercial "cures" are simply combinations of antacids and painkillers which don't really get to the root of the problem. Likewise, a "hair of the dog" merely compounds the damage. A hangover is your body's way of telling you it is horribly out of balance and needs help. Your aim should be to restore lost vitamins and minerals and to give the body the fuel it needs to regain its equilibrium.

First of all, take a large glass of fresh, unsweetened, orange or grapefruit juice. It will replace some of the vitamin C you have lost. Run a hot bath which will, in itself, help to sweat some of the alcohol out of your system. Aromatherapist Robert Tisserand recommends adding two drops of lavender, two drops of juniper and one drop of rosemary essential oil into the water. In addition, he says, stir one drop of fennel and juniper essential oils into 600 ml of warm water and mix thoroughly. Soak cotton pads in the solution, squeeze them out and place them on your forehead, temples and liver area.

Although the temptation is to race for the strongest cup of coffee you can brew, resist it and try peppermint tea instead. It will soothe the stomach and quell any queasiness. And although you might have cravings for greasy fry-ups, stick to simple wholesome food for breakfast. Honey boosts energy and encourages the body to rid itself of the alcohol. Because it tops up your blood sugar levels it will make you feel more human. Pour it on yogurt with a sprinkling of wheatgerm or on porridge. Both will help to settle the stomach. Follow with dry rye toast—the carbohydrate will help flagging energy levels. If you have the stomach for it, apparently chicken soup will help your body restore its levels of salt and potassium which the alcohol has stripped from the bloodstream.

It might sound an unappealing mixture, but be grateful you don't live in parts of the world which opt for more draconian measures. In Russia they drink salted cucumber juice, while South Americans swear by raw fish marinated in a spicy sauce. In this country [the UK] the old folk remedy for a hangover was an unappetizing cocktail of black bread soaked in water or roast onions and snails.

Apart from nutrition there are some additional remedies that are worth trying. Herbal remedies can flush out the by-products of alcohol. Try mixing a teaspoon each of dandelion leaves, yarrow, meadowsweet, balm and chamomile in boiling water and leave to infuse for five minutes. Then strain the mixture and sweeten it with honey before drinking. Herbalist Penelope Ody of the Herb Society suggests evening primrose oil as a useful hangover cure. "Take a large dose (2–3 g) on the morning after to bring rapid relief," she says.

GP and homeopath Dr. Andrew Lockie, and author of *The Family Guide to Homeopathy* (Hamish Hamilton), underlines the point that alcohol "destroys vitamins and minerals, particularly A, B, C, D, K, folic acid, bioflavonoids, iron, manganese, potassium and the amino acid cysteine." He recommends taking a high-dose multivitamin and mineral supplement. Also, he points out, homeopathy has a number of remedies for the effects of overindulgence. *Nux vomica* is perhaps the best known, recommended when the head aches and the victim feels "dull, dizzy and irritable." If the hangover is due to rich food as well as alcohol try *Pulsatilla;* for excessive flatulence and nervous exhaustion, particularly following solitary drinking, try *sulphur;* if the hangover makes you feel more depressed and irritable than normal, *Avena* could help; and *zinc* can help if you feel trembly, lethargic, apprehensive and sensitive to noise. There is even a remedy geared for beer-drinkers who suffer nausea and vomiting—*Kali bichrom.* Choose remedies labeled 6c (sixth potency)—this is the strength of homeopathic remedies most suitable for acute and DIY use. They should be readily available from chemists and health-food shops.

Unfortunately there is no instant cure for the hangover—yet. But while you are suffering, bear in mind one small piece of cheerful news. Jill Nice points out that "it is rumored that only the truly healthy feel the agonies of a hangover."

The Natural First-Aid Kit for Christmas

Ten essential items for the party season—all readily available from most good chemists and health-food stores.

1. Peppermint tea bags. Peppermint soothes the stomach and quells queasiness—ideal after too much food and alcohol.
2. Bach Rescue Remedy. The "first-aid" preparation made from various flower essences. Useful for any Christmas disaster—after an accident or shock, or even try it during a family row. Simply take a few drops in any drink.
3. Multivitamin and mineral supplements. Take a good-quality preparation (Biocare, Solgar and Quest are all excellent) throughout the Christmas season to help your body with all the stresses and strains.
4. Vitamin B complex and vitamin C. Takes doses of these vitamins in addition to your multivitamin and supplement before you head out for a night's drinking, and again in the morning, to replace the vitamins you have lost.
5. Lavender oil. Essential oil of lavender is nature's great soother. Pop a couple of drops in a hot bath the morning after the night before to help a hangover. Add to a warm (not hot) bath last thing at night to soothe frayed nerves. Dab a drop on temples and wrists to combat headaches, and a few drops on your pillow will help you sleep.
6. Calendula lotion or cream. A gentle healing preparation for any unexpected accidents, cuts and bruises.
7. An eye mask. Buy one which can be either cooled in the fridge or warmed in hot water to soothe raw sore eyes. Eye drops are also a wise investment to soothe eyes after late nights in smoky atmospheres.
8. Orange essential oil. The great mood-lifter. If you're feeling a bit flat, try putting a few drops of orange oil in an oil burner or a bowl of hot water and let the scent permeate the room.
9. *Nux vomica*. The homeopathic remedy most commonly needed at this time of year—take it if you are suffering the ill effects of overeating and alcohol, particularly if you have indigestion, are feeling irritable, stuffy and in need of air.
10. Chamomile tea. When your nerves are at screaming pitch, chamomile can soothe and de-stress. Leave a couple of teabags to stew for five minutes, strain and then sit back, sip and unwind.

Life After Christmas

Straight after Christmas, the festivities continue with the wild and raucous celebrations for the New Year. In olden times the two festivals were all part of the same Yuletide package—it was just one long holiday. Nowadays, New Year seems to be the more sociable festival. We tend to stay at home for Christmas or be with close family but, come New Year, we venture back into the world, socializing at parties or, increasingly, taking breaks away. Whatever you do and wherever you spend the New Year, doubtless you will carry on the custom of New Year Resolutions. That's great but, as I said right back at the beginning of this book, this can be a tough time of year to carry out certain resolutions, however good they may be. I would suggest that rather than using New Year as a kind of Lent, where you give up smoking, drinking, fatty foods, whatever—starting in the cold light of day on January 1—that you take the resolution process a little more deeply and a little more slowly.

Something I do every year which I find really useful is to make a long list of everything I want to achieve, everything I want to do. It might sound excessive or extremely indulgent but aim for 100 things—or at least fifty to start with (you can always add on). Sit down and write out everything you want in your life—from tiny little things like having a haircut or getting a leaking window fixed, through larger endeavors like learning to drive, traveling around France or losing weight, right up to the real biggies such as shifting job, getting married, having a baby, moving abroad.

Look at your list and really think about it. Do you really want these things? Do you want them now? Are some of them things you'd like to do later on in life? Is there anything missing from your list? Is there anything there because you feel it ought to be there? Because someone else wants it there? Edit your list if you need to and perhaps divide it into "Things I want to do this coming year" and "Things I want to do in my life."

It can be highly enlightening to do this exercise with your partner or family (no conferring until you've all completed your lists). When my husband and I tried it we were surprised to find how similar our lists were. However, we were also surprised at where they differed. He wanted to visit places, to do things I had no inkling of, and vice versa. Use your lists as the starting point for some healthy discussion about what you are both seeking in life. It can bring tricky topics out into the open and give you a chance to say what you really feel. Equally it's a chance for children to express what they want and for the whole family to work out what can be feasibly agreed upon.

Above all, though, it's fun. Let your imagination really go and you will be surprised with what you come up with. Drop your limiting beliefs ("I can't afford it"; "I don't dare do it"; "I'm too old/too young/too unfit"; "it's frivolous"; "it's dangerous"; "it's insane"). After all, no one is saying you *have* to carry out every single thing on your list.

Now comes the practical part. Look down your list and pick out the ones you can do something about immediately. Make a "to do" list and schedule a day when you will sort it all out (e.g., book your hair appointment; find a plumber in the *Yellow Pages*; get the dog booked in to training classes). Better still, schedule a precise time you will make your arrangements (e.g., between 10–11 a.m.)—that way you will really do it. Then look at your longer-term projects and decide when in the year would be the best time to start them. How long will they take? If you want to lose weight, remember that you should aim for no more than one to two pounds (half to one kilogram) a week weight loss. If you've got a lot of weight to lose, it's not a quick-fix number. You will need to schedule in a fair few months possibly. It's the same with getting fit—you won't turn into Jane Fonda overnight. So be realistic. That way you will get results. If you want to learn a language, think about how much time you really need to devote to it, not just the evening class but the homework and practice too. Check back on the time-management tips and learn how to "eat elephants" so that you schedule in the time you need every week. If you want to go on a long trip, then work out how you might do it. If you saved so much money each week, how long would it take? Almost anything is possible—if you are prepared to be flexible, inventive and realistic.

Using Affirmations

One technique which can be really useful at this time of year, when you are thinking about new beginnings, is that of affirmations. Affirmations are very simple things: they merely involve putting your intention into positive terms and repeating it to yourself as often as possible. It's like lines for grownups. You will find almost every self-help book and personal development guru will advocate their use. If you want to look into them in more depth I would suggest Louise Hay's books *You Can Heal Your Body* and *You Can Heal Your Life* as a starting point.

People generally either love the idea of affirmation or loathe them. I must admit I found myself very skeptical to begin with (especially after reading that if I wanted to rid myself of constipation I should endlessly recite "I love my beautiful bowels"). However, I did try (other ones I hasten to add) and have found them very useful. Here's how they work.

The theory behind positive affirmations is that we create our own reality by our thoughts. So if you are constantly thinking "Life's awful," then sure enough life probably will oblige and indeed be awful. If you think "I'm fat and ugly," your subconscious will do its darndest to make sure you stay fat and ugly—or at least appear so to yourself. Our subconscious will work as hard as it can to create the world we believe in. It's a scary thought but it does seem to make sense. So the idea is to reprogram your subconscious by bombarding it with bright positive messages. The subconscious then begins to believe what it keeps hearing and so obediently tries to bring whatever you are affirming into existence. It's a kind of verbal equivalent of the treasure map we looked at earlier.

So, for example, if you are fed up with failing at everything you do you could alter the thought from "I fail" to "I succeed." Make your statement a little over the top and totally positive. So, rather than say "I never fail" or "I don't fail any more," turn it round and say something like "I always succeed in everything I do." Yuk—does that sound horribly Californian? If so, then good. The most effective affirmations are the ones that really ring your bell, the ones that make you cringe and feel downright uncomfortable. Many affirmation devotees have favorite formulae for phrasing affirmations. The woman who taught them to me suggested starting with "It is safe, fun and exciting for me, (insert your name) to be totally (whatever you want—successful, healthy, relaxed, loved.)" Once you have decided upon your affirmation (only use one at a time for maximum effectiveness), write it out in large, clear letters and stick it up where you can see it often during the day. I tend to have one on my computer, one on the fridge and one on the bathroom mirror. Then, in addition, write out your affirmation at least twenty times a day for at least a week. Each time you write it out, pause for a moment and see if you feel a response to the affirmation. Often you will find, especially at the beginning, that you will want to contradict or ridicule the affirmation. That's good. So your affirmation sheet might look something like this:

I, Jane, now choose to become fit and healthy (but I'm a lazy slob).
I, Jane, now choose to become fit and healthy (no chance).
I, Jane, now choose to become fit and healthy (but I've never been able to get fit before, I've always given up, why should it change?).

Toward the end of the week you may well find you have exhausted your fund of negative thoughts and more positive ones start creeping in: "Well, maybe"; "Perhaps I could"; "It would be great to feel fit," and so on. With any luck by the time you finish the exercise you will be really getting into the idea—answering yourself with things like "Yes, I *can* be totally healthy"; "I can look and feel great"; even, who knows, "I could run a marathon."

Some people suggest that you split your twenty daily affirmations into three groups, each starting with a different personal pronoun followed by your name: for example, the first six or seven affirmations starting with "I, Jane . . ."; the next starting "You, Jane . . ."; and the third starting "She, Jane . . . ," adapting the rest of the sentence to fit the personal pronoun you're using. This can seem really weird, but the reasoning is that we are not only giving subconscious messages to ourselves throughout the day; we also take them in from other people. So using all three pronouns reinforces the message—as if we were hearing it from other people, not just from ourselves.

Affirmations like this may seem silly but, in my experience, they really do work. Use them with your list of things you want to do in the New Year if you find you have blocks. They could make your world a happier, more positive place.

January

After the bright lights and festive fare of Christmas, January often seems cold, dark and gloomy. Even the countryside appears dead and quiet: the birds have eaten all but the last few berries; the fields seem empty and barren; the world a frozen, empty place. Venturing out isn't just cold and miserable. With icy roads, it can be downright dangerous as well. It seems as if there is nothing to look forward to now until the far-off days of spring. And yet the Native Americans call the major part of January the Renewal Time so there must be something good about it. Look around you and watch for those tiny signs of renewal, of new life, of new hope. There's the bright yellow forsythia in the garden and the subtle yet beautiful flowers of the hellebores. See the early bulbs breaking through the hard earth, shoots of bright, young, fresh green. If you cannot see them yet, then believe in them—they will come.

This period after Christmas can be a tough time so I recommend you take it easy in January and be gentle on yourself. After the excesses of Christmas and New Year you are probably feeling like a break from all the rich food and drink—not a bad idea. However, it's not a good time of year to launch into a full detox or stringent diet (your body still needs the strength from good nutrition to combat the evil cold) but get yourself back to a sensible, healthy eating pattern by taking solid, nourishing food with warming spices and herbs to keep your taste-buds interested.

In the old days, this phase after the great Yuletide festival was the time they purified their surroundings to make room to bring luck into the house. There were many rituals to call in good fortune: from sprinkling holy water, to sealing up the whole house and fumigating it with scented branches of juniper. In farming communities they would sweep out and purify the stables and barns in the same way. And once all the cleaning and purifying was done, there would be ceremonies to bring in all the new luck and blessings for the year to come.

It's a lovely idea and one we can continue today. We have already looked at several ways of cleansing your environment (space clearing in SPRING and feng shui in SEPTEMBER), but there are some additional touches which are nice at this time of year. This time we are going to call on the power of the elements.

Cleansing With the Elements

Denise Linn, the well-known workshop leader and author on things marvelous and mystical, is a great believer in space clearing. Before her workshops she always makes sure the room she's working in is totally cleansed and purified. And she sees no reason why everyone shouldn't use similar techniques in their homes. The ideas here are just a taster—she has now written a whole book on the subject called *Sacred Space* which is well worth buying if you'd like to do more.

"Your home can be a sanctuary within which you can retreat and recharge," says Denise, "an oasis of peace amidst turmoil. Homes can be places of healing and regeneration." What a lovely idea. She believes that by simple processes such as chanting and lighting candles, by introducing color and using essential oils, you can transform your home. But how can such tiny changes possibly have an effect? Denise says it all comes down to how we alter the subtle energy in our homes. Ancient cultures have known for millennia what modern physics is just discovering, that everything around us, whether it's the dog, a tree or the kitchen table, is actually made up of energy. All the atoms and molecules that make up life are in constant motion, endlessly creating energy.

"Your home is not just a composite of materials thrown together for shelter and comfort," she says. "Every cubic centimeter, whether solid or seemingly empty space, is filled with infinite vibrating energy fields." While the science remains mind-bogglingly baffling, almost everyone would understand the theory in practice. When there has been a terrible argument, the room seems heavy and tense—we use the phrase "you could have cut the air with a knife." The mood during a lively party is different again. Denise says that by learning how to shift the energy of our environment to suit our needs we can find life much easier and happier.

She agrees with the feng shui experts that one of the fastest ways to cleanse the energies in a home is simply by cleaning it. Not only does the general straightening of the clutter make a psychological difference in feeling but whenever your home is cleaned there are subtle shifts in the energy fields. The deeper the cleaning the better—wash the windows, vacuum under the bed. I know you've done this once before in the course of this book but that was several months ago now and, ten to one, the clutter has had time to build up again, those magazines and papers have multiplied and your clothes seem to have been breeding. So have another clear out. Go through your drawers and cupboards and apply the motto "use it, love it or get rid of it."

Dawna Walters who started up The Holding Company (a marvelous shop which specializes in clever ways to store everything you can possibly think of) is, perhaps surprisingly, also a fan of giant clear-outs. Her advice is to look at your wardrobe and give away anything that you haven't worn for two years; anything that has been too small for two years or anything which has a stain. Be ruthless and give unwanted or unused items to charity shops. Banish piles of magazines from corners and hoards of clothes from cupboards. Give all those old paperbacks you'll never read again to the next jumble sale. Fling away old make-up—it goes off and, anyhow, you will always want to buy something new. Open the windows and let light stream into the house. Sounds familiar? Exactly the same advice that we've heard before. So surely there must be something in it . . .

Denise Linn uses many of the traditional ceremonies of the Native Americans, updated to fit in with modern life. One of the most powerful ways of introducing good energy into the house, she avers, is by using the power of the four elements, fire, air, water and earth.

FIRE: THE ENERGIZER

The use of fire in the home for spiritual cleansing and dedication is one of the oldest, surest and most immediate of space-clearing techniques according to Denise. Fire brings energy into the house, and one of the simplest and most lovely methods is to use candles. First choose a color that suits your purpose. Blue will help you achieve peacefulness and balance; reds or yellow will bring lively energy. If you are seeking love or wish to conceive a child, burn a pink candle in your bedroom. A green candle is helpful for money and abundance. Yellow candles can bring joy and conviviality; they also help concentration. To gain the maximum benefit, first of all you need to focus your intention, so that before you light the candle you are very clear as to why you are lighting it. Then concentrate intensely while lighting the candle. It's very similar to the way you make a wish before blowing out the candles on a birthday cake.

If you can have a real fire in your home, do so. A fire can bring warmth, strength and a feeling of peace. Also, hanging cut-lead crystals in your windows will help to bring the fire energy of the sun into your home. Children, in particular, love the rainbows that dance round the room from crystals. So do cats: my usually very dignified black cat turns into a kitten careering and leaping when the beams skitter around the walls. Try as well to hang mirrors in strategic places so that the sunshine can be reflected into your home.

WATER: THE PURIFIER

Water, the next element, is the great purifier and has been used in spiritual ceremonies since ancient times right up to modern baptism services. Water is excellent for clearing a room of negative emotions. After an argument, the air in a room might seem thick and almost charged with negative energy. The fastest way to neutralize this residual energy is to mist the room. "Spraying your home with water is one of the simplest and most effective techniques for shifting your home's energy and to cleanse residual emotions," says Denise, who explains that the fine spray also creates a negative-ion-rich environment such as you find next to a waterfall, or by the sea or in a pine forest.

The key is to use spring water in a fine spray and lightly spray all over the room. You can also use the Bach flower remedies in a mister—Denise suggests using Rescue Remedy after an argument or illness; Cherry Plum for calm, quiet courage; Star of Bethlehem to clear tension; Water Violet for tranquillity, poise and grace. Equally you could try combining aromatherapy with misting water. Use lemon-grass in the kitchen; lavender in the living room and geranium in the bedroom.

AIR: THE TRANSFORMER

While water heals, cleanses and rejuvenates, the element of air transforms. Air changes all that it encompasses. A simple way to enliven a room is to light a stick of incense. But choose a scent that you like and which feels appropriate for the room. Aromatherapy can also be a powerful medicine for the home. Our bodies react emotionally and powerfully to different scents, and the smells in your home can contribute to or detract greatly from the way you feel about it. Use oils in vaporizers or diffusers, in a bowl of hot water or on a ring that fits on your light bulb. Try the following: orange, lemon and grapefruit are uplifting and refreshing; geranium balances mood swings; chamomile is excellent after an argument; pine is refreshing and cleansing; rosemary helps with studying. The following oils work well in combination: lavender, rose geranium and ylang-ylang for the bedroom; rosemary, peppermint, basil and bergamot in the study; orange, mandarin and bergamot in the living-room; lemon and grapefruit in the kitchen; peppermint and pine in the bathroom.

EARTH: THE STRENGTHENER

The next element, earth, is grounding and strengthening. It brings stability, ancient wisdom and power into our lives. Introducing earth into your home will generate an energy which is serene and stable. You will feel more certain of your direction in life.

Salt is one of the most powerful ways of bringing earth into the home. Salt has the ability to neutralize negativity and to cleanse the energy field that surrounds us, the aura. It is a powerful purifier—in the ocean it acts as an antiseptic to destroy bacteria and it has been used in rituals for centuries. In the past, church bells were anointed with salt and water to bless them. An ancient baptism ritual saw the baby rubbed with salt to repel demons. We still throw a pinch of salt over our shoulders to "hit the devil in the eye." If you ever feel as if you are being thrown off balance by outside influences in your life, try the following. Take salt and make a large ring that goes around the periphery of your room, including all the corners. Then make a smaller circle of salt right around your bed. Just a small trickle will be effective.

Crystals and semi-precious stones can also help to bring the earth element into your home. Although crystals or any stone are not magical in themselves, they do seem to act as catalysts for energy. The following stones can all be used in the home: Citrine apparently clears thoughts, promotes confidence, and helps communication and decision-making; Tiger's Eye is grounding and focusing; Rose Quartz is excellent for helping children and family and for aiding creativity and love; Smoky Quartz helps promote wisdom and abundance; Coral fosters physical strength and determination.

Using Sound for Space Clearing

• Music can dramatically affect a room's energy. Music by Bach or Albinoni are good for soothing your senses and your soul. So is flute music. African drumming conjures creativity, life force and strength. Gregorian chant promotes a powerful dynamic energy.

• Singing and chanting can clear the energy in a room. Sing songs that fill you full of joy and power. Ohm is the most powerful yet simple spiritual chant. Feel it vibrating through your body. Look back at the ideas for introducing sound therapy into your life and, if you didn't try them before Christmas, try them now.

• A squeaky toy can insert humor into a room where people have been very serious and the atmosphere needs lightening.

• Clapping dissipates energy and so can clear a room of unwanted negative energy. To disperse stagnant energy, clap all the way from the floor up to the ceiling with your arms spread apart after each clap. Work all round the room, taking especial care on the corners.

Using Color in the Home

Color can have a subtle but powerful effect on the energy and mood of your home.

Red can be extremely vitalizing and stimulating and can help overcome depression, inertia, fear or melancholy. A study at the University of Texas found that simply looking at the color red could increase strength and muscle activity. A red dining-room will stimulate appetite, but avoid red if you are trying to diet. Red in the bedroom can make your love life passionate and exciting but it can make it difficult to rest and relax (a soft pink would be better or, as we discussed in the feng shui section, introduce your passion in manageable bite-sized pieces—a rich ruby red velvet cushion or two, or a sensual shawl or throw). Meanwhile, red in a living-room will stimulate movement and activity.

Orange fosters optimism, confidence, self-motivation, enthusiasm and socializing. Orange is good in rooms used for group gatherings. It doesn't have to be that virulent Sixties-style orange—think instead of a warm pumpkin color which could transform a room into a great family room, a room where things get done.

Yellow stimulates the intellect and communication. It is associated with mental discrimination, organization, attention to detail, academic achievement, administration and harmony. Yellow is good for concentration and clarity of thought and so is an excellent color for use in a home office. Yellow kitchens generate a feeling of well being. It is also a good color for a young child's room. Again, it doesn't have to be bright "daffodil" yellow, although I once had a kitchen in that color—it was so popular I could never shift people out from it into the dining-room. But equally, try shades of pale gold, of dusky sandy colors, soft cowslip or brazen buttercup.

Green stimulates feelings of balance, harmony, peace, hope, growth and healing. A good color for any room, it is restful yet energizing. Green is perfect for bathrooms—use either a bright spring green or a clean leaf green.

Blue helps you to attain inner peace and to live out your ideals. It stimulates inspiration, creativity, patience and composure. Blue has been used for pain reduction in hospital tests. It's an excellent color for a bedroom, especially for hyperactive children and for any room where you want to have a feeling of peace.

Purple is calming, soothing and comforting and stimulates spiritual awareness and intuition. Dilute it to lavender or violet for a bedroom or meditation room. Lavender rooms are excellent for convalescence.

White is purifying and healing. However, an all-white room can feel too sterile. Too much white can make a house feel unapproachable.

Geopathic Stress: Is It Harming Your Health?

Have you tried all the space-clearing and feng shui exercises and yet still feel that something is dragging you down? There is growing interest in the world of natural health in the concept of geopathic stress. The idea is that harmful energy fields radiating from deep under the earth might be ruining your life and proving hazardous to your health. Many complementary health practitioners are convinced that abnormal energy fields generated by deep underground streams, large mineral deposits or faults in the substrata of the earth could be seriously compromising the health of millions. They call the condition geopathic stress (GS) and suggest it can be a major contributing factor in everything from migraines to cancer, from nightmares to divorce. But is this a genuine health crisis or merely alarmist conjecture? I am not, to be honest, totally convinced yet myself, even after researching the matter quite deeply. But I think it is something you should be aware of so that, if it makes sense to you, you can pursue your own investigations.

The evidence suggests that geopathic stress certainly *does* exist. In Germany it has been researched since the Twenties and is taken very seriously. Experiments have shown that bacteria grow abnormally when grown over underground currents of water, while mice inoculated with disease will fall ill far more rapidly when kept over a subterranean vein of water. Now builders in Germany and Austria test sites before building, and many will routinely give guarantees that new buildings do not have lines of "bad" energy passing through them.

However, in the UK even organizations such as The Building Research Establishment, who advise on radon gas and other environmental problems, are barely aware of it. And yet, according to Geraint Jones-David, a management consultant turned geopathic stress detective, it is possible that over four million people in the UK could be affected, with fifteen to twenty percent of houses suffering from geopathic stress. He and his wife, Sylvia, diagnose and treat the problem from their clinic in Carmarthen.

"It's far more prevalent than you imagine," he says, and points out that, although harmful energy in itself does not cause cancer, ME, MS, or any of the numerous other diseases and complaints that have been associated with it, it appears to lower the body's immune system so that if a predisposition to disease is present, the condition is more likely to develop. Sometimes, he says, the effects are very obvious. One local therapist had three clients all suffering from cancer, all from the same village. She called in Jones-David, who found that a line of geopathic stress ran straight through the three people's houses. On questioning them, he found that other neighbors also suffered from cancer. The opposite side of the street, where no one was ill, had no geopathic stress.

It sounds terrifying, but practitioners reassure that even if your house *does* suffer GS, your health need not necessarily be affected. Wilma Tait, a healer and GS consultant, promises, "GS comes up through the earth in thin bands or small spirals, so it will only affect you if you are sleeping directly on top of it or sitting in it all day. It is very easy to move your desk or your bed to avoid it."

Tom Williams states that geopathic stress can be measured with a geological instrument called a geo-magnetometer, yet none of the practitioners I spoke to used one. Instead they all dowse for geopathic stress using rods or a pendulum. And herein lies that first major problem, as Williams explains. He was a director of nursing services for twenty-two years before he left to study complementary medicine. Now he runs the Healthshare Foundation (a natural healthcare clinic) in Newton Abbot and studies the effects of the environment on health, in particular geopathic stress. While he has no doubts that geopathic stress *does* exist and *can* cause health problems, he admits that dowsing can prove an uncertain means of detection. "Dowsing does depend on the operator which is somewhat of a problem," he says. "It's like two people looking at a color, they might see it quite differently."

I asked two consultants to check my house for geopathic stress. Geraint Jones-David came armed with metal dowsing rods and walked around the house, both inside and out, watching for the rods to cross indicating the presence of GS. He pinpointed four lines running through the house and tow lines crossing in the living room providing a clear "black spot." The levels weren't serious, he said, but I should move my bed to avoid a line running through it which could cause problems.

On the other hand, Wilma Tait was able to check my house over the phone using a pendulum. It took just a few minutes for her to give the house the all-clear: "No, it's clear. No negative energy. No radon gas. No geopathic stress."

Bemused, I asked a further two consultants for their analyses: the first (dowsing over the phone again) said no, quite clear but that I could do with a feng shui consultant! The second, dowsing over a plan of the house, showed several lines intersecting the house but in different places from those Geraint Jones-David found.

So who was right? And, if I *did* suffer from GS what would it cost to cure it? Wilma Tait charges 60 pounds and offers a two-year guarantee against GS—she "clears" both the house and its inhabitants by psychic healing. Geraint Jones-David agrees the harmful energy can be neutralized in this way but also takes a more pragmatic approach: he sells neutralizers which employ magnets to attract the harmful energy and then feed it back through the earth current in the electrical circuit of your house. They cost from 200-700 pounds. In addition, his wife Sylvia, a reflexologist, then treats patients for the damage geopathic stress has caused in their bodies (sessions cost 50 pounds).

It's an expensive business. And some people are suggesting that not all the cures actually work. A BBC1 *Watchdog* report focused on a GS neutralizer named RadiTech manufactured by a company called the Dulwich Health Society. The machine was tested by a government lab which pronounced that it couldn't work because the wires inside weren't connected to anything. At 72 pounds, Watchdog decided it was "worst buy" of the week.

Jane Thurnell-Read, a complementary health practitioner who has written a book on geopathic stress, also thinks there is a problem with neutralizing devices. "There are various proprietary devices on the market which claim to neutralize geopathic problems," she says. "However, it has been my experience that no one device can address the full range of geopathic energies . . ."

Tom Williams disagrees. He has a RadiTech device himself and swears by its efficacy. As evidence, he recalls the time when his wife inadvertently unplugged the machine and started to suddenly experience bad nightmares. When they discovered the RadiTech wasn't on and replugged it, the nightmares vanished.

He's not alone. Hundreds of people swear to the amazing results of GS clearing (whether via machines or human intervention). Both Wilma Tait and the Jones-Davids have files bulging with testimonials from satisfied and grateful customers who claim that GS clearing has improved their health and even saved their marriages (GS can apparently cause irritability and fuel disagreements as well as making children hyperactive and destructive). And Tom Williams is satisfied that GS is the missing factor in many patients who seem resistant to almost all treatment, those who constantly feel ill or under par and those with serious ailments.

But he feels more research needs to be done to take the

"mumbo-jumbo" out of the field. Also he suggests that in order to receive unbiased advice, "you need to look for a dowser who has no interest in selling you anything."

I quite agree. I'm not the only person who has been given contradictory readings by dowsers. One woman answered an advertisement for a device to divert harmful energy. She sent a check and waited for a parcel. Instead she received a message on her answerphone saying that her house had very severe geopathic stress and needed urgent attention. The cost would be 100 pounds. In the interim she had had the house checked by a local dowser who found no GS at all.

My first reaction to all this contradictory evidence was to say forget the whole thing, ignore the problem. Geopathic stress seems to be a complete minefield and potentially a very expensive one. Even if you correctly diagnose GS, there is no guarantee that the device you buy to cure it will do so. However, experts like Tom Williams and Jane Thurnell-Read warn that we ignore geopathic stress at our peril. "Geopathic stress will become more of a problem in the future," warns Thurnell-Read. "Levels of electromagnetic pollution from televisions, computers and so forth are rising which, in turn, affects our ability to cope with geopathic stress."

But, as Tom Williams readily admits, "In this field you are working on the edge of the area of credibility." And, if, as seems possible, geopathic stress is contributing to widespread illness and lack of well being, then that simply isn't good enough. There seems no doubt that we should follow the lead of Germany and investigate geopathic stress thoroughly and scientifically. Much more research is needed.

DETECTING GEOPATHIC STRESS

If you think geopathic stress might be affecting your home there is some DIY detection you can try for yourself.

• Wilma Trait says GS is most probably affecting people who complain of constantly feeling tired and below par. "Everything is an effort. They are easily depressed and irritable." They constantly suffer from colds while illnesses, aches and pains will not respond to any treatment. Children become disruptive and badly behaved.

• Because GS comes up in thin lines it can easily affect just one person in the house—a line can pass through one side of the bed or one armchair. It is quite possible only one member of the family could be affected.

• Tom Williams suggests that if you suspect you suffer from GS, to try putting cork tiles under your bed or favorite chair for a few weeks and to see whether you start to feel better. The tiles, he explains, seem to neutralize the rays for a limited period. If you do start to feel better, try moving your bed or chair.

• Geraint and Sylvia Jones-David advise you to watch where your pets sleep. Cats adore GS and will often choose to sleep on a bad spot, while dogs will avoid it at all costs. If the cat always makes a beeline for your favorite armchair, try moving it to the dog's favorite spot.

• Babies are apparently very sensitive to GS. If your baby constantly rolls over to one corner of the cot, he or she may be attempting to escape GS. Move the cot to another part of the room and see whether the baby stays where it is put.

• Jane Thurnell-Read says that if you feel you are affected by GS, you should try the following: switch on a hairdryer and run it all over you with the side of the dryer touching your body. "It sounds crazy," admits Thurnell-Read, "but if you do it once a week it does seem to help."

Delving into the Past: Looking for Clues

Having sorted out your environment and hopefully given yourself a clear, clean place in which to live and work, you are ready to look deeper into your self. This is a time of year that is well suited to the deeper, more mystical forms of therapy. Not everyone will feel comfortable with them and, as always, if these "soul" therapies make you feel uneasy, then they're not for you—or at least not for now. Never do anything you feel uncomfortable with; it's just not worth it. Not that anything awful would happen; it's more likely that nothing would happen at all. You would simply feel so tense or critical that the therapy wouldn't have a real chance. So leave it out.

The therapies I'm going to outline now are still quite controversial. You may well have read about past life therapy in the press and had a good laugh. It is less likely that you will have read about rebirthing in the same way, but it is often greeted with just as much ridicule. However, both of these therapies have had wonderful results for some people.

REBIRTHING: BREATHING BACK TO BABYHOOD

Rebirthing is a form of therapy which aims to take you back to early childhood, to birth and even, in some cases, to your very conception and beginning. Whereas Freud maintained that our "problems" don't begin until the Oedipal stage at around four years of age, more recent psychological thought acknowledges that a newborn child already internalizes feelings about its emotional environment and that even pre-birth experiences can affect later thought patterns. Rebirthing is at the forefront of the early-life scrutineers, averring that the birth experience is at the very heart of modern psychological trauma. Although originally "discovered" back in the Sixties, rebirthing is now finding itself literally "born again" with a recent upsurge of interest.

Its technique is simple. The key lies in "conscious connected breathing," breathing in and out without pausing between the inhale and exhale—a procedure which rebirthers believe can connect you to very early memories, bringing them into the conscious mind to be acknowledged and safely reintegrated. You simply lie on a couch or on the floor in a warm room and the rebirther will help you to breathe properly. It's not a particularly comfortable form of breathing and when I first tried it it felt as if I were hyperventilating; my head became dizzy and my hands and feet cramped. But you soon go past that stage and then the images start to arrive. Sometimes they are clear, like old home movies; sometimes they are more like vague feelings, dusty long-forgotten memories. Usually you will simply be left to breathe in this way for about an hour and a half.

At the end of that time, soft music will gently bring you back. When you emerge the real work begins. Sometimes you can find strong emotions surfacing as you remember old hurts—tiny things that mean nothing to an adult but that can cause heartbreak to a child. Beyond those hurts lie memories of birth inaccessible to our conscious brain but which our subconscious minds still dwell on. Rebirthing teaches that we make lifetime decisions based on such early experiences: say my male obstetrician hurt me while delivering me I might subconsciously go through life thinking "men hurt me" and end up attracting men who do precisely that, fulfilling the prophecy.

The rebirthing process tries to bring those unconscious memories into consciousness and then set about changing them. Homework comes in the form of affirmations, those positive statements we talked about last month, that have to be written out twenty times a day for at least a week, noting your responses as you go along. I remember one which ran "I, Jane am innocent," which *sounded* innocuous enough but brought up all kinds of old memories including my guilt as a ten-year-old for not visiting my dying father enough in hospital. I lay on my bed and sobbed in a way I haven't cried since I was a child.

I discovered mainly psychological benefits, but rebirthing appears to have profound effects on the physical level too. Practitioners claim particular success with stress-related disorders and nervous complaints such as asthma and eczema. One rebirthee even found it cured a trapped nerve in her spine. "I could hardly walk but the rebirther insisted I go to the session," she relates. "When I arrived, she made me sit down and write out ten reasons why it was useful for me to be ill at that time. That in itself made me realize how I have used illness as an excuse for avoiding unpleasant situations. Then I lay down and did the breathing. When I got up the pain had quite literally vanished and it hasn't come back over a year later."

Impressive, but she was by no means wholehearted in her praise of rebirthing. "It did have an incredible effect on me but it was a very scary process," she continues. "I went through agony. At times my body cramped so badly that I thought I was going to die." Rebirthers say that cramp is the result of old traumas being held in the body, but critics of the therapy put it down to hyperventilation.

Uncontrolled hyperventilation increases the amount of carbon dioxide leaving the body which, in turn, alters the body's acid balance. It can result in a variety of symptoms ranging from dizziness, cramp and mild hallucination to palpitations, spasm and chest pain. But rebirthers insist that their technique, practiced correctly, isn't technically *hyper*ventilation: if the breathing is kept rhythmical and relaxed it is *super*ventilation and can cause no harm.

For maximum results, ten sessions are recommended. But the rebirthing experience need not end there: you could opt for "wet" rebirthing (in a bath with a snorkel) or you could switch to a rebirther of the opposite sex for a further ten sessions. Then there are one-day seminars, weekend workshops and week-long or month-long trainings—all recommended and none of them cheap. I stopped after the ten sessions having felt I had done something very worthwhile. However, for some people rebirthing becomes a whole new way of life; others, more critically, hail it as a pseudo-religion, tantamount to a mini-cult.

If rebirthing is a religion, its gospel is love and forgiveness. You forgive others for what they've done to you, and you forgive yourself for absolutely everything. By taking charge of your whole life you can create your own reality, drawing to you whatever you need or desire. But rebirthing has its high priests and priestesses as well and none more admired and adored than Sondra Ray, founder of the Loving Relationships Training (LRT), a weekend workshop which utilizes rebirthing to transform lives. The weekend teaches you how to attract better relationships, better work, better health, more money and more joy. It asks you to clear up your relationships, to forgive your parents, to get straight with your partner, to get even with God. It can even, promises Ray, change your relationship with that big bugbear Death. "All death is suicide," states Ray confidently. "The belief that death is inevitable has killed more people than any other cause." To avoid the grim reaper we are advised to go on frequent fasts, to cut down on sleep, to chant and meditate, to (naturally) attend lots of workshops and have lots of rebirthing, and even to shave our heads every ten years.

She appears totally sincere and many of rebirthing's devotees really do believe they're going to live forever. Unfortunately, however, all the goodwill and head shaving in the world cannot halt the hand of fate. One "immortal," totally convinced of his physical eternity, was knocked down by a car on his way to an

immortality workshop. He died. I have been on an LRT training
and found it interesting although I must say it did not really
change anything in my life. My husband, on the other hand,
absolutely hated it, particularly the emphasis on immortality and
our relationship with God and spirit.

So is rebirthing merely a cranky con promising eternal life for
your cash or is it a genuinely helpful therapy? It depends very
much on what kind of person you are and how you use it. The
purely pragmatic might find its New Age psychobabble off-putting;
the gullible and the lonely might lean on it as an all-pervasive
and expensive crutch. But if you take some of its more wacky
prescriptives with a liberal pinch of salt, the actual process can
cause quite remarkable changes.

When I first started investigating rebirthing (many years ago) I
was initially highly skeptical and even keen to expose it as yet
another trendy scam. However, I took the whole ten sessions
and did my homework assiduously. Call it coincidence, but my
life really seemed to shift. My self-esteem grew and I obtained a
new job, a new relationship and a new living situation within a
few weeks. Many years on, I honestly feel like a different person.
I still have moments of doubt and anguish and I haven't prized
out all my skeletons by any means, but however it worked (be
it the breathing, the affirmations or simply because I *wanted* to
change my life), it really did make a difference. One day I mean
to go back and have another session or so (maybe even the "in
a bath with a snorkel" variety!).

PAST LIFE THERAPY: BACK INTO THE MISTS OF TIME

If you think rebirthing sounds weird, try to get your head around
past life therapy. It demands you ask those weird, unnerving
questions like "Have we lived before?" Have we walked, talked,
loved and lost in other times, in other places, in other bodies?
Reincarnation is a beguiling philosophy, and it is small wonder
that, from ancient times right up to the present day, people have
been fascinated with the perennial question: is this lifetime all
we are allotted or do we continue, time and time again?

Until the last few years, past life regression remained little more
than a parlor game, with ancient personae simply being "re-

vealed" to the querent: now, however, it has transformed into therapy, with its advocates claiming they can cure anything from migraines to severe psychological trauma.

The sea-change came about as hypnotherapists found that, under trance, their clients would sometimes shift far farther back than expected. Back through childhood, back into the womb, and then, unexpectedly, back farther still—into other lifetimes. Some dismissed the phenomenon as over-fertile imagination; others began to pursue these other "lives" to see whether they might have any therapeutic use.

"You can regress a person right back to childhood and they will still resist treatment," says Denise Linn, who is an expert in the field (quite aside from her other work). "But, if you take them back to a *past* life, you often see that the same pattern exists in the past. It can become so strongly embedded in the psyche that it will be manifested physically in the present life."

Dr. Roger Woolger, a Jungian psychotherapist and another acknowledged expert in the field firmly believes that our emotional problems, psychological hang-ups and even our physical weaknesses and recurrent illnesses have their roots in our past lives. If you are asthmatic in this life, he suggests, you could have died struggling for breath; if you have psychosexual problems, there might be memories of abuse or rape in your psyche; and if you permanently have problems shifting weight, your subconscious might simply be remembering lifetimes when food was short and starvation a real possibility. The theory ignores factors such as genetic weakness, parental conditioning or environmental effects and puts all our problems down to one factor alone: the past.

Frankly I found the whole concept far-fetched. But, like most people, I possessed a niggling curiosity behind the solid skepticism. Could I, under trance, access former lifetimes; would I suddenly find a reason for my fascination with medieval architecture or my love of the Greek islands? I went along to one of Denise Linn's weekend workshops to find out.

Lying on the floor, wrapped in a blanket, I listened to Denise's voice instructing us to close our eyes and regulate our breathing. Using standard techniques for inducing deep relaxation and a light hypnotic state (in which you remain quite aware and conscious) she made us systematically relax each part of our bodies and then visualize ourselves in a beautiful, safe, place. "Imagine a door in front of you," she said. "As the door opens you will walk into a 'time tunnel' full of mist." I imagined the tunnel and walked through the mist until Denise's voice instructed me to stop. "Look down at your feet as the mist clears and tell me what you see," she said. To my eternal surprise, I "saw" in my imagination a pair of short, stumpy, very hairy and very dirty feet. The experience was strange, to say the least. I was fully aware of my surroundings; I could hear noises in the hall in which I was lying and the distant sound of traffic outside. It was as if I were in the middle of a very vivid daydream. Images just seemed to pop into my head. Sometimes they seemed so realistic I could almost *feel* the clothes I was wearing or the cold wind blowing. Following Denise's instructions I looked at my clothing and at the place in which I was standing. My mind's eye came up with harsh cloth rags and a muddy track with deep furrows. It appeared I was a peasant in medieval England; it was winter and I was very cold and very miserable.

Denise then suggested I find out more about my life, asking me to imagine my home and family (I was a man, married with a horde of children). It was not a cheerful experience; most of my life was spent trying to keep warm and endeavoring to find enough food for the family to survive. When I finally "experienced" my death (from a fever) it felt like an enormous relief.

But was this a true past life I was imagining and could my medieval hunger really be the underlying reason for my lifelong battle with my weight or was it simply my subconscious enjoying a free romp?

Throughout the weekend I experienced other "lives" (as an ancient Greek athlete, seventeenth-century herbalist, Victorian housewife). It was great fun and I would gladly go through the experience again but, to be quite honest, I still retained my doubts. I envisaged nothing that I could not have read about or seen in films or documentaries and there were no great revelations or feelings of *déjà vu*. And, sad to say, re-experiencing life as a starving peasant did not alter my relationship with food one iota.

But, say the therapists, whether you experience true past lives or whether it is simply your imagination is unimportant and does not affect any therapeutic outcome. Neil French of the International Association of Hypno-Analysts says that although his organization looks for answers to problems in *this* life, they have investigated the past life phenomenon in some depth. "Under hypnosis our patients go back to earlier experiences, childhood and traumatic moments," he explains. "And frequently people *appear* to go back to past lives as well. But we don't leave it there, we go back further to find out where they might have obtained the information. And, in every case, the patient him or herself has realized that it was not a true life experience."

However, despite the evidence against past lives, he does not dismiss their use as a therapeutic tool. "You can utilize the phenomenon," he says. "A patient of mine under hypnosis saw a sword being thrust into his entrails. He relived it horrifically and was very upset by it but it did have a therapeutic effect. Perhaps it works symbolically. Say someone was claustrophobic and they 'went back' to being locked up alive in a catacomb. Well, if they really believe that, then their claustrophobia would probably vanish, even if it were not a real past life experience."

John Butler, of the British Society of Hypnotherapists, is equally skeptical but even more cautious. "It's a very contentious area," he comments. "The problem is that there are no controls and pretty well anyone can set up as a therapist: in this field there are certainly a fair number of cowboys." He is also concerned that delving into past lives might cause more problems than it solves. "Aren't there enough problems in *this* life to deal with?" he points out. "I worry that by sifting through, say twenty lives, you might just complicate the situation. Also there's a danger that you might start living in the past, dwelling on a former personality which is perhaps more interesting than your present persona." While he does not dismiss reincarnation out of hand, he advises extreme caution before taking the plunge.

Real or not, there's no denying the vicarious pleasure of "discovering" your possible past selves. At the least it can be great fun, and many people swear it has offered startling insights into their present problems. Take it with a hefty pinch of salt, don't expect miracles and, if you have serious problems, look for your answers in this life, not the last.

February

The year starts to turn in February. Outside it may still be cold and damp, dreary and dark, but there are signs that life will begin again. The first flowers, crocuses, snowdrops, aconites are stoically pushing up through the hard earth. Brave buds are forming on the trees. Tractors buzz around the fields spreading muck and ploughing the earth in dark deep furrows. In the Native American system the Renewal Time gives way to the Cleansing Time—the world is being purified, perfected before the cycle of life starts all over again. February starts with the great Celtic festival of Imbolc or Candlemas. It falls on February 2 and the world actually derives from "sheep's milk," because in the olden days the first lambs were not born until after the festival.

Imbolc: Celebration of Hope and Trust

Although we do not commonly celebrate it nowadays Imbolc is a lovely festival and one worthy of resurrection. In the pagan calendar it is very important, as pagan priestess Shan explains.

"It is the festival of hope, of trust, of dreaming of better times to come. Everything around us is black and cold but under the earth the new seeds are stirring." She celebrates the festival by lighting lots of little candles or tiny nightlights to symbolize the "tiny hopes and dreams that keep us going when life is hard." Children are given tiny gifts which I think is a lovely idea. Children love festivals and for young minds which only have the memory of a few years it often seems like a very long time from Christmas to Easter. Little Imbolc gifts can bridge the gap. Adults, says Shan, should allow themselves some serious pampering around this time. "Have a massage, a sauna, a new hairstyle or a manicure," she suggests. I'd certainly agree with that. I'm a bit lax when it comes to beautifying but, come February, I suddenly get the overwhelming urge for a facial (preferably something involving delicious aromatherapy and a neck massage) or a decadent pedicure (so what that no one will see your toes under all those woolly socks—it just *feels* so good).

But above all else, Imbolc is a festival of trust. Life may have seemed dead and ended to our ancestors, but they held onto their faith that the sun would return and the fields return to abundance. While we do not have those immediate pressing worries, we still need trust in our lives. Imbolc is about keeping faith—in ourselves, in those we love and in the world to provide what we need. Shan also suggests that Imbolc is a good time to indulge in dreams. "Even if you have been hurt or let down, the one thing no one can take away from you are your dreams," she says. "When the outer part of your life seems difficult or is not helping you, go to the inner part of life. Renew yourself with dreaming. By dreaming you will begin to bring the outer world back to you."

I think those are very wise words. At this time of year it can be tough to go out there and fight the world, to take life head-on. Sometimes we need to hide away a little, to retreat and nourish our inner world. Which is why this time of year can be the perfect time to get away, to escape. It's a good time to have a holiday in the sun. But, equally, it can be a wonderful time simply to take time out, to stop the world and retreat.

Retreating: A Holiday for Your Soul

Sometimes all you want is just to run away and hide; to find a secret spot in which to curl up and escape from the sheer madness of everyday life. It's more than just needing a rest: it's nearer a sense that your whole being needs recharging, that your very soul is desperate for a break. When that feeling erupts, most of us imagine we need a holiday but maybe what we are really crying out for is a retreat.

Retreats were an accepted part of life in the past: you simply took yourself off to a monastery or convent and spent time in contemplation and prayer, often fasting and keeping silent throughout your vigil. It was a time spent with God and your soul, a true religious experience.

Perhaps surprisingly, there are still simple religious retreats to be found all over the country but, in the Nineties, retreating has expanded way beyond the convents and monasteries and is fast becoming a boom industry. Roman Catholic or Tibetan Buddhist, Zen Christian or pure agnostic, there is a retreat tailored for every belief system and plenty that don't even expect faith of any kind. You can retreat in the time-honored tradition of solitude and silence or join with like-minded people on activity retreats, learning yoga or meditation, practicing healing, or even swimming with the dolphins. There are as many different retreats as there are days in the year, but the aim is always the same: to take a step outside your ordinary life, to put the world on pause for a while.

As Stafford Whiteaker, author of *The Good Retreat Guide,* explains, "A retreat is an inward exploration that lets your feelings open out, and gives you access to both the light and dark corners of your deepest feelings and relationships. It is simply the deliberate attempt to step outside ordinary life and relationships and take time to reflect, rest and be still. It is a concentrated time in which to experience yourself and your relationships to others and, if you are fortunate, to feel a sense of the eternal."

I experienced my first retreat at a time of huge stress. After the stresses and strains of moving house, of coordinating builders and coping with the shock of a fire, I felt in dire need of some spiritual solace. But would I find "the eternal" via meditation in

Devon or worship with the brothers in Inverness? The choices were myriad, but after days of deliberation I found myself en route to Gaunts House in the rolling Dorsetshire countryside. Gaunts hosts a vast variety of courses (all of which are retreats in their own right), but I chose to visit at a quieter time. Gaunts House appealed because it is totally nondenominational. Whatever your belief, or even if you think you have no belief, you are equally welcome. It was established about six years ago with the aim of finding "right ways for living now and in the future," and its regular community of around twenty people try to live in harmony with themselves, one another and the wider congregation of the planet.

As I was welcomed to the beautiful old mansion, my spirits began to lift. A board in the hall detailed the day's activities. If I wanted to join the community in early-morning meditation or for daily discussions I was very welcome. Equally, if I simply wanted to lose myself in the 2,000 odd acres of estate that was just fine.

I stretched back on my bed, shut my eyes and breathed a deep sigh of relief. All around me was peace and quiet: no ringing phones, no crashing builders. There was nothing to do for a few days but relax.

A lake beckoned beyond the trees and I set out to explore. Within minutes I found myself deep in the heart of a magic wooded wonderland, a carpet of bluebells stretching as far as the eye could see (this wasn't in February, I hasten to add). Quite overcome, I sat down on a tree stump and just drank it in. All around me were the busy sounds of the wood: birds twittering, leaves rustling, the faint trickle of water. I watched a squirrel rushing about its business and studied the perfect newness of a freshly emerged ivy leaf. Time truly seemed to stand still.

Over the next few days I sank deeper into the quiet life. Sometimes I simply wandered over the fields, watching the hares leap and the pheasants stroll leisurely past. One morning I sat under a tree and read a book; one afternoon I curled up in front of a blazing fire and dozed for a couple of hours. If I wanted to be totally alone, I could simply head for the open countryside or climb the tower stairs to the peaceful shrine room. If I felt like company, there was always someone working in the ground-floor kitchens or offices who would willingly share a cup of tea or a chat. I was taken totally at face value: no one asked me what I did for a living; no one questioned me about my life.

On one of my walks I stumbled across the walled garden. Three people were working steadily, in a quiet and calm race against the spring. Within minutes I found myself on my knees with a trowel, planting out cabbages and broccoli. It was hard work but utterly engrossing. We worked mostly in companionable silence, like monks in their kitchen garden. The air was fresh and sweet, the earth rich and deep and all around the birds sang for joy. My fellow gardeners told me that some people choose to spend their whole retreat up to their arms in compost and I can quite understand why.

Meals are communal but informal affairs—vegetarian and tasty—but equally you can wander into the kitchens and fix yourself tea and toast at any time of day or night. And there is usually something going on in the evening if you fancy a break from all that introspection. One night I found myself stretching and relaxing in a gentle yoga class which ended up with us all munching crumpets and drinking tea until almost midnight; on another I discovered the delights of circle dancing, swirling round the room in a traditional jig one minute and then switching to slow hypnotic dances which were almost moving meditations. I realized then that these evening activities weren't, in fact, "breaks" from the retreat routine but instead a very fundamental part of the process.

By the end of my short stay I felt as if I had been at Gaunts for months. The serenity of the place and the warmth of its inhabitants touched a deep chord in my inner being. I found myself re-evaluating my life and almost laughing at what I saw. The sheer size of Gaunts and the enormity of the task facing its overstretched gardeners put my household moans and worries firmly into perspective. And the quiet philosophy of so many of Gaunts' inhabitants soothed my soul. They see no difference between the physical, the mental and the spiritual: God is in everything and by changing ourselves, they believe, we can take that first step toward changing the world. It's a philosophy that gives a sense of peace but also a profound sense of responsibility—our very personal thoughts and actions can affect the larger whole. I left Gaunts a different person.

Since then I have "run away from the world" on several occasions. I couldn't recommend it highly enough. It reaches deeper than a holiday. On holiday there are expectations of what you should do, what you should see, where you should eat, how brilliant a suntan you should take back, how many postcards you should write, how much you're enjoying yourself. On retreat there are no strictures, no rules and no feelings of "I should . . ." You give yourself permission simply to be, to think (or not to think), to watch the world going by. Such periods of tranquility can often help you make decisions, put things in perspective and even gain an insight into what you really want from life. Do try it.

Find Happiness

Retreating from the world may not solve all your problems, and it may give you even more choices and decisions to make. It might not even make you happy. But then what is true happiness? Ask anyone if they are happy, *really* happy and few would say an emphatic yes. Most of us are just content or getting by or coping OK. And we have this weird habit (particularly in Britain) of not liking to say that we're doing great. It's as if extreme politeness doesn't allow us to parade our joyfulness. But equally, most of us are still pursuing happiness as if it were some mythical unicorn.

Hopefully, having carried out some of the suggestions in this book you will have a better idea of what it would take to make you happy in life. You might even feel that things are, indeed, getting better. With any luck your health and fitness will be improved, your emotions will have become more peaceable, and you will have gained a better idea of what you want from life and work. Before we finish, let me suggest just one final thought: you may already be much happier than you think you are.

After all, what is it that stands between us and happiness? Surely only our expectations and the demands of the modern world. We are living in a world which is speeding up by the second, in which we are taught to always want more, want better, want best. We have become achievement junkies, obsessed with keeping up, with doing better, with improving ourselves and our lot.

There is only one true way to stop all the speed and chatter and that is to stop projecting all our hopes into the future, to stop dwelling on the past and to learn how to live right here and now, in the moment. This is nothing new—every meditator knows the rule. But we need to take this sense of the moment out of the half-hour meditation slot and plug it into our everyday lives. It's a case of taking delight in the little wonders of life— all those "tiny things" that symbolize Imbolc. The miraculous curve of a rainbow, the wonder and delight of stretching your body and feeling your muscles almost sing; of staring deep into the eyes of someone you love and thinking how special they are, rather than criticizing some small defect. It's like going back to childhood when the world was full of wonder and everything seemed new and fresh. We need to take on board that if we always want more, there will never be an end in sight.

Television presenter Angus Deayton summed it up pretty well in a television documentary he presented some time back called *In Pursuit of Happiness*. He suggested that people imagine they would be happy if they had a swimming pool. However, he pointed out, once they have the swimming pool, they want a bigger pool. Then, he laughed, they would want a sea. Then an ocean. Then a larger ocean. In other words, once you get on that treadmill, you will never stop; you will always set yourself up for disappointment because there is always something better, someone richer, more beautiful, more successful.

And yet we refuse to see it: we have all become experts at postponing happiness. We can't catch the wonder of the moment because we're never focusing on the present. When I first thought about this I surreptitiously glanced at the sixteen-page tome of "Things to Do" stabbed onto my noticeboard and felt a bit squirmy. I've got a great job, a wonderful house, good health, a super husband, but am I satisfied? Am I hell. I'll be happy when I get the house fixed . . . life would be brilliant if I could lose that extra stone . . . if only I had a new car, a few days without a deadline, a holiday booked in Bali, the prospect of a trolley-dash round Armani. Like the majority of the Western world, I'm projecting happiness off into the future. And yet happiness is not a miraculous God-given state of being; it is simply a series of great moments. Tack enough together and you have a free-fall run of happiness. And the good news is that anyone can choose to have them. It's all down to how you look at life.

Fiona Arrigo agrees. As a psychotherapist she spent years watching people hunt desperately for happiness in a hectic world. Then she ran Stop the World, a center in Somerset, where she gently persuaded people to stop panicking and start living. Then she realized that she was falling into the same snare herself and so packed it all in to focus on her needs. Last time I spoke to her she was living the good life in Ireland with her family, working with people on a one-to-one basis, pampering them and helping them decide what they really need in life. By the time this book is published, doubtless she will be doing something else. Hopefully it will be another version of Stop the World which was a totally wonderful package. Learning how to have real moments of joy was all part of the treatment.

"We are so caught up in looking to the future that we have lost the gift of magic," says Fiona. She says the first thing we need to do in pursuit of true joy is to work out if we are avoiding it and, if so, why? Unfortunately, most of us seem to be looking at life with long-vision glasses. We are often so fixated on our long-term goals and ambitions that we ignore the potential happy moments under our own noses.

ARE YOU AVOIDING HAPPINESS?

Answer the following questions, honestly:

• Do you constantly have to be doing something? Are you a workaholic who claims you can never find the chance to take time off? Do you get nervous when you're doing nothing? When you go on holiday, do you have to be doing things, seeing sights, visiting shops, trying every new sport? When you're "relaxing" at home, do you tend to have the TV or radio on all the time? Do you do several things at once?
• Do you rely on "habits" to get you by? Are you addicted to smoking, drinking, eating, tranquilizers? People who are hungry for more lasting joy often use addictions to get a temporary hit of happiness.

• Are you cynical, pessimistic, or sarcastic? This is a classic cover-up for pain, hiding a deep disappointment in people and in life itself. Are you judgmental? It's impossible to feel happiness with people if you are constantly judging and disconnecting from them.

• Do you live your life through others? Do you make your partner, your children, your friends, the center of your life rather than your own self?

If you answered yes to any of these questions, the odds are that you are not giving yourself the chance for happiness in your life

But why would anyone in their right mind turn down a dose of joy? Easy. Firstly, we are afraid of real happiness because these stabs of sheer happiness can be very confrontational. When you stop doing too much and take time to have a real sense of joy, you will undoubtedly come face to face with emotions, revelations or realities of which you simply weren't aware.

The second reason for avoiding happiness is that we are often scared of intimacy. It's not a case of sharing deep, dark secrets but about making meaningful connections with people, even with complete strangers. Try to communicate with the people you meet, however fleetingly. Aim to get past everyday banalities and become "intimate," and who knows what might happen. At the very least, you will have passed a few moments being pleasant rather than paranoid and that, in itself, has to be worth the effort.

HOW TO CATCH HAPPINESS: A FEW POINTERS

1. Take time to be by yourself and work out what you really want from life. Ask yourself some simple home truths.

   • Am I happy? What would make me happy?
   • What do I need to do in my life to be free?
   • What parts of myself, both in the past and the present, have I hidden from others for fear they would disapprove of me? What parts do I bury even from myself?
   • What are *my* values and beliefs? If I lived them 100 per-

cent, how would that look in my life? How would the people close to me react?

- Am I living where and how I want to live or where and how someone else wants me to live? What would I have to change to have my lifestyle congruous with my desires?

2. Concentrate on your feelings, says Fiona. "You have to go through a very honest self-evaluation of what makes you feel good in the world—from what hours you keep, to what food you eat to what music you like."

Don't live your life by rules and regulations, she continues. "What was good for you last week or last year may not be good for you now. You need to have the courage to live for you, to be true to your self, not to your boss, not to your lover, not to your image. But, above all, be gentle with yourself. This is a very deep process and shouldn't be seen as yet another task to get through."

3. Fiona suggests active forms of meditation to get into real moments. "Just breathing consciously, following your breath in and out, brings you right into the present," she says. Whatever you are doing, whether it is writing a report or lazing in the garden, making love or cooking a curry, concentrate on what you are actually doing. Say to yourself, "*Right now* I am lying underneath the trees . . . *right now* I am listening to the birds . . . *right now* I am breathing deeply . . . *right now* I am stretching." Take deep relaxing breaths between each "right now." Keep going for about five minutes for best benefits and practice this at least once a day. Always end with the phrase "Right now, I am right here, right now."

4. Keep a journal or diary—not of events but of your feelings, your observations, any moments of sheer joy, however fleeting. You don't have to write every day but make sure you are honest and record your thoughts without censorship.

FINDING HAPPINESS AT WORK

You don't need to resign from your job in order to find happiness. However, you might need to change your attitude. The key to finding happiness at work is in your attitude to what you do. If you constantly put down your work, think it's not important or not good enough, then you will always hate what you do. And yet there is normally *something* valid or valuable about what you do. I've done some pretty boring or unglamorous jobs in my time. I've served up food in a hospital canteen; mucked out kennels and mixed tripe at a boarding kennels; served in a department store and even sat filing each and every day. I looked for things I liked about my job or worked out ways to do the job even better or more efficiently. It became a kind of game.

As an example, a friend and I once had jobs selling tickets for shows at Earls Court. It was pretty mindless, and most of our fellow ticket vendors had faces like hatchets. We, however, set ourselves a challenge to see how fast we could clear the queues and how many punters we could get to smile at us. The job became hilarious as we tried to outdo each other in the niceness stakes; the hours raced by and our co-workers were stunned at how many people we had served and how many had complimented us on our friendly service.

Arrigo agrees. "Whatever you are doing, whether it is mopping a floor, working in a bank or running ICI, throw yourself into what you are doing at that moment. If you're always thinking, 'I should get a promotion; I should be a therapist; I should marry a millionaire; you will always postpone happiness. Be aware, accept life and flow with it." That's not to say you should be content with your lot and never aim higher: simply that life and work will be much happier if you concentrate on getting the most out of what you're doing rather than permanently bemoaning your fate.

FINDING HAPPINESS IN LOVE

Whatever happened to the equation love equals happiness? Divorce rates have never been higher and newspapers run stories about couples who are still in love after fifty years as if they were talking about aliens landing in London. The wonder of first love and the thrill of the chase gives way to boredom, familiarity and, sadly, often a fair dose of contempt.

But there is nothing to say that you have to follow the pattern. A relationship is a dynamic, always changing, partnership. You have the ability to turn it into whatever you so desire. Not by changing your partner but by making a little effort with a little imagination. Above all, start communicating—seriously.

Instead of slumping in front of the television with tray of food, set the table and talk. Have cozy evenings with quiet music, candles and a fire. Wrap up warm and go for walks together. Give each other little surprise presents. They don't have to be elaborate or expensive, just thoughtful. Perhaps a book or tape he or she has wanted, a favorite food, or some nice bath goodies. Or choose a bouquet of unusual flowers (a tiny posy of violets, a bunch of sweet-scented bluebells, an armful of bendy twigs and catkins).

Fiona Arrigo thinks these are sweet ideas but feels the whole issue of happiness in relationships revolves around daily commitment. Above all, she warns that we are always trying to change our partners. Once again we're off in Neverland, imagining our partner will one day transform from Mr. Average into a suave superhero who is lean, tough, caring, and sharing all at the same time. "You have to get back into the moment," says Arrigo. "Choose to be where you are every minute, accept that and give your whole being to the person and the moment." In other words, look for the good bits rather than pouncing in on the bad.

FINDING HAPPINESS FOR YOURSELF

Our modern society is so geared to speed and efficiency that we rarely think about taking time for ourselves. And women, in particular, are adept at throwing away happiness. We are too self-sacrificing, too desperate to try to do it all and to do it all perfectly that we never give ourselves time and peace away from the hurly burly. Try to make time for yourself—a few hours or even minutes every day just for you, enjoyed in perfect peace and quiet. Use this little space to do what you want to do, not what anyone else wants you to do or what you feel you *ought* to be doing.

Fiona Arrigo persuades people to start to pamper themselves. "Take a long luxurious bath; go for a gentle walk; curl up with a book; sleep; do nothing," she advises. "People always say there isn't time to have a massage or sit and talk, but we can create the time because we are in charge of ourselves."

Happiness is basically a choice. Look at the world with jaundiced, jaded, cynical eyes and it will irritate the hell out of you. You will always be yearning for a future life of impossible perfection. However, try shifting your perspective and see the beauty in small things, the joy in other people and the world will suddenly seem a brighter place. Who knows, you might even find you're happier than you think.

Endings—and Beginnings

How you view a year can depend on many things. If things are going wrong it can seem to last forever; if things are going well, it can race past like a greyhound. You often hear people say how much they hate January, or how they wish it could be summer all the time, or how they can't wait until Christmas. But by working with the different seasons and energies of the year we can learn to take each season, each month as it comes, appreciating its individuality, adapting ourselves to its rhythms—going with it rather than fighting against it.

I hope you have enjoyed this book and that it might have helped in some small way. I also hope that it will continue to be useful to you in the years that come.

Review the Year

Now the tasks and tests are over, at least for now. But, before we close I'd like you to take another look at the questionnaire with which we began this journey. Don't look at your original answers, in fact don't even think back to when you first looked at these questions. For that reason I've set them out again here. Take the time, once again, to go through and write down your thoughts and feelings. Don't censor what you're writing and don't refer back. Just put down what you would answer now if you were coming on these questions for the first time.

YOUR HEALTH

1. Are you happy with your health? Do you consider yourself a healthy person?
2. Do you like your body? What do you like about it? If not, why not? Do you feel comfortable with your body? If not, what parts feel uncomfortable?
3. Are you happy with your weight? If not, why not? What would your ideal weight be?
4. Do you consider yourself to be fit? How fit are you really? Would you like to be fitter?
5. Do you incorporate regular exercise in your life? How much and how often?
6. Is your body flexible? Can you easily bend and stretch or do you have aches and pains?
7. Do you have good posture? Does your body feel comfortable and easy at all times?
8. Do you suffer from stress and tension in your body? Do you find you hold tension in your shoulders, neck muscles or jaw? Or do you suffer from nervous tension in your stomach? Do you get headaches or migraine when you are tense? What are the physical symptoms of stress you suffer?
9. How do you sleep? Do you suffer from insomnia or interrupted sleep? And what are your dreams like? Any recurring? Nightmares? No dreams at all?
10. Think about your diet. What kind of food do you eat? How much of it? Be honest. Write down a typical day's food. Do you eat much chocolate, sweets or cakes? Do you often or occasionally eat convenience food, prepackaged food, junk food or takeaways?
11. What do you drink? How much tea, coffee and fizzy soft drinks do you consume? How much alcohol?

12. Have you had any accidents? Do you suffer pain or discomfort as a result?

13. Do you smoke? How much? Do you take any recreational drugs?

14. Do you live in a very polluted area? Do you spend much time traveling on roads? How is your breathing?

15. Are you on any medication? How much and what for? Do you understand your drugs: what they are for; how they work; any side effects?

16. Do you feel happy with your GP? Can you talk to him/her about your problems? Or do you feel dissatisfied with your health care?

17. Do you feel in control of your body and your health?

18. How are your senses? Do you have clear eyesight or do you need glasses/contact lenses? How is your hearing? Your sense of taste? Your sense of smell? Do you ever think about how you feel or touch things? Would you say your senses are acute or dull?

19. Do you worry about your health? Are you scared of becoming ill or of being out of control of your body?

20. List the five things you would like to change about your health.

YOUR PSYCHE: EMOTIONS AND FEELINGS

1. Do you consider yourself a happy person? Or are you more generally unhappy? What is it that makes you feel discontent with your life?

2. Are you fearful? What frightens you?

3. Do you express your feelings? Can you freely express grief, sadness, anger, frustration, love, gratitude, joy, etc. Are there any emotions you cannot express?

4. Did you have a happy childhood? Were you loved? Did the members of your family get on with each other?

5. How did you cope with adolescence? What were your feelings around puberty?

6. Have there been any major traumas in your life? Any death, divorce, abuse?

7. Are you on good terms with your family—both immediate and extended?

8. Do you have a good relationship with your partner? Is it a partnership of equals or do you feel discontented with it? If you don't have a partner does that cause you unhappiness?
9. Do you ever suffer from depression? When? Any triggers?
10. Do you have solid friends you can talk to and confide in?
11. Do you ever do things just for the hell of it? Do you take time off to play?
12. Do you have hobbies or interests outside work you really enjoy?
13. If you spend time on your own how do you feel? Do you enjoy it or do you feel slightly uncomfortable or downright unhappy?
14. Do you ever feel trapped by your life?
15. Have you got good self-esteem? Do you believe you are a worthwhile, interesting, valuable person? Or do you feel that you don't really matter that much; that other people are far more exciting and interesting than you are?
16. Can you be assertive if you need to be? Can you stand up for your rights, or do you let people walk all over you?
17. Do you have a good sex life? Are you happy with your sexuality? Is there anything you would like to change?
18. Do you feel in control of your life?
19. Are you scared of your emotions?
20. List five things you would like to change in your emotional life.

YOUR LIFE PATH

1. Do you feel as if you are in the right niche? Are you happy with your career or your life path?
2. Do you feel fulfilled?
3. Is there something you have always yearned to do with your life?
4. Do you have enough money or is money a constant worry?
5. Do you feel secure?
6. Do you wake up in the morning and feel raring to go, as if each day is a new challenge, or do you wish the world would go away?
7. Do you feel creative in your life? Whether it's in your work,

your family and home, artistic pursuits or new ideas and challenges?

8. Can you adapt well to change or does it frighten you?
9. If you could do anything in life what would it be?
10. Do you feel that your outward persona matches your inner self?
11. Do you feel respected in your life work?
12. Do you have good relationships with your fellow workers? Do you get on well with your boss, your colleagues, your employees?
13. Is your work a joy or a battleground?
14. Do you work with people who support one another, or do you work in an environment which thrives on "creative conflict," pitting people against each other? Do you enjoy your work environment?
15. Are you ever bored with your work?
16. Are you doing the best you can, or are you underused and understretched?
17. Does your work environment harm your health in any way?
18. Do you switch off when you leave work or do you never have a break? Do you take work home with you and work at weekends? How do your family and friends see your work? Does your work compromise your relationships? Are you a workaholic?
19. Does your work give you stress? How do you deal with it?
20. If you could change your work in any way, how would you do it? What career did you want as a child? What is your ideal career? Do you want to work at all?

YOUR SOUL

1. How do you feel at the idea of spirit or soul? Is it an alien concept; something rather embarrassing; something frightening or is it something you feel quite comfortable with?
2. Do you express your spirituality? Do you have any kind of religion, whether organized or not?
3. Do you fear the unknown?
4. Are you scared of eternity, of death?

5. Do you believe in luck, chance, random events?
6. Do you ever have the feeling that your life is being overseen in any way?
7. Do you blame the misfortunes of life on something beyond your control—on karma, God, fate, past life?
8. Do you give yourself time to dream, to think, to muse?
9. Do you meditate or practice any form of visualization or relaxation techniques?
10. Do you feel as if your life has purpose?
11. Does life fill you with a sense of complete joy sometimes?
12. Do you have time to be on your own?
13. Do you ever escape into nature—whether the local park or countryside? Where do you feel happiest: by the sea, in the mountains, in a forest? Or do you feel happier in the city, surrounded by people, or in a quiet cozy room?
14. Do you feel safe?
15. Do you live in the now or are you living in the past or projecting into the future?
16. Do you ever stop and just do nothing?
17. Do you feel as if life is just one long trial and that there is nothing you can do to change it?
18. Do you take enough holidays and days off?
19. Do you believe that you deserve good health, great relationships and a wonderful life?
20. If you could do something just for you, what would it be?

Once you've finished, think about how you've changed in the last year. What has happened to you? Good things? Bad things? Has it been a good year or not so good? Then look back at your original answers and see how you've fared.

It can be quite surprising to discover what you wrote a whole year ago. We often have a tendency to forget the bad things. People who have tried this often find that they have, in fact, made quite wonderful progress. It might not be anything huge or apparently life-changing, but you might find that you are more flexible than you were at the beginning, that you have a little more courage, or a slightly more optimistic view on life.

Give yourself a metaphorical pat on the back for having done something positive with this year. I firmly believe that we are not generous enough when it comes to praising ourselves. If you have done well, feel good about it. If it has been a bad year, then look over it carefully and be honest. Was it *all* bad? Were there any good things about it?

I looked back at one year and all I saw was a series of deaths in the family, ghastly things going wrong with the house, lots of illness and arguments. When I scanned right through the year, I realized I had forgotten about the fact that I had also got married, had been given a wonderful puppy, had had lots of lovely weekends with good friends and had enjoyed a great holiday. And those were just the big events. It's easy to focus on the bad and forget the good. But equally, take a look at the bad things in life and work through those too. Make sure you are not repressing any grief or anguish from unpleasant or sad past situations. If so, seek some help.

I hope that I have given you some guidelines and useful suggestions for living in greater harmony with yourself and with the natural year. It's an ongoing quest so do keep up with it. Shift your diet with the seasons, keep exercising and keep in touch with your inner self and you shouldn't go far wrong. By now you should be far more in touch with all aspects of your self, even with the seasonal shifts of the year. You should intuitively find yourself knowing what to do when. Trust your feelings. Remember we are all natural beings—just as natural as the trees, the fields and the sky.

I wish you good health, true moments of happiness and a deep sense of abiding peace.

Further Information

Introduction to the Natural Year

Traditional Chinese Medicine (TCM)
* Traditional Chinese Medicine/Acupuncture: American Association of Oriental Medicine, 433 Front Street, Catasauqua, PA 18032; tel: (610) 266-1433

Ayurveda
* Ayurvedic Institute, 11311 Menaud NE, Suite A, Albuquerque, NM 87112; tel: (505) 291-9698

Naturopathy/Nutritional Therapy
* American Association of Naturopathic Physicians, 601 Valley Street #105, Seattle, WA 98105; tel: (206) 298-0126 and referrals— (206) 298-0125.
* American Naturopathic Medical Association, PO Box 96273, Las Vegas, NV 89193; tel: (702) 897-7053
* Bastyr University of Natural Health Sciences, 14500 Juanita Drive NE, Bothell, WA 98011; tel: (425) 823-1300
* National Institute of Nutritional Education, 1010 S. Joliet Street 107, Aurora, CO 80012; tel: (303) 340-2054

Spring

Exercise
Chi Kung

*   The International Chi Kung/Qi Gong Directory, 2730 29th St., Boulder CO 80301; tel: (303) 422-3131 or contact James MacRitchie, founding president of the group, PO Box 19708, Boulder, CO 80308

Yoga

*   International Association of Yoga Therapists, 20 Sunnyside Avenue, Suite A243, Mill Valley, CA 94941; tel: (415) 332-2478 or (800) 858-9462
*   Integral Yoga Teachers' Association, Route 1 Box 1720, Buckingham VA 23921; www.moonstar.com/~yoga. Also try www.yogacite.com and www.yogajournal.com as good sources of information about teachers.

Tai Chi
Look in your local health center or sports center for local classes. Or contact:
*   Alexander Krych, c/o Belvidere Post Office, Belvidere, NJ 07823-2018; tel: (908) 475-1619; 74640.2154@compuserve.com

Psychocalisthenics
Psychocalisthenics is an amazing system which exercises every muscle in the body in about ten minutes.
Arica Institute, Inc., 145 Palisade Street, Suite 401, Dobbs Ferry, NY 10522; tel: (914) 674-4091.

Space Clearing
Karen Kingston Promotions, Inner Space, 1623 Stanford Street, Santa Monica, CA 90404; tel: (310) 264-1843

Aromatherapy
*   American Aromatherapy Association, PO Box 3609, Culver City, CA 90231
*   Aromatherapy Institute of Research, PO Box 2354, Fair Oaks, CA 95628; tel: (916) 965-7546

Bodywork

- American Massage Therapy Association, 820 Davis Street, Suite 100, Evanston, IL 60201-4444; tel: (847) 864-0123
- Associated Bodywork and Massage Professionals, 28677 Buffalo Park Road, Evergreen, CO 80439-7347; tel: (303) 674-8478
- The Feldenkrais Guild, PO Box 489, Albany OR 97321; tel: (541) 926-0981
- Reiki Alliance, PO Box 41, Cataldo, ID 83810; tel: (208) 682-3535
- Trager Institute, 21 Locust Avenue, Mill Valley, CA 94941; tel: (415) 388-2688

Herbalism

- American Herbalists Guild, PO Box 1683, Sequel, CA 95973; tel: (408) 484-2441
- American Botanical Council, PO Box 201660, Austin, TX 78720; tel: (512) 331-8868

Dance
Biodanza

Denise Melo, 1104 Willingham Way, Moore, OK 73160; tel: (405) 794-0500

Summer

Counseling

- American Counseling Association, 5999 Stevenson Avenue, Alexandria, VA 22304; tel: (703) 823-9800

Bodywork for Emotions

Although the prime aim of osteopathy and chiropractic is to heal the body, some people do find that emotions are released through these healing practices. Anyhow, these are useful numbers to have:

Chiropractic

- American Chiropractic Association, 1701 Clarendon Boulevard, Arlington, VA 22209; tel: (703) 276-8800

• World Chiropractic Alliance, 2950 North Dobson Street, Suite One, Chandler, AZ 85224-1802; tel: (800) 347-1011

Osteopathy
• American Osteopathic Association, 142 East Ohio Street, Chicago, IL 60611; tel: (312) 280-5800
• American Academy of Osteopathy, 3500 DePauw Boulevard, Suite 1080, Indianapolis, IA 46268-139; tel (317) 879-1881

Rolfing
The Rolf Institute, 205 Canyon Boulevard, Boulder, CO 80302-4920; tel: (303) 449-5903

Hellerwork
Hellerwork International, 406 Berry Street, Mount Shasta, CA 96067; tel: (530) 926-2500

Zero Balancing
The Zero Balancing Association, Box 1727, Capitola, CA 95010; tel: (408) 476-0665

SHEN Therapy
International SHEN Therapy Association, 3213 W Wheeler, Suite 202, Seattle, WA 98199; tel: (206) 298-9468

Sound Therapy
Sound Healers Association, PO Box 2240, Boulder, Co 80306; tel: (303) 443-8181

Biodynamic Therapy
Association for Humanistic Psychology, 45 Franklin Street, Suite 315, San Francisco, CA 94102; tel: (415) 864-8850

Watsu
Worldwide Aquatic Bodywork Association (WABA), PO Box 889, Middletown, CA 95461; tel: (707) 987-3801

Autumn/Fall

Feng Shui
William Spear, 24 Village Green Drive, Litchfield, CT 06759; tel: (860) 567-8801, fengshuime@aol.com

Stress
Flower Essences
* Flower Essence Society, PO Box 459, Nevada City, CA 95959; tel: (916) 265-9163

Meditation
Check your local health center for classes. If there is no one in your area, TM has teachers all over the USA.
* TM—Maharishi University of Management, Fairfield, Iowa 52557; tel: (515) 472-1134

Art Therapy
American Art Therapy Association, 1202 Allanson Road, Mundelein, IL 60060

Winter

Geopathic Stress
* The Geo Group, PO Box 602, Medina, WA 98039; chuckp @geo.org Offer a geopathic survey service. Website: http://www.geo.org

Space Clearing with the Elements
Denise Linn runs workshops around the U.S.A. There is also a range of videos and tapes. DLinnl@aol.com

Rebirthing
Rebirth International, PO Box 118, Walton, NY 13856; tel: (607) 865-8254

Past Life Therapy
International Association of Past Life Therapists, 19744 Beach Blvd, Suite 356, Huntington Beach, CA 92648; tel: (714) 536-1953

Retreating
Retreats International, Box 1067, Notre Dame, IN 46556; tel: (219) 631-5320

Further Reading

Chinese Medicine/Philosophy

Accolla, Dylana and Yates, Peter, *Back to Balance* (Newleaf)

Mole, Peter, *Acupuncture* (Element)

Reid, Daniel, *Guarding the Three Treasures* (Simon & Schuster)

————, *The Tao of Health, Sex, and Longevity* (Fireside)

Walter, Derek, *Chinese Geomancy* (Element)

Ayurveda

Chopra, Dr. Deepak, *Perfect Health* (Bantam Books)

Morningstar, Amadea, *The Ayurvedic Cookbook* (Lotus Press)

Morrison, Judith H., *The Book of Ayurveda* (Gaia)

Rhyner, Hans H., *Ayurveda: The Gentle Health System* (Sterling)

Verma, Dr. Vinod, *Ayurveda: A Way of Life* (Weiser)

The Native American Tradition/Shamanism

Meadows, Kenneth, *Earth Medicine: A Shamanic Way to Self-Discovery* (Element)

————, *The Medicine Way* (Element)

————, *Where Eagles Fly* (Element)

Summer Rain, Mary, *Earthway* (Pocket Books)

Naturopathy (and Detoxing)

Chaitow, Leon, *Body Tonic* (Gaia)

Helvin, Marie, *Bodypure* (Headline). Don't let the fact it's a celebrity book put you off; it's co-written by Louise Atkinson who really knows her detoxing.

Turner, Roger Newman, *Naturopathic Medicine* (Thorsons)

Natural Healthcare (General)

de Vries, Jan, *How to Live a Healthy Life* (Mainstream Publishing)

Godefroy, Christian H, *Super Health* (Piatkus)

Haas, Dr. Elson, *Staying Healthy with the Seasons* (Celestial Arts)

Kloss, Jethro, *Back to Eden* (Back to Eden Books)

Lockie, Dr. Andrew, *The Family Guide to Homeopathy* (Hamish Hamilton)

Murray, Michael and Pizzorno, Joseph, *The Encyclopaedia of Natural Medicine* (Optima)

Needles, Robin, *You Don't Have to Feel Unwell* (Gateway Books)

Northrup, Dr. Christiane, *Women's Bodies, Women's Wisdom* (Piatkus)

Null, Gary, *The 90s Healthy Body Book* (HCI)

Olsen, Kristin, *The Encyclopedia of Alternative Healthcare* (Piatkus)

Vogel, Dr. H. C. A., *The Nature Doctor* (Mainstream Publishing)

Ritual

The following offer a general, nondenominational and more psychological approach to ritual:

Imber-Black, Evan and Roberts, Janine, *Rituals for Our Times* (HarperCollins)

Roose-Evans, James, *Passages of the Soul: Ritual Today* (Element)

St. Aubyn, Lorna, *Rituals for Everyday Living* (Piatkus)

These see ritual from a pagan perspective but can easily be adapted for non-religious use:

Budapest, Zsuzsanna E., *Grandmother Moon* (HarperCollins)

———*The Grandmother of Time* (HarperCollins)

Campanelli, Pauline, *Wheel of the Year* (Llewyllyn Publications)

Green, Marion, *A Calendar of Festivals* (Element)

King, John, *The Celtic Druids' Year* (Blandford)

Shan, *Circlework* (House of the Goddess)—not always stocked by bookshops—for mail order write to the House of the Goddess, 33 Oldridge Road, London SW12 8PN.

Nutrition

Davies, Dr. Stephen and Stewart, Dr. Alan, *Nutritional Medicine* (Pan Books).

If you are considering finding a nutritional therapist read:

Lazarides, Linda, *Principles of Nutritional Therapy* (Thorsons)

The following give interesting ideas on how to boost the health-giving potential of your diet:

Carper, Jean, *The Food Pharmacy* (Positive Paperbacks)

Haas, Dr. Elson M., *A Diet for All Seasons* (Celestial Arts)

Mindell, Earl, *The Food Medicine Bible* (Souvenir Press)

Van Straten, Michael and Griggs, Barbara, *Superfoods* (Dorling Kindersley)

If you are interested in how to protect yourself from hereditary family weaknesses read:

Simopoulos, Dr. Artemis P., Herbert, Dr. Victor, and Jacobson, Beverly, *Genetic Nutrition: Designing a Diet Based on Your Family Medical History* (Macmillan)

Exercise

Brown, Carolan, *Bodywatch* (Headline)

Douillard, John, *Body, Mind and Sport* (Bantam)

Heaner, Martica, *Curves* (Hodder)

Aromatherapy

There are loads of books on aromatherapy but, to my mind, you won't do much better than the following:

Worwood, Valerie Ann, *The Fragrant Pharmacy* (Bantam Books). The author has now written a companion, *The Fragrant Mind* (also Bantam), which looks at how aromatherapy can affect your personality, mind, moods and emotions. Fascinating. Also recommended are:

Davies, Tricia, *A-Z of Aromatherapy* (C. W. Daniels)

Hopkins, Cathy, *The Joy of Aromatherapy* (Angus and Robertson)

Mojay, Gabriel, *Aromatherapy for Healing the Spirit* (Gaia)

Tisserand, Robert, *The Art of Aromatherapy* (C. W. Daniels)

Acupressure/Shiatsu

Ferguson, Pamela, *The Self-Shiatsu Handbook* (Newleaf)

Harvey, Eliana and Oatley, Mary Jane, *Acupressure* (Headway)

Liechti, Elaine, *Shiatsu* (Element)

Herbs

Chinese

Lu, Henry C., *Chinese System of Food Cures* (Sterling)

Reid, Daniel, *A Handbook of Chinese Healing Herbs* (Simon & Schuster)

Tang, Stephen and Craze, Richard, *Chinese Herbal Medicine* (Piatkus)

Teeguarden, Ron, *Chinese Tonic Herbs* (Japan Publications)

Western

Campion, Kitty, *A Woman's Herbal* (Vermilion)

Grieve, M., *A Modern Herbal* (Penguin)

Mindell, Earl, *The Herb Bible* (Vermillion)

Ody, Penelope, *The Herb Society's Complete Medicinal Herbal* (Dorling Kindersley)

Nice, Jill, *Herbal Remedies* (Piatkus)

Robbins, Christopher, *The Household Herbal* (Bantam Books)

Williams, Jude C., *Jude's Herbal Home Remedies* (Llewellyn Publications)

Polarity Therapy

Stone, Dr. Randolph, *Health Building* (CRCS)

Tibetan Medicine/Philosophy

Donden, Dr. Yeshi, *Health Through Balance* (Snow Lion)

Rinpoche, Akong Tulku, *Taming the Tiger* (Rider)

Weight Loss

Brock, Eve, *Think Slim* (Vermilion)

Chopra, Dr. Deepak, *Perfect Weight* (Rider)

Colclough, Beechy, *It's Not What You Eat It's Why You Eat It* (Vermilion)

Chiropractic/Osteopathy

Chaitow, Leon, *Osteopathy: A Complete Health Care System* (Thorsons)

Howitt Wilson, Dr. Michael B., *Thorsons Introductory Guide to Chiropractic* (Thorsons)

Zero Balancing
Smith, Dr. Fritz Frederick, *Inner Bridges* (Humanics Ltd.)

Self-Esteem
Cleghorn, Patricia, *The Secrets of Self-Esteem* (Element)
McKay, Matthew and Fanning, Patrick, *Self-Esteem* (New Harbinger Publications)
Markham, Ursula, *How to Deal with Difficult People* (Thorsons)

Sound Therapy
Goldman, Jonathan, *Healing Sounds* (Element)

Play
Holden, Robert, *Laughter: The Best Medicine* (Thorsons)

Careers
One book that is invaluable is:
Bolles, Richard Nelson, *What Color Is Your Parachute? A Practical Manual for Job Hunters & Career-Changers* (Ten Speed Press)

Feng Shui/Space Clearing
Kingston, Karen, *Creating Sacred with Feng Shui* (Piatkus)
Linn, Denise, *Sacred Space* (Rider)
Rossbach, Sarah, *Feng Shui* (Dutton)
Rossbach, Sarah, *Interior Design with Feng Shui* (Dutton)
Spear, William, *Feng Shui Made Easy* (Thorsons)
Walters, Derek, *Feng Shui: The Chinese Art of Designing a Harmonious Environment* (Simon & Schuster)

Time Management
Adair, John, *Effective Time Management* (Pan)
Atkinson, Jacqueline, *Better Time Management* (Thorsons)
Gitlin, Marek, *Making Time Work For You* (Sheldon)

I Ching
Dening, Sarah, *The Everyday I Ching* (Simon & Schuster)
Hook, Diana ffarington, *The I Ching and You* (RKP)
Wilhelm, Richard, *I Ching* (trans.) (RKP)

Nine Star Ki
Sachs, Bob, *The Complete Guide to Nine Star Ki* (Element)

Becoming Psychic/Developing Intuition
Burns, Litany, *Develop Your Psychic Abilities* (Bantam)
Furlong, David, *Develop Your Intuition and Psychic Powers* (Bloomsbury)
Lawrence, Richard, *Journey Into Supermind* (Souvenir Press)
———*Unlock Your Psychic Powers* (Souvenir Press)

Stress
Holden, Robert, *Stress Busters* (Thorsons)
Kenton, Leslie, *10 Day De-Stress Plan* (Ebury Press)
Markham, Ursula, *Managing Stress* (Element)
Ruhnke, Amiyo and Wurzburger, Anando, *Body Wisdom* (Newleaf)
Tisserand, Maggie, *Stress: The Aromatic Solution* (Hodder & Stoughton)
Quinn, Kaleghl, *Reclaim Your Power* (Mandala)

Floating
Hutchinson, Michael, *The Book of Floating* (Quill)

Art Therapy
Frings Keyes, Margaret, *Inward Journey: Art as Therapy* (Open Court)
McNiff, Shaun, *Art as Medicine* (Piatkus)

Dreamworking
Godwin, Malcolm, *The Lucid Dreamer* (Element)
Goodison, Lucy, *The Dreams of Women* (Women's Press)
Green, Celia, *Lucid Dreams* (IPR)
Hunt, Harry T., *The Multiplicity of Dreams* (Yale)

Light Therapy
Downing, Dr. Damien, *Day Light Robbery* (Arrow)
Liberman, Jacob, *Light: Medicine of the Future* (Bear & Co.)

Mindfulness
Kabat-Zinn, Jon, *Full Catastrophe Living: How to Use the Wisdom of Your Body and Mind to Face Stress, Pain and Illness* (Piatkus)

Kabat-Zinn, Jon, *Mindfulness Meditation for Everyday Life* (Piatkus)

Affirmations
Hay, Louise, *You Can Heal Your Body* (Eden Grove)
————*You Can Heal Your Life* (Eden Grove)
Gawain, Shakti, *Living in the Light* (Eden Grove)

Geopathic Stress
Thurnell-Read, Jane, *Geopathic Stress* (Element)

Rebirthing
Leonard, Jim and Laut, Phil, *Rebirthing: the Science of Enjoying All of Your Life* (Trinity Publications)
Ray, Sondra, *Celebration of Breath* (Celestial Arts)
————*Loving Relationships* (Celestial Arts)

Past Life Therapy
Rossetti, Dr. Francesca, *Psycho-Regression* (Piatkus)
Woolger, Roger J., *Other Lives, Other Selves* (Crucible)

Retreating
The following lists hundreds of retreats in the UK, Ireland, France and Spain:
Whiteaker, Stafford, *The Good Retreat Guide* (Rider)

INDEX